Thieme

Synopsis of Foot and Ankle Surgery

Simon Lee, MD
Associate Professor;
Foot and Ankle Section Chief;
Fellowship Director
Department of Orthopaedics
Rush University Medical Center
Chicago, Illinois, USA

Christopher E. Gross, MD
Professor
Department of Orthopaedics
Medical University of South Carolina
Charleston, South Carolina, USA

351 Illustrations

Thieme
New York • Stuttgart • Delhi • Rio de Janeiro

Library of Congress Cataloging-in-Publication Data is available from the publisher.

MIX
Paper | Supporting responsible forestry
FSC™ C016779

Thieme Publishers New York
333 Seventh Avenue, 18th Floor
New York, NY 10001, USA
www.thieme.com
+ 1 800 782 3488, customerservice@thieme.com

Illustrations: Graeme Chambers at Illumina Medical Illustration Ltd/© Thieme
Cover design: © Thieme
Cover image source: © Thieme
Typesetting by TNQ Tech Private Limited, India

Printed in India by Replika Press Pvt. Ltd. 5 4 3 2 1

DOI: 10.1055/b-006-160175

ISBN: 978-1-62623-724-7

Also available as an e-book:
eISBN (PDF): 978-1-62623-725-4
eISBN (epub): 978-1-63853-494-5

Important note: Medicine is an ever-changing science undergoing continual development. Research and clinical experience are continually expanding our knowledge, in particular our knowledge of proper treatment and drug therapy. Insofar as this book mentions any dosage or application, readers may rest assured that the authors, editors, and publishers have made every effort to ensure that such references are in accordance with **the state of knowledge at the time of production of the book.**

Nevertheless, this does not involve, imply, or express any guarantee or responsibility on the part of the publishers in respect to any dosage instructions and forms of applications stated in the book. **Every user is requested to examine carefully** the manufacturers' leaflets accompanying each drug and to check, if necessary, in consultation with a physician or specialist, whether the dosage schedules mentioned therein or the contraindications stated by the manufacturers differ from the statements made in the present book. Such examination is particularly important with drugs that are either rarely used or have been newly released on the market. Every dosage schedule or every form of application used is entirely at the user's own risk and responsibility. The authors and publishers request every user to report to the publishers any discrepancies or inaccuracies noticed. If errors in this work are found after publication, errata will be posted at www.thieme.com on the product description page.

Some of the product names, patents, and registered designs referred to in this book are in fact registered trademarks or proprietary names even though specific reference to this fact is not always made in the text. Therefore, the appearance of a name without designation as proprietary is not to be construed as a representation by the publisher that it is in the public domain.

Thieme addresses people of all gender identities equally. We encourage our authors to use gender-neutral or gender-equal expressions wherever the context allows.

We would like to dedicate this text to those who nurture our creativity and form the bedrock of our every endeavor. We also thank those whose graceful presence fills our lives with warmth and curiosity. In their soft, subtle ways, they infuse these pages with a whimsical touch of inspiration.

Simon Lee, MD
Christopher E. Gross, MD

Contents

23. Pediatric Disorders of the Foot and Ankle 299

Ian S. MacLean, David Zhu, Charles P. Hannon, and Monica Kogan

Foreword

When I started my orthopaedic residency, in 1985, there were certainly no quick references or online options for the middle-of-the-night questions for a junior resident on-call. There were some handbooks (pocket sized) that we carried around as interns, which served to keep us out of trouble on our general surgery and internal medicine rotations. For orthopaedics, it was a wasteland. Although the options for basic information have got better when taking general orthopaedic trauma call, references for the common questions and issues faced by the beginning clinician in foot and ankle are still lacking. As someone who has trained junior residents on the foot and ankle service for 30+ years, this has continued to be a problem. We had to provide information off the cuff, which was appropriately nuanced for someone just beginning to understand the clinical intricacies and perils of a foot and ankle surgeon. This hole in offerings for the junior foot and ankle clinician is surprising when the clinical progress in foot and ankle surgery has exploded in the last 20 years. It is in this background that I am excited for this book.

As with any basic textbook, the authors have started with the basics for aspiring ankle and foot surgeons. The basis for our surgical expertise begins with anatomy. Anatomy then translates to surgical approaches to do the surgeries that we need to perform to help our patients. The challenges of foot and ankle, before worrying about pathology, begin with an understanding of normal biomechanics. The authors then focus on the basics of imaging, history taking, and examination, which will allow the interested reader to begin to understand the complex pathologies that we see in the ankle and foot. As to the pathologies, all of the common and some uncommon conditions are covered in the subsequent chapters.

As my trainees and mentees have heard me say many times over the last decade, as foot and ankle surgeons, we have at our fingertips, the best science, tools, and intellects that we have seen in the history of focused inquiry in the space. Although we are eternally grateful to the educational giants who came before us, the present time is our time. It is educational offerings, like this book, that will allow a speedy introduction for the smart, talented trainees of today into the interesting and fascinating complexities in the treatment of foot and ankle maladies. I see this book as the beginning of a satisfying journey for the reader. There is no doubt that this can be a valuable resource for an outstanding future career.

W. Hodges Davis, MD
Medical Director
OrthoCarolina Foot and Ankle Institute
Atrium Health
Charlotte, North Carolina, USA

Preface

Many orthopaedic surgery residents find that foot and ankle is one of the most complex subspecialties in terms of anatomy, biomechanics, and the variety of surgeries that are performed. Reading comprehensive, in-depth foot and ankle surgery texts is not always feasible for a resident on a brief rotation. Therefore, the purpose of the present textbook is to provide a concise, easy-to-read resource covering the fundamentals of care for common foot and ankle disorders. The target audience for the textbook includes medical students, residents, nurses, and physician assistants.

In the rapidly evolving world of orthopaedic foot and ankle surgery, it is imperative for the budding health care providers to be armed with a profound and comprehensive understanding of the intricacies of our discipline. This manual was crafted by the thought leaders in foot and ankle surgery. It is designed to illuminate the intricate art and science of foot and ankle surgery. With each chapter, readers will find themselves immersed in anatomy, pathophysiology, and nonoperative and surgical solutions.

To those learning foot and ankle orthopaedics, may this manual serve as an anchor in your formative years, instilling in you the passion, expertise, and vision to take care of our patients.

Simon Lee, MD
Christopher E. Gross, MD

Contributors

Samuel AbuMoussa, MD, MS
Physician
Department of Orthopaedic Surgery
Medical University of South Carolina
Miami, Florida, USA

Craig Chike Akoh, MD
Partner
Department of Orthopaedic Surgery
Regenerative Orthopaedics and Spine Institute
Stockbridge, Georgia

Annunziato Amendola, MD
Professor and Director of Sports Medicine
Department of Orthopaedic Surgery
Duke University
Durham, North Carolina, USA

D. Anthony Barcel, MD
Orthopaedic Surgeon
Department of Orthopaedics
Carolina Orthopaedics and Neurosurgical Associates
Spartanburg, South Carolina, USA

Gonzalo F. Bastias, MD
Chief of Foot and Ankle Surgery
Department of Orthopedic Surgery
Hospital del Trabajador
Santiago, Region Metropolitana, Chile

Thomas B. Bemenderfer, MD, MBA
Orthopaedic Surgeon
South Bend Orthopaedics
OrthoAlliance
Granger, Indiana, USA

Clayton C. Bettin, MD
Orthopaedic Foot & Ankle Surgeon
Department of Orthopaedic Surgery
University of Tennessee - Campbell Clinic
Memphis, Tennessee, USA

Adam D. Bitterman, DO
Assistant Professor
Department of Orthopaedic Surgery
Donald and Barbara Zucker School of Medicine at Hofstra, Northwell
Hempstead, New York, USA

Natalie R. Black, MD
Resident Physician
Department of Orthopaedic Surgery and Rehabilitation
University of Texas Medical Branch
Galveston, Texas, USA

Joseph Chavarria, MD
Assistant Professor
Department of Orthopedics
Baylor Scott and White Healthcare
Frisco, Texas, USA

Jie Chen, MD, MPH
Assistant Professor
Department of Orthopaedic Surgery and Rehabilitation
University of Texas Medical Branch
Galveston, Texas, USA

Jocelyn Compton, MSc, MD
Department of Orthopedics
Orthopedic and Fracture Specialists
Portland, Oregon, USA

Austin R. Davidson, MD
Orthopedic Foot & Ankle Surgeon
Department of Orthopaedic Surgery
OrthoTennessee
Knoxville Orthopedic Clinic
Knoxville, Tennessee, USA

Tobin Eckel, MD
Associate Professor
Department of Orthopaedic Surgery
Walter Reed National Military Medical Center
Bethesda, Maryland, USA

Kent Ellington, MD
Orthopedic Surgeon
OrthoCarolina
Foot and Ankle Institute
Charlotte, North Carolina, USA

Fred T. Finney, MD
Consultant
Attending
Peachtree Orthopedics
Atlanta, Georgia, USA

Derrick Foge, MD
Board Certified Orthopedic Spine Surgeon, Fellowship Trained
Department of Orthopedic Surgery
Orthopedic Physicians Alaska
Anchorage, Alaska, USA

Austin T. Fragomen, MD
Professor of Clinical Orthopaedic Surgery;
Fellowship Director, Limb Lengthening & Complex Reconstruction
Department of Orthopaedic Surgery
Hospital for Special Surgery
New York, New York, USA

Katherine Gavin, MD
Associate Professor
Department of Orthopaedic Surgery
University of New Mexico
Albuquerque, New Mexico

Nicholas Genovese, MD
Orthopedic Resident
Department of Orthopedics
Rutgers New Jersey Medical School
Jersey City, New Jersey, USA

Eric Giza, MD
Professor of Orthopaedic Surgery;
Chief, Foot & Ankle Surgery
Department of Orthopaedics
University of California, Davis
Sacramento, California, USA

Christopher E. Gross, MD
Professor
Department of Orthopaedics
Medical University of South Carolina
Charleston, South Carolina, USA

Gregory P. Guyton, MD
Division Chief
Orthopaedic Foot and Ankle Service MedStar Union Memorial Hospital
Baltimore, Maryland, USA

Charles P. Hannon, MD, MBA
Consultant
Associate Professor
Division of Hip and Knee Surgery
Department of Orthopedic Surgery
Mayo Clinic
Rochester, Minnesota, USA

Thomas M. Hearty, MD, DPT
Associate Division Head Surgery
Division of Surgery, IHA Medical Group Trinity Health
Ann Arbor, Michigan, USA

Kenneth J. Hunt, MD
Associate Professor and Chief – Foot and Ankle Surgery;
Vice Chair – Quality, Patient Safety and Outcomes
Department of Orthopaedic Surgery
University of Colorado School of Medicine
Aurora, Colorado, USA

Todd A. Irwin, MD
Fellowship Director
Foot and Ankle Institute
OrthoCarolina;
Adjunct Associate Professor
Department of Orthopaedic Surgery
Atrium Health Musculoskeletal Institute, Wake Forest School of Medicine
Charlotte, North Carolina, USA

Carroll P. Jones, MD
Orthopedic surgeon
OrthoCarolina
Charlotte, North Carolina, USA

Benjamin Jong, MD, FRCS(C), BSc (Kin)
Clinical Instructor
Department of Orthopaedics
University of British Columbia
White Rock, British Columbia, Canada

Phillip T. Kirn, MD, PharmD
Orthopedic Surgeon
Jacksonville, Florida, USA

Monica Kogan, MD
Residency Director
Department of Orthopaedic Surgery
Rush University Medical Center
Chicago, Illinois, USA

Ethan Krell, MD
Orthopedic Research Fellow
Department of Orthopedics
Rutgers New Jersey Medical School
New York, New York, USA

Christopher D. Kreulen, MD, MS
Professor
Department of Orthopaedics
University of California, Davis
Sacramento, California, USA

Brian C. Lau, MD, FAAOS
Assistant Professor
Department of Orthopedic Surgery
Duke University, Urbaniak Sports Science Institute
Durham, North Carolina, USA

Simon Lee, MD
Associate Professor;
Foot and Ankle Section Chief;
Fellowship Director
Department of Orthopaedics
Rush University Medical Center
Chicago, Illinois, USA

Anthony Lin, BS
Orthopedic Research Fellow
Department of Orthopaedics
Rutgers New Jersey Medical School
Forest Hills, New York, USA

Johnny L. Lin, MD
Assistant Professor
Department of Orthopedic Surgery
Rush University Medical Center
Chicago, Illinois, USA

Sheldon S. Lin, MD
Associate Professor
Department of Orthopedics
New Jersey Medical School – Newark
Newark, New Jersey, USA

Benjamin B. Lindsey, MD
Department of Orthopaedics
OrthoSC
Conway, South Carolina, USA

Ian S. MacLean, MD
Assistant Clinical Professor
Department of Orthopedic Surgery
Virginia Commonwealth University
Richmond, Virginia, USA

Jayenth Mayur, MD
Orthopedic Research Fellow
Department of Orthopedics
Rutgers New Jersey Medical School
New York, New York, USA

Benjamin J. Miller, MD, MS
Professor and Vice Chair of Faculty Affairs
Department of Orthopaedics and Rehabilitation
University of Iowa
Iowa City, Iowa, USA

Randal Morris, BS
Biomedical Engineer
Department of Orthopaedic Surgery and Rehabilitation
University of Texas Medical Branch
Galveston, Texas, USA

Maximilian Muñoz, MD
Orthopedic Research Fellow
Department of Orthopedics
Rutgers New Jersey Medical School
Morristown, New Jersey, USA

Vinod K. Panchbhavi, MD, FACS, FAOA, FABOS, FAAOS
Professor and Chief
Department of Orthopedic Surgery
University of Texas Medical Branch
Galveston, Texas, USA

Phinit Phisitkul, MD
Orthopaedic Surgeon
The Center Neuroscience, Orthopaedics & Spine (CNOS)
Dakota Dunes, South Dakota, USA

Michael S. Pinzur, MD
Professor, Orthopaedic Surgery
Loyola University
Maywood, Illinois, USA

Steven M. Raikin, MD
Emeritus Professor
Department of Orthopaedic Surgery
Rothman Orthopaedic Institute
Philadelphia, Pennsylvania, USA

S. Robert Rozbruch, MD
Professor of Clinical Orthopaedic Surgery;
Chief, Limb Lengthening & Complex Reconstruction
Department of Orthopaedic Surgery
Hospital for Special Surgery
New York, New York, USA

Michael Russell, MD, MBA, MPH
Orthopedic Surgeon
Department of Orthopedics, University of Iowa
Iowa City, Iowa, USA

Augustine M. Saiz Jr., MD
Assistant Professor
Department of Orthopaedic Surgery
UC Davis
Sacramento, California, USA

Adam P. Schiff, MD
The Alan R. Kohlhaas, MD Director of Orthopaedic Education
Residency Program Director and Vice-Chair of Education
Loyola University Medical Center
Maywood, Illinois, USA

Lew C. Schon, MD, FACS, FAAOS
Director of Orthopaedic Innovation
Institute of Foot and Ankle Reconstruction
Mercy Medical Center
Baltimore, Maryland, USA;
Professor of Orthopaedics
New York University Langone
New York, New York, USA;
Professor of Orthopaedics & BME
Johns Hopkins School of Medicine
Baltimore, Maryland, USA;
Associate Professor of Orthopaedics
Georgetown School of Medicine
Washington, D.C., USA;
Adjunct Professor and Fischell Literati Faculty
University of Maryland Orthopaedics & Fischell Department of Bioengineering
University of Maryland
College Park, Maryland, USA

Scott B. Shawen, MD, FAOA, FAAOS
Section Chief, Orthopaedic Foot & Ankle Surgery
Department of Orthopedic Surgery
Foot & Ankle Institute, OrthoCarolina
Charlotte, North Carolina, USA
Associate Professor
Department of Orthopaedic Surgery
Wake Forest Universiy
Winston Salem, North Carolina, USA

Thomas I. Sherman, MD
Orthopaedic Surgeon & Foot and Ankle Surgical Specialist
Orthopedic Associates of Lancaster
Lancaster, Pennsylvania, USA

Natalie V. Singer, MD
Assistant Professor
Department of Orthopedic Surgery
Albany Medical Center
Albany, New York, USA

Justin Tsai, MS, MD
Clinical Assistant Professor
Orthopedic Surgery
Donald and Barbara Zucker School of Medicine at Hofstra/Northwell
Staten Island, New York, USA

Emily C. Vafek, MD
Physician
Department of Orthopedic Surgery
Orthopedic Partners
North Franklin, Connecticut, USA

David M. Walton, MD
Associate Professor
Department of Orthopedic Surgery
University of Michigan
Ann Arbor, Michigan, USA

Keith L. Wapner, MD, FAAOS, FACS, FAOA
Emeritus Professor, Orthopedic Surgery;
Emeritus Chief, Division of Foot and Ankle Surgery
University of Pennsylvania;
Adjunct Professor, Orthopedic Surgery
Drexel College of Medicine;
Past President, American Orthopedic Foot and Ankle Society
Philadelphia, Pennsylvania, USA

John Yanik, MD
Orthopaedic surgeon
EmergeOrtho
Asheville, North Carolina, USA

David Zhu, MD
Department of Orthopaedic Surgery
Illinois Southwest Orthopedics
Glen Carbon, Illinois, USA

1 Foot and Ankle Anatomy

Jie Chen, Natalie R. Black, Randal Morris, and Vinod K. Panchbhavi

Abstract

The foot and ankle comprise one of the most functionally important structures in the human body. Key to understanding the complex pathology and debilitating conditions is a solid foundation in foot and ankle anatomy. Containing 26 bones, 30 joints, and more than 100 tendons, ligaments, and muscles, the foot is intricate in design. The ankle is a constrained joint whose stability is afforded by a complex interplay between various ligaments, and our understanding of this interplay continues to evolve. This chapter outlines the unique anatomy of this fascinating region, emphasizes high-yield facts, and provides common test questions.

Keywords: foot, ankle, anatomy, bones, ligaments, tendons, joints

1.1 Ankle

1.1.1 Arthrology

Distal Tibiofibular Joint (Syndesmosis)

- Articulation between the convex medial side of distal fibula and the concave lateral aspect of distal tibia (▶ Fig. 1.1).[1]
- Allows for small degree of external rotation and proximal to distal translation of the fibula against the tibia.
- Serves to keep the ankle mortise intact by maintaining the spatial relationship of the distal tibia and the distal fibula.
- Borders of the ankle mortise includes the tibial plafond superiorly, medial malleolus medially, and the lateral malleolus laterally.
- Stabilized by syndesmotic ligaments (see below). See Figure 1.2

Ankle Joint

- Hinge-type joint between the distal tibia, distal fibula, and talus.
  - Primarily acts in plantar and dorsiflexion, but also components of internal and external rotation.
- Normal range of motion (ROM) is around 20 degrees dorsiflexion and 50 degrees plantar flexion.
- The talar dome has a biconcave surface with a central sulcus.
  - The talus is wider anteriorly than posteriorly, leading to increased instability in plantar flexion.
  - Ankle chondrocytes are uniformly horizontally aligned and stiff, have decreased permeability, are less responsive to catabolic mediators, and synthesize proteoglycans at a greater rate, which leads to increased repair capacity. Thus, there is a **lower incidence of primary ankle degenerative joint disease (DJD) compared to the knee and hip.**
  - Medial and lateral stability is provided by the robust deltoid ligament and strong lateral ligaments including the anterior talofibular ligament and calcaneofibular ligament.

1.1.2 Ligaments

Syndesmosis

- Four syndesmotic ligaments (▶ Fig. 1.2)[2,3]:
  - Injury here indicates "**high ankle sprain.**
  - Anterior inferior tibiofibular ligament (AITFL).
    - Origin: tibial anterolateral tubercle.
    - Insertion: fibular anterior tubercle.
    - Weakest syndesmotic ligament.
  - Posteroinferior tibiofibular ligament (PITFL).
    - Origin: tibial posterior tubercle.
    - Insertion: posterior lateral malleolus.

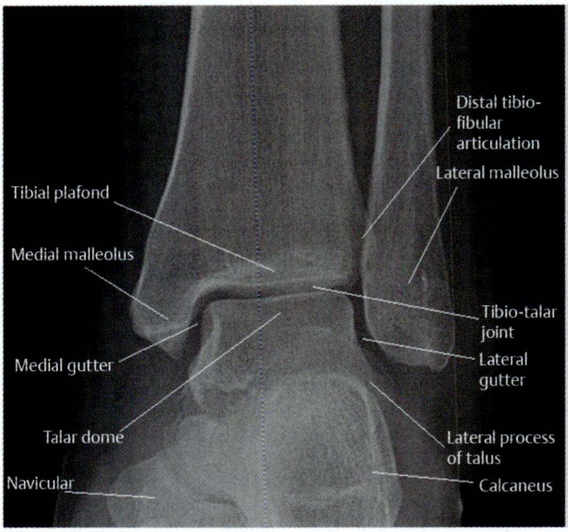

Fig. 1.1 Ankle osteology.

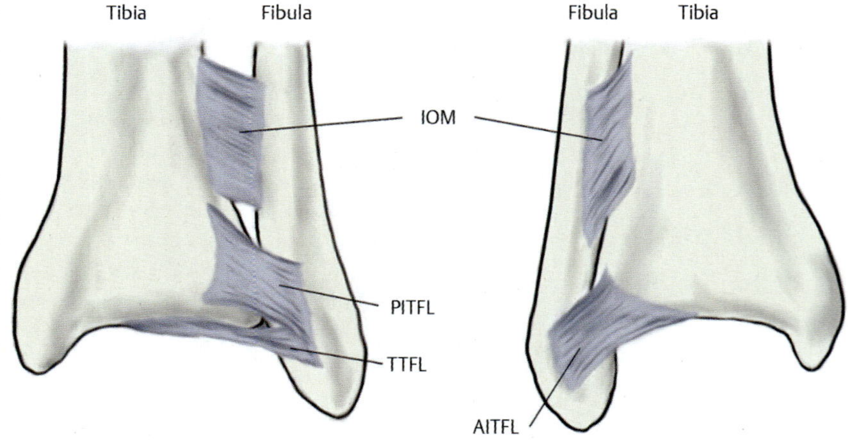

Fig. 1.2 Ankle syndesmosis.

  - Strongest syndesmotic ligament.
- Interosseous ligament (IOL).
- Inferior transverse ligament (ITL).

Lateral Ligaments

- Anterior talofibular ligament (▶ Fig. 1.3):
  - Attaches the anterior distal fibula to the talar neck.
  - **Resists inversion in plantar flexion.**
  - Most commonly injured in "low ankle sprains."
- Calcaneofibular ligament:
  - Attaches the distal fibula to the calcaneus, crossing the subtalar joint.
  - Runs deep to the peroneal tendons.
  - **Resists inversion in neutral or dorsiflexion.**

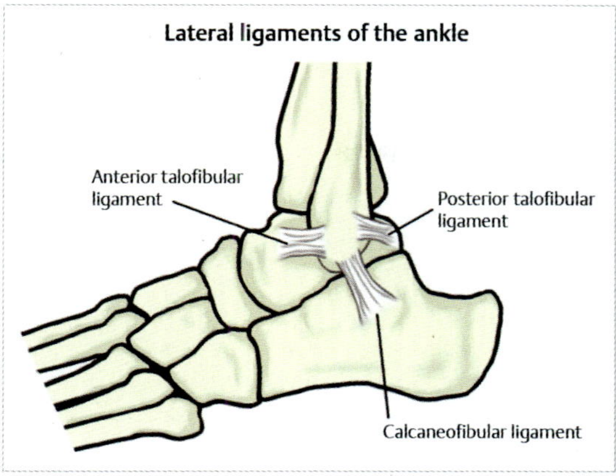

Fig. 1.3 Ankle lateral ligaments.

  - Second most commonly injured in low ankle sprains.
- Posterior talofibular ligament:
  - Attaches the posterolateral distal fibula to the posterolateral talus.
  - Strongest lateral ligament.
  - Rarely torn.
- Lateral talocalcaneal ligament:
  - Attaches the talar lateral process to the lateral calcaneus.

Medial Ligaments

- Thickest and strongest ligaments in the ankle (▶ Fig. 1.4).
- Superficial deltoid:
  - Four parts: anterior tibiotalar, tibionavicular, tibiocalcaneal, and posterior tibiotalar.
  - Origin on the anterior colliculus of the medial malleolus.
  - Resists ankle eversion.
- Deep deltoid:
  - Origin on the posterior colliculus of the medial malleolus.
  - Resists external rotation and lateral translation.
  - Stronger than the superficial deltoid.
- Spring ligament.
- Calcaneonavicular ligament.
  - Connects the sustentaculum tali of the calcaneus to the plantar navicular.
  - Plays important role in maintaining the medial longitudinal arch by acting as a sling to support the talar head.

1.2 Hindfoot

1.2.1 Osteology

Talus

- Around 60% covered with articular cartilage (▶ Fig. 1.1).[4]
- No tendinous attachments.
- Divided into the talar head, neck, body, and posterior and lateral processes.
- Blood supply is through three main arteries: posterior tibial artery, dorsalis pedis artery, and perforating peroneal artery.
  - Dominant blood supply to the body is through the artery of the tarsal canal, a branch of the posterior tibial artery.
  - Retrograde blood flow from the neck places the body at risk of avascular necrosis with talar neck fractures.
- The lateral process is at risk of fracture in **snowboarders**.
  - Attachment site of the lateral talocalcaneal ligament.

Calcaneus

- Largest bone in the foot:
  - Posterior projection for Achilles tendon attachment acts as a lever

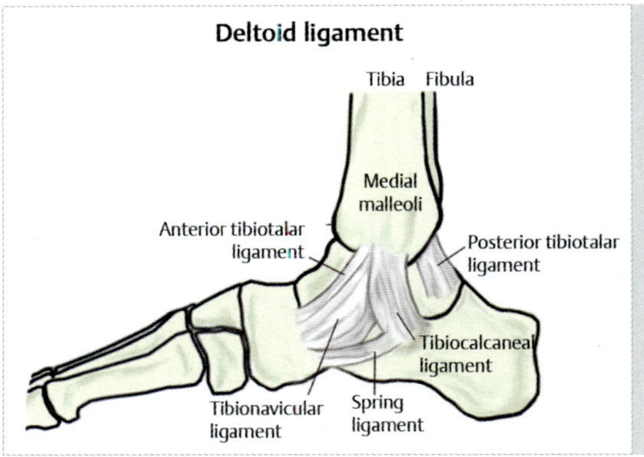

Fig. 1.4 Medial ankle ligaments.

arm to increase force of plantar flexion.
  - Comprising the body, sustentaculum tali, and several articular facets (anterior, middle, and posterior).
    - The body includes the tuberosity, medial and lateral processes, and the peroneal tubercle.
- Calcaneal tuberosity is the attachment site for the Achilles tendon:
  - Medial and lateral processes serve as origins for the abductor hallucis and the abductor digiti minimi.
- Peroneal tendons pass through the peroneal tubercle:
  - The sustentaculum tali is a medial projection that supports the anteromedial talus.
    - **The flexor hallucis longus (FHL) tendon runs beneath.**
- Articular facets for the subtalar joint and calcaneocuboid joint.

Navicular

- Named for its "boat" shape.
- Articulates with the talus proximally, cuboid laterally, and three cuneiforms distally.
- Blood supply is mainly through the branches of the dorsalis pedis.
- **Prone to stress fractures, tenuous blood supply in the middle third.**
- Insertion of the posterior tibial tendon medially.

Cuboid

- Wedge-shaped bone with three articular surfaces.
- Posterior articulation with the calcaneus.
- Medial articulation with the lateral cuneiform.
- Anterior articulations with the fourth and fifth metatarsals.
- Inferior groove for passage of the peroneus longus tendon.

1.2.2 Arthrology

Subtalar Joint

- The talus and calcaneus articulate through three processes: posterior, middle, and anterior articular processes.
- The **posterior process is the largest and the most commonly injured.**
- The middle facet located on the sustentaculum tali.
- Primary motion is inversion/eversion.

Transverse Tarsal Joint (Chopart's Joint)

- Comprises the talonavicular and calcaneocuboid joints.
  - Along with the subtalar joint, the main function is to allow flexibility and stability during the gait cycle.
    - When the subtalar joint is inverted during push-off, the axes of the talonavicular and calcaneocuboid

joint are not aligned and functionally "locked," allowing for creation of a stiff lever arm for push-off. This action is facilitated by the posterior tibial tendon.
  - When the subtalar joint is everted during heel strike, the axes of the talonavicular and calcaneocuboid joint are aligned and functionally "unlocked," allowing for a supple foot, which accommodates the ground reaction forces.

1.3 Midfoot

1.3.1 Osteology

Cuneiforms

- Medial, middle (intermediate), and lateral cuneiforms (▶ Fig. 1.5):
  - Trapezoid-shaped structures.
  - Wider plantarly than dorsally to provide strength to the "Roman arch" configuration of the tarsometatarsal joints.
  - *Medial cuneiform:* Partial insertions of the tibialis anterior, peroneus longus, and posterior tibial tendon.
  - *Intermediate cuneiform:* Shortest; allows for the base of the second metatarsal to "key" in.
- Articulations between the cuneiforms, navicular, cuboid, and metatarsal bases 1 to 3.

Tarsometatarsal Joint (Lisfranc Complex)

- The midfoot and its articulations allow for transference of force from the hindfoot to the forefoot during gait (▶ Fig. 1.6). It provides both the stability and the flexibility needed for normal walking.
- Comprises three columns.
  - *Medial:* First metatarsocuneiform joint.
  - *Middle:* Second and third metatarsocuneiform joint.
    - Most rigid of the columns to allow for stable push-off.

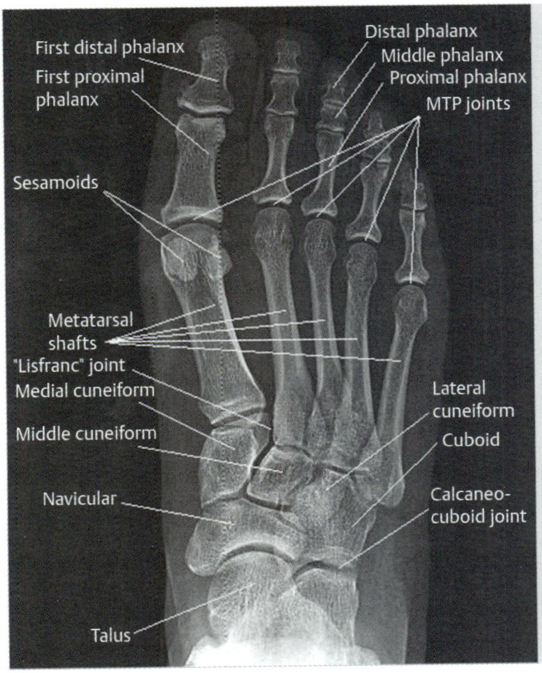

Fig. 1.5 Foot osteology.

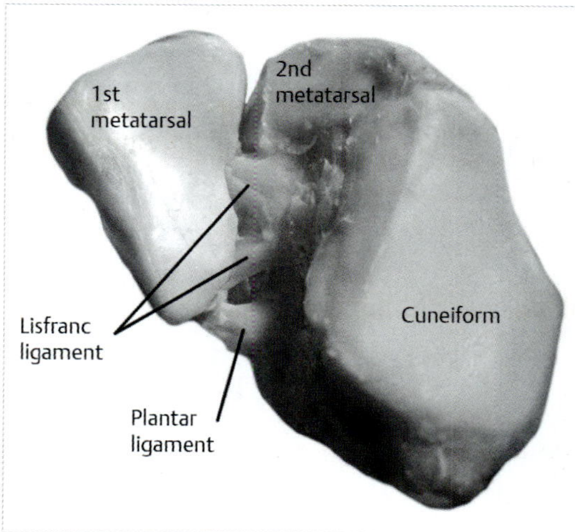

Fig. 1.6 Lisfranc ligament.

  - *Lateral:* Fourth and fifth metatarsocuboid joint:
    - Most mobile of the columns to allow for flexibility when walking on uneven surfaces.
- Osseous anatomy creates a "Roman arch" structure in which the base of the second metatarsal acts as the "keystone" as it articulates with the recessed middle cuneiform.
- Tarsometatarsal ligamentous stability is provided by three layers:
  - **The interosseous layer is the strongest and contains the Lisfranc ligament, which connects the medial cuneiform to the plantar aspect of the second metatarsal.**
  - Plantar ligaments between the medial cuneiform and the second and third metatarsals help provide transverse stability.
- Dorsal ligaments are the weakest.
- Intermetatarsal articulations:
  - Intermetatarsal ligaments run between the second and fifth metatarsal bases, but there is no ligament connecting the first and second metatarsal bases.
- Cuneiforms are connected by plantar, dorsal, and IOLs.
- Allows for a minimal amount of gliding.
- Naviculocuneiform and intercuneiform articulations:
  - Minimal motion.

1.4 Forefoot

1.4.1 Osteology

Metatarsals

- Each metatarsal has a base, shaft, neck, and head.
- Distal intermetatarsal ligaments between metatarsals 2 and 5 provide length and alignment stability.
- First metatarsal:
  - Shortest and widest of the metatarsals.
  - Bears up to 50% of the weight of the forefoot.
  - The metatarsal head has a crista that separates the two sesamoids (▶ Fig. 1.7).
- Second metatarsal:
  - Longest of the metatarsals and most prone to stress fractures.
- Third metatarsal:
  - **Rarely fractures in isolation.**
- Fourth and fifth metatarsals:
  - Flexible articulation with the cuboid.
- The fifth metatarsal base has a tenuous blood supply in the watershed area, leading to risk of nonunion. Vascularity

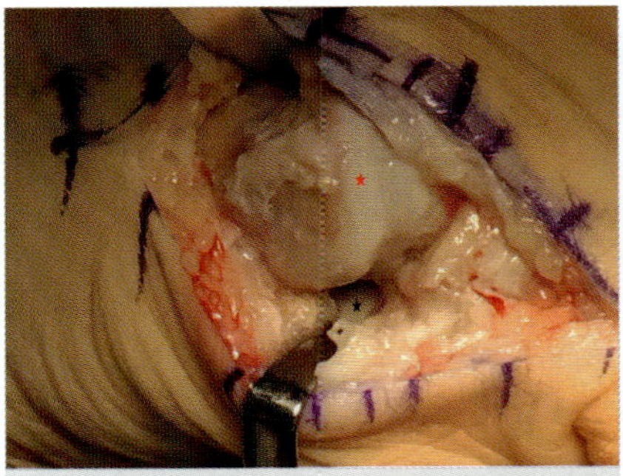

Fig. 1.7 Medial approach to the first metatarsal head showing the metatarsal–sesamoid articulation. *Black star:* The medial sesamoid. *Red star:* The metatarsal head.

is through the metaphyseal vessels and diaphyseal nutrient artery.

Phalanges

- Long bones in the foot distal to the metatarsals.
- The great toe contains two phalanges (proximal and distal).
- The small toes contain three phalanges (proximal, middle, and distal).

Joints

- *Metatarsophalangeal (MTP):* Between the metatarsal and the proximal phalanx.
  - *Proximal interphalangeal (PIP;* ▶ Fig. 1.8*):* Between the proximal and middle phalanges.[3,5,6,7]
  - *Distal interphalangeal (DIP):* Between the middle and distal phalanges.[3,5,6,7]
  - *Interphalangeal (IP):* Between the proximal and distal phalanges (great toe).

Plantar Plate

- Protects the metatarsal heads from pressure and prevents toe overextension.
  - ***Turf toe:*** **Injury caused by hyperextension of the plantar plate and metatarsophalangeal joint (MTPJ) sesamoid damage.**

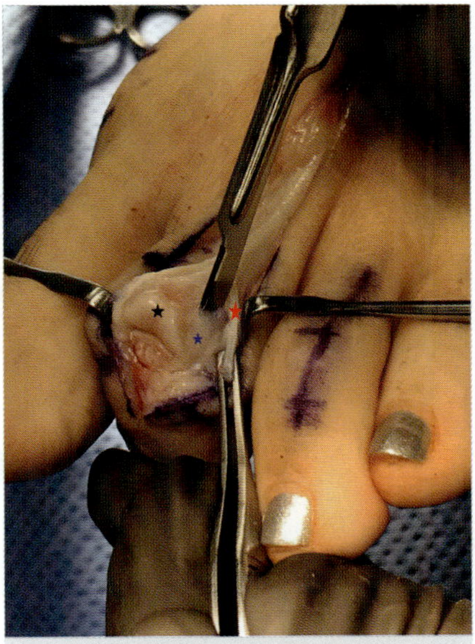

Fig. 1.8 Lesser toe proximal interphalangeal (PIP) joint. *Black star:* The head of the proximal phalanx. *Red star:* The split extensor tendon. *Blue star:* The collateral ligament.

- Strong supporting ligament of the toes.
- Located on the ball of the foot.

1.5 Muscle Anatomy

1.5.1 Leg Compartments

Anterior Compartment

- *Neurovascular contents:* Deep peroneal nerve and anterior tibial vessels (▶ Fig. 1.9).
- *Muscle innervation:* Deep peroneal nerve
- Tibialis anterior:
  - *Origin:* Proximal lateral tibia.
  - *Insertion:* Medial cuneiform and plantar base of the first metatarsal.
  - *Action:* Ankle dorsiflexion and foot inversion.
- Extensor hallucis longus (EHL):
  - *Origin:* Medial fibula and interosseous membrane.
  - *Insertion:* Great toe distal phalanx.

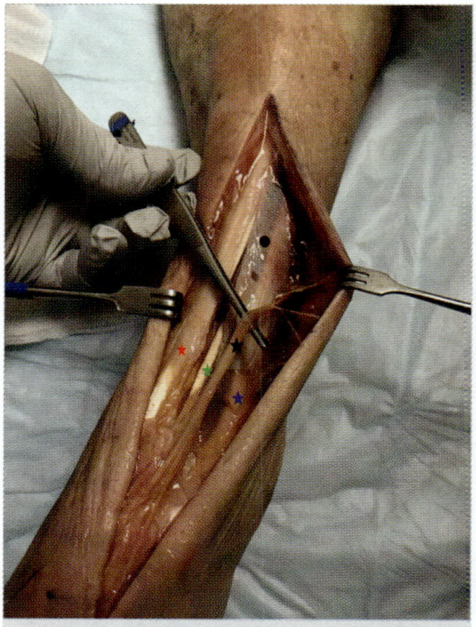

Fig. 1.9 Anterior ankle exposure. *Black star:* The superficial peroneal nerve. *Red star:* The tibialis anterior tendon. *Green star:* The extensor hallucis longus tendon. *Blue star:* The extensor digitorum longus tendon. *Black circle:* The extensor retinaculum.

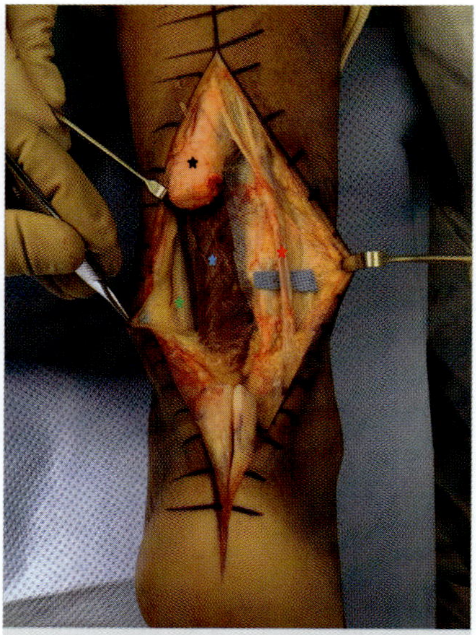

Fig. 1.10 Posterior leg with the Achilles tendon cut/reflected and fascia to deep posterior compartment incised. *Black star:* The Achilles tendon. *Red star:* The plantaris. *Green star:* The flexor digitorum longus tendon. *Blue star:* The flexor hallucis longus muscle belly.

  - *Action:* Great toe dorsiflexion and extension.
- Extensor digitorum longus:
  - *Origin:* Lateral tibial condyle and proximal fibula.
  - *Insertion:* Middle and distal phalanges 2 to 4.
  - *Action:* Dorsiflexion and extension of digits 2 to 4.
- Peroneus tertius:
  - *Origin:* Distal fibula and interosseous membrane.
  - *Insertion:* Fifth metatarsal base.
  - *Action:* Dorsiflex and foot eversion.

Lateral Compartment

- *Neurovascular contents:* Superficial peroneal nerve.
- *Muscle innervation:* Superficial peroneal nerve.
- Peroneus longus:
  - *Origin:* Fibular head and proximal lateral fibula shaft.
  - *Insertion:* Plantar medial cuneiform and base of the first metatarsal.
  - *Action:* Foot eversion, ankle plantar flexion, and supports the arch of the foot.
- Peroneus brevis:
  - *Origin:* Distal lateral fibula shaft.
  - *Insertion:* Fifth metatarsal base.
  - *Action:* Foot eversion and ankle plantar flexion.

Superficial Posterior Compartment

- *Neurovascular contents* (▸ Fig. 1.10): sural nerve.
  - *Muscle innervation*: Tibial nerve.
- Gastrocnemius:
  - *Origin:* Medial and lateral femoral condyles.

- *Insertion:* Posterior calcaneus as the Achilles tendon.
  - The Achilles tendon is the largest tendon in the body. **Rupture can be misdiagnosed as ankle sprain in up to 25% of cases.**
- *Action:* Ankle plantar flexion.

- Soleus:
  - *Origin:* Proximal posterior fibular head and medial tibial shaft.
  - *Insertion:* Posterior calcaneus as the Achilles tendon.
  - *Action:* Ankle plantar flexion.
- Plantaris:
  - *Origin:* Supracondylar line of the lateral femur.
  - *Insertion:* Calcaneus.
  - *Action:* Weak ankle plantar flexion.

Deep Posterior Compartment

- *Neurovascular contents (▶ Fig. 1.11):* Tibial nerve, posterior tibial vessels, and peroneal vessels:
  - *Muscle innervation*: Tibial nerve.
- Popliteus:
  - *Origin:* Lateral surface of the lateral femoral condyle.
  - *Insertion:* Proximal posterior tibia.
  - *Action:* Internal rotation of the tibia/knee during initiation of knee flexion.
- FHL:
  - *Origin:* Inferior posterior fibula.
  - *Insertion:* Great toe distal phalanx.
  - *Action:* Great toe plantar flexion (▶ Fig. 1.12).
- Flexor digitorum longus (FDL)

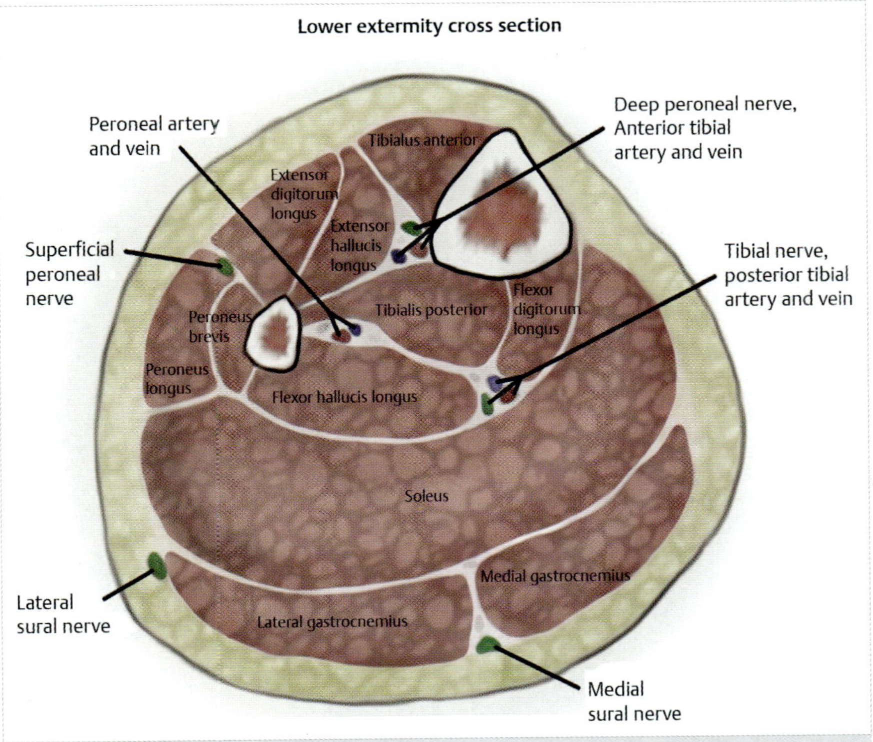

Fig. 1.11 Lower extremity cross-section.

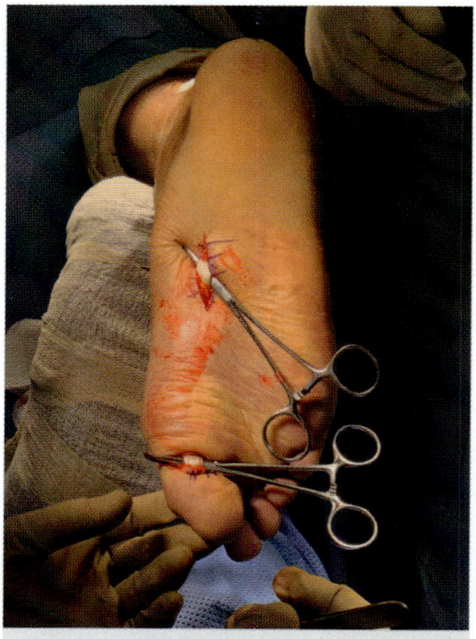

Fig. 1.12 Flexor hallucis longus at its distal insertion and at the knot of Henry.

 - *Origin:* Posterior tibia.
 - *Insertion:* Distal phalanges 2 to 5.
 - *Action:* Toes 2 to 5 plantar flexion.
- Tibialis posterior (TP):
 - *Origin:* Posterior tibia, fibula, and interosseous membrane.
 - *Insertion:* Plantar navicular cuneiforms and metatarsals.
 - *Action:* Foot inversion, adduction, and ankle plantar flexion. Primary source of dynamic arch support.
 - **Posterior tibial tendon insufficiency is the most common cause of adult-acquired flatfoot deformity.**
- Posterior tibial tendon has three terminal limbs:
 - *Anterior limb:* Insertion on the first cuneiform and navicular tuberosity.
 - *Middle limb:* Insertion on cuneiforms 2 to 3, cuboid, and metatarsals 2 to 4.
 - *Posterior limb:* Insertion on anterior sustentaculum tali.

1.5.2 Layers of the Foot

Compartments

- Nine compartments described by Manoli and Weber (controversial).
- Medial.
- Superficial.
- Lateral.
- Adductor.
- Calcaneal.
- Four interosseous.

Plantar Fascia

- Divided into three bands.
- Central band or plantar aponeurosis:
 - Originates at the medial calcaneal tuberosity and divides to insert on each toe (flexor tendon sheaths superficially and deep transverse metatarsal ligaments deep).
- Medial band.
- Lateral band:
 - Stabilizes the arch, especially during toe-off, via the **windlass mechanism** and protects deeper structures of the foot.
- Common injuries include **plantar fasciitis** and **fibromatosis.**

First Plantar Layer

- **Most superficial layer.**
- Muscles:
 - Abductor hallucis.
   - *Origin:* Medial process of calcaneal tuberosity.
   - *Insertion:* Base of the proximal phalanx of the great toe.
   - *Innervation:* Medial plantar nerve.
   - *Action:* Abduction of the great toe.
 - Flexor digitorum brevis (FDB).
   - *Origin:* Medial process of calcaneal tuberosity.
   - *Insertion:* Middle phalanges of toes 2 to 5.
   - *Innervation:* Medial plantar nerve.
   - *Action:* Flexion of toes 2 to 5.
 - Abductor digiti minimi (ADM).
   - *Origin:* Medial and lateral processes of calcaneal tuberosity.

- *Insertion:* Lateral base of the fifth toe proximal phalanx.
- *Innervation:* Lateral plantar nerve.
- *Action:* Abduction of the fifth toe.

Second Plantar Layer

- Muscles:
  - Quadratus plantae:
    - *Origin:* Plantar calcaneus.
    - *Insertion:* Lateral tendon of the FDL.
    - *Innervation:* Lateral plantar nerve.
    - *Action:* Aids toe flexion (with FDL).
  - Lumbrical muscles:
    - *Origin:* Branches of the FDL.
    - *Insertion:* Proximal phalanges.
    - *Innervation:* Medial and lateral planter nerves.
    - *Action:* Flexion of the MTP joints and extension of the IP joints.
- Tendons:
  - **FDL.**
  - **FHL.**
    - ***Knot of Henry:* The FDL crosses over the FHL at the level of the navicular, and the tendons are connected via multiple attachments.**
- Neurovasculature:
  - **Terminal branches of the tibial nerves.**
  - Medial and lateral plantar nerves.
  - Medial plantar artery.
  - Lateral plantar artery.

Third Plantar Layer

- Muscles:
  - Flexor hallucis brevis (FHB):
    - *Origin:* Cuboid and lateral cuneiform.
    - *Insertion:* Proximal phalanx of great toe.
    - *Innervation:* Medial plantar nerve.
    - *Action:* Flexion of the great toe MTP joint.
- Adductor hallucis:
  - Oblique and transverse heads:
    - *Origin:* Two to four metatarsals (oblique) and lateral four MTP (transverse).
    - *Insertion:* Proximal phalanx of the great toe.
    - *Innervation:* Lateral plantar nerve.
    - *Action:* Adduction of the great toe.
    - **Implicated in hallux valgus deformity.**
  - Flexor digiti minimi brevis (FDMB):
    - *Origin:* Fifth metatarsal base.
    - *Insertion:* Proximal phalanx of the small toe.
    - *Innervation:* Lateral plantar nerve.
    - *Action:* Flexion of MTP of the small toe.

Fourth Plantar

- **Deepest layer.**
- Muscles:
  - Dorsal interosseous muscle:
    - *Origin:* Adjacent metatarsals.
    - *Insertion:* Lateral proximal phalanx 2 to 4 and medial proximal phalanx 2.
    - *Innervation:* Lateral plantar nerve.
    - *Action:* Toe abduction.
  - Plantar interosseous muscle:
    - *Origin:* Medial metatarsals 3 to 5.
    - *Insertion:* Medial proximal phalanxes 3 to 5.
    - *Innervation:* Lateral plantar nerve.
    - *Action:* Toe adduction, MTPJ flexion, and LPJ extension.
- Tendons:
  - Travel through the fibro-osseous tunnels.
  - Peroneus longus.
  - TP.

Dorsal Layer

- Extensor digitorum brevis (EDB):
  - *Origin:* Dorsolateral calcaneus.
  - *Insertion:* Proximal phalanxes 2 to 4.
  - *Innervation:* Deep peroneal nerve.
  - *Action:* MTPJ 2 to 4 extension.
- Extensor hallucis brevis:
  - *Origin:* Dorsolateral calcaneus.
  - *Insertion:* Proximal phalanx of great toe.
  - *Innervation:* Deep peroneal nerve.
  - *Action:* MTPJ great toe extension.

1.5.3 Neural Anatomy

There are five main nerves that supply the foot and ankle (▶ Fig. 1.13).

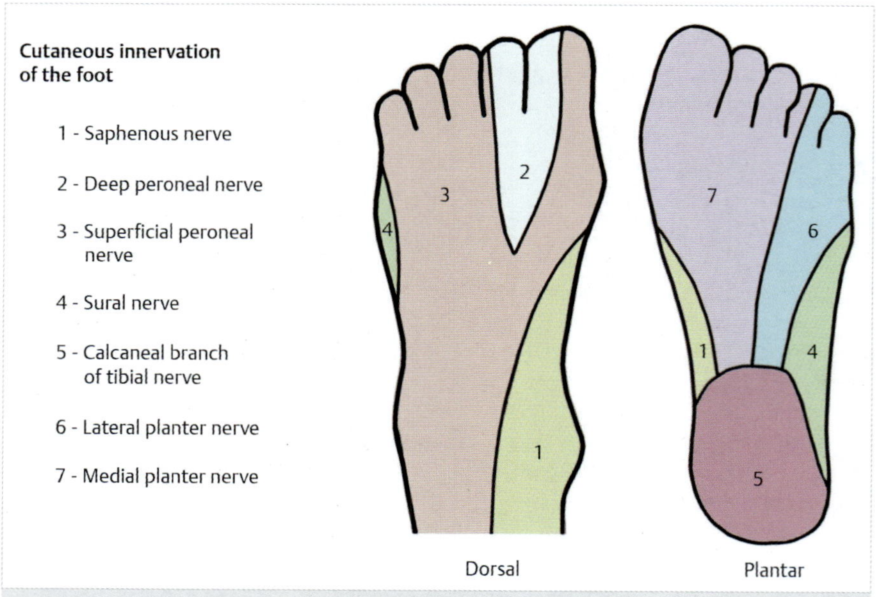

Fig. 1.13 Cutaneous innervation of the foot.

Tibial Nerve

- Runs posterior to the medial malleolus into the tarsal tunnel, then divides into the medial calcaneal branch and medial and lateral plantar nerves.
- Medial calcaneal branch:
  - Supplies sensation to the plantar heel.

Medial Plantar Nerve

- Sensation to the medial plantar foot and toes, motor to the abductor hallucis, FDB, medial lumbricals, and FHB.

Lateral Plantar Nerve

- Sensation to the plantar lateral foot and toes, motor to the abductor digiti minimi (via **Baxter's nerve,** which is the first branch and is often implicated in heel pain), quadratus plantae, lateral lumbricals, adductor hallucis, FDMB, and dorsal and plantar interosseous muscles.

Superficial Peroneal Nerve

- Dorsal foot and medial great toe sensation. **Can be injured during the lateral approach to the ankle and also the anterolateral arthroscopy portal.**

Deep Peroneal Nerve

- Sensation to the first dorsal webspace and motor to the EDB and EHL.

Sural Nerve

- Dorsolateral foot sensation.

Saphenous Nerve

- Medial foot sensation.

1.5.4 Vascular Anatomy

- Three major arteries in the foot and ankle:
  - *Posterior tibial artery:* Supplies the medial malleolus and calcaneus.

Two terminal branches are the medial and lateral plantar arteries. These have further branches that anastomose to form the **deep plantar arch**.
- *Anterior tibial artery:* Supplies the medial and lateral malleolus along with the dorsum of the foot. Also gives way to the **dorsalis pedis** artery in the foot.
- *Peroneal artery:* Supplies the posterior talus, lateral malleolus, and the calcaneus via a perforating artery that goes through the interosseous membrane.

Bones with tenuous blood supply include the talus, navicular, and the base of the fifth metatarsal.

1.6 Key Testing Facts

- The anterior talofibular ligament is the most commonly injured ligament in ankle sprains.
- Artery of the tarsal canal, a branch of the posterior tibial artery is the major arterial supply to the talus.
- Posterior tibial tendon insufficiency is the most common cause of adult acquired flatfoot deformity.
- The Flexor hallucis longus tendon runs beneath the sustentaculum tali.
- The insertion of the tibialis anterior is the medial cuneiform and the base of the first metatarsal The contents of the tarsal tunnel from anteromedial to posterolateral: tibialis posterior, FDL, posterior tibial artery, posterior tibial vein, tibial nerve, and FHL

References

[1] Van Heest TJ, Lafferty PM. Injuries to the ankle syndesmosis. J Bone Joint Surg Am. 2014; 96(7): 603–613

[2] Boyer MI. AAOS Comprehensive Orthopaedic Review. 2nd ed. Rosemont, IL: American Academy of Orthopaedic Surgeons; 2014

[3] Hunt KJ, Phisitkul P, Pirolo J, Amendola A. High ankle sprains and syndesmotic injuries in athletes. J Am Acad Orthop Surg. 2015; 23(11):661–673

[4] Thompson JC. Netter's Concise Orthopaedic Anatomy. 2nd ed. Philadelphia, PA: Elsevier Saunders; 2010

[5] Manoli A, II, Weber TG. Fasciotomy of the foot: an anatomical study with special reference to release of the calcaneal compartment. Foot Ankle. 1990; 10(5):267–275

[6] Miller MD, Thompson SR, Hart JA. Review of Orthopaedics. 6th ed. Philadelphia, PA: Elsevier Saunders; 2012

[7] Pomeroy G, Wilton J, Anthony S. Entrapment neuropathy about the foot and ankle: an update. J Am Acad Orthop Surg. 2015; 23(1):58–66

2 Surgical Approaches to the Foot and Ankle

Natalie V. Singer and David M. Walton

Abstract

Surgical approaches to the foot and ankle can be intimidating due to the complex anatomy, which was outlined in the previous chapter. The following surgical approaches are intended to describe the fundamental exposures utilized in foot and ankle surgery. A solid understanding of these approaches allows a surgeon to adapt to patient-specific factors such as deformity, previous incisions, or the combination of procedures. This is not a comprehensive list. Many of these approaches can be modified for the utilization of specific techniques or multiple procedures. In these situations, certain structures can act as an anatomical reference from which other structures and hazards can be identified.

Keywords: ankle, foot, surgical approach, dissection, techniques

2.1 Ankle Approaches

- **Direct anterior:**
  - *Uses:*
    - Tibiotalar arthrodesis, total ankle arthroplasty, hemi-talar allograft, talar open reduction and internal fixation (ORIF), pilon ORIF, incision and drainage (I & D) of ankle, and supramalleolar osteotomy.
  - *Position:*
    - Supine with bump under ipsilateral hip.
  - *Superficial landmarks:*
    - Proximal: palpate the tibial crest.
    - Distal: The medial to lateral midpoint of the foot can be assessed by manipulation of the Chopart joint. The midpoint should be over the lateral portion of the talonavicular joint.
    - Incision: The length of the proximal aspect of the incision is specific to the application of the approach and is started 1 cm (one fingerbreadth) lateral to the tibial crest. This is carried along a projected straight line to the midpoint of the foot (▶ Fig. 2.1a).
  - *Superficial dissection:*
    - The skin and subcutaneous tissue are sharply dissected. As the proximal aspect of the tibiotalar joint is approached, the superficial peroneal nerve (SPN) will be encountered. Blunt dissection is used to carefully free the crossing branches toward the distal aspect of the wound.
    - The extensor retinaculum is immediately deep to the subcutaneous tissue. From medial to lateral, the tibialis anterior (TA) and extensor hallucis longus (EHL) are palpable and distinguishable with flexion and extension of the first metatarsophalangeal (MTP) joint.
    - With the SPN retracted and protected, the extensor retinaculum is sharply incised and the sheath is opened proximally and distally[1] (▶ Fig. 2.1b).
  - *Deep dissection:*
    - The interval between the TA and the EHL is developed.
    - The deep neurovascular bundle containing the anterior tibial artery and deep peroneal nerve is directly deep to the EHL tendon. Along with the EHL, the bundle is carefully retracted laterally and the TA is medially, exposing the joint capsule and periosteum (▶ Fig. 2.1c).
    - In line with the incision, the capsule and periosteum are sharply incised with care to avoid injury to the cartilage.
    - The ankle joint is exposed in subperiosteal fashion medially and laterally (▶ Fig. 2.1d).

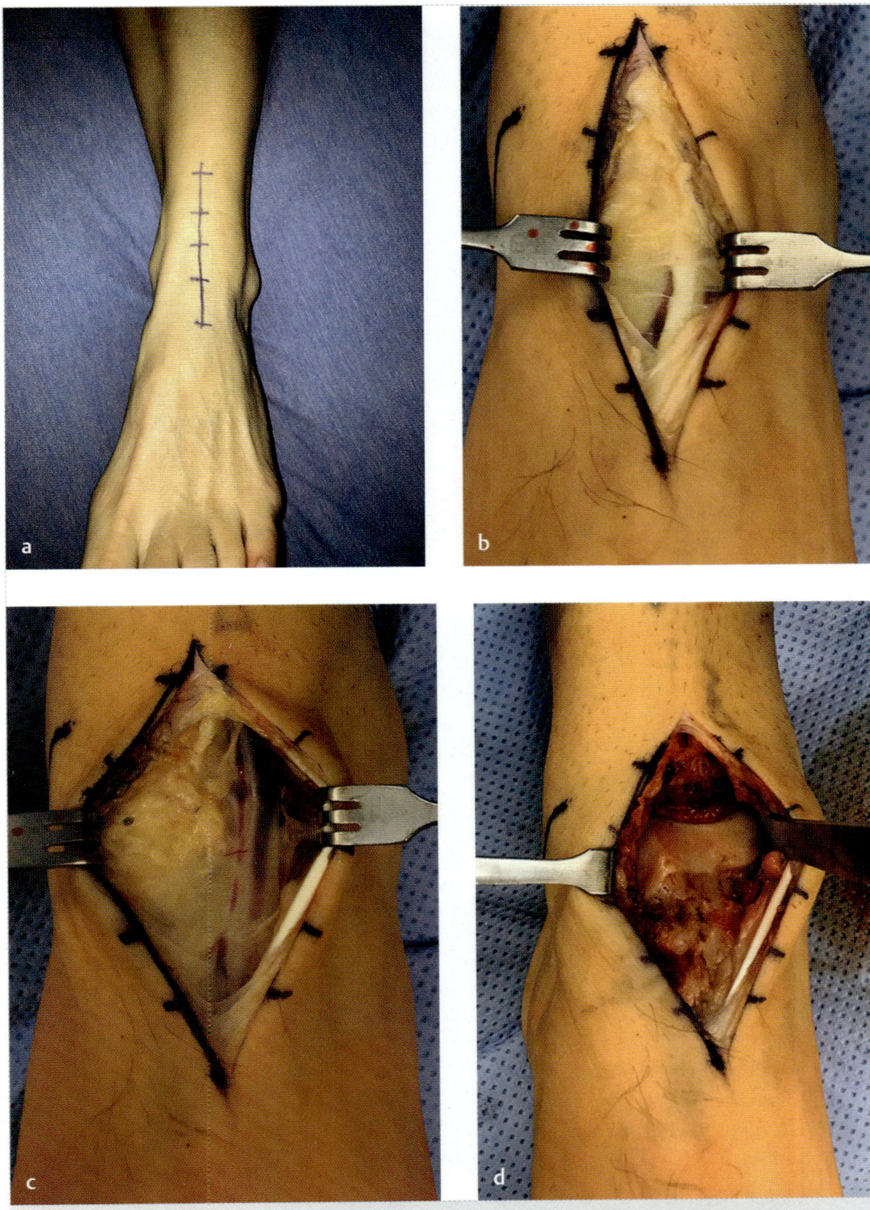

Fig. 2.1 Anterior ankle approach. **(a)** Incision centered over the ankle joint. **(b)** Superficial dissection with the extensor hallucis longus (EHL) tendon visible. **(c)** Once EHL tendon sheath opened, encounter the neurovascular bundle deep to this. **(d)** Ankle joint exposed after capsular incision and periosteal elevation.

- *Hazards:*
  - SPN:
    - It crosses superficially from lateral to medial proximal to the tibiotalar joint line.
  - Deep neurovascular bundle:
    - Anterior tibial artery and deep peroneal nerve are immediately deep the EHL tendon.
- *Technique pearls:*
  - The SPN often has multiple branches at this level and careful distal dissection can allow greater excursion and less traction throughout the procedure.
  - The extensor retinaculum can alternately be opened directly over the TA. With the TA retracted medially and sharp dissection through the deep TA sheath to the tibia, this reliably places the neurovascular bundle laterally.
  - The extensor retinaculum is ideally opened through thick portions of the retinaculum for ease with closure, this will help prevent bowstringing of the tendons.
- *Anatomical reference:*
  - EHL and TA.

- **Posterolateral:**
  - *Uses:*
    - Posterior malleolus fractures, trimalleolar fractures, os trigonum excision, (FHL).
  - *Position:*
    - Prone with towels under the tibia allowing the ankle to dorsiflex to neutral and to avoid injury to the posteromedial neurovascular bundle.
    - Bump placed under the contralateral hemi-pelvis.
  - *Superficial landmarks:*
    - Medial: the medial border of the Achilles tendon.
    - Lateral: the posterior fibula.
    - Incision: make a longitudinal incision placed midway between these two landmarks. As you travel distally, you can curve toward the tip of the lateral malleolus (▶ Fig. 2.2a).
  - *Superficial dissection:*
    - The skin and subcutaneous tissue are sharply incised in line with the incision. Care should be taken to avoid the sural nerve throughout the incision.
    - In the proximal portion of the wound, The "sural" nerve may be found traversing from medial to lateral along with the short saphenous vein. Distally the sural nerve courses laterally inferior to the fibula.
    - The deep fascia of the ankle is then encountered and should be sharply divided in line with the incision.
    - With gentle retraction, the peroneal retinaculum can be identified laterally. Deep in the wound is the FHL fascia.
    - The peroneal retinaculum can be released to mobilize the peroneal tendons (▶ Fig. 2.2b).
  - *Deep dissection:*
    - The FHL fascia is sharply incised in line with the incision and opened proximally and distally.
    - The FHL muscle belly lies on the posterior tibia and its identity can be confirmed with flexion and extension of the hallux (▶ Fig. 2.2c).
    - Retracting the FHL medially and the peroneal tendons laterally will expose the posterolateral 2/3 of the tibia (▶ Fig. 2.2d).
    - Care should be taken to maintain retractors lateral to the FHL as the neurovascular bundle lies just medial to it.[2]
    - Releasing the FHL muscle fibers off the fibular origin can enhance proximal exposure.
    - Retracting the peroneal tendons allows access to the posterior aspect of the fibula.
  - *Hazards:*
    - Sural nerve and small saphenous vein course parallel to the incision;

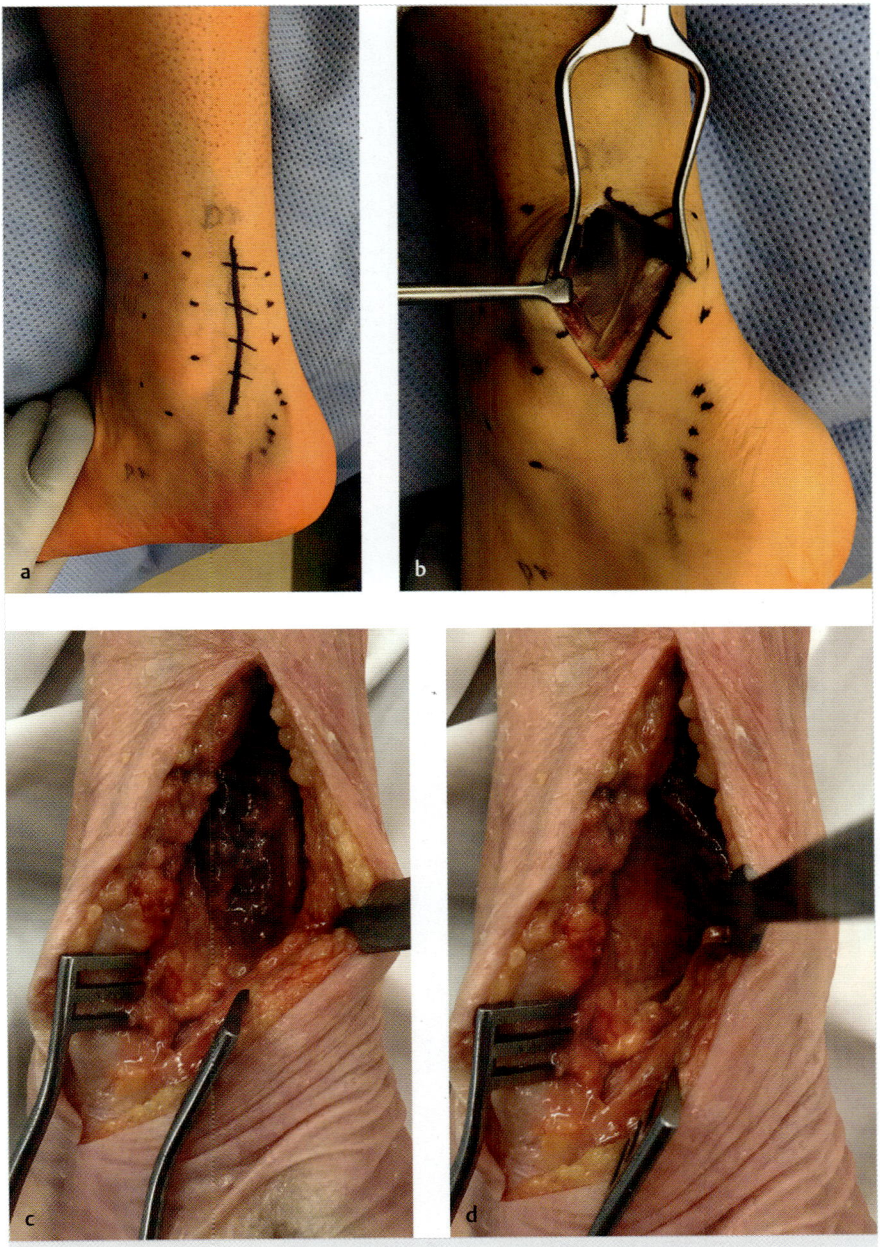

Fig. 2.2 Posterolateral ankle approach. **(a)** Incision centered between the lateral edge of the Achilles tendon and the fibula. **(b)** Superficial dissection with peroneal tendons retracted exposing the flexus hallucis longus (FHL) fascia. **(c)** FHL muscle belly laying on posterior tibia. **(d)** Posterior tibia exposed after retraction of the FHL medially and peroneal tendons laterally.

however, these can cross from medial to lateral at the proximal aspect. Injury commonly leads to painful paresthesias or a painful neuroma.
    - Posteriorly, the tibial nerve and artery lie medial to the FHL and can be injured with aggressive or poorly placed retraction.
    - Peroneal artery: During elevation of the FHL, the peroneal artery is at risk as it courses anteriorly between the FHL and the peroneus brevis along the posterior aspect of the syndesmosis.
  - *Technique pearls:*
    - The incision can be adjusted medially or laterally to give more access to the structures of interest.
    - The distal aspect of the incision can be curved laterally to gain greater exposure to the distal fibula.
  - *Anatomical reference:*
    - FHL and peroneals.
- **Lateral:**
  - *Uses:*
    - Ankle fracture, ankle arthrodesis, fibular osteotomy, Broström procedure, and peroneal work.
  - *Position:*
    - Supine with bump under the ipsilateral hip.
    - Lateral position.
  - *Superficial landmarks:*
    - The distal fibula: Outline the lateral malleolus and then palpate the fibular shaft in a stepwise fashion proximally, marking the midline as you go.
    - Incision: Longitudinal over the midline of the fibula, angled anteriorly over the distal aspect of the malleolus (▸ Fig. 2.3a).
  - *Superficial dissection:*
    - The subcutaneous tissue is sharply divided.
    - The SPN passes from posterior to anterior, but its location is variable; effort should be made to identify and carefully protect it (▸ Fig. 2.3b).
  - *Deep dissection:*
    - The deep fascia over the lateral compartment is incised and opened proximally (▸ Fig. 2.3c).
    - The peroneal muscles are bluntly dissected and retracted posteriorly to expose the proximal fibula.
  - *Hazards:*
    - SPN: It courses from posterior to anterior approximately 5 cm proximal to the ankle joint or 7-10cm proximal to the tip of the fibula.[3]
    - The short saphenous vein courses in line with the posterior aspect of the fibula. This is more commonly encountered with posterolateral fibular exposure.
  - *Technique pearls:*
    - While the SPN has a commonly described level for which it crosses the fibula, it varies significantly. Therefore, sharp dissection to bone is discouraged prior to identifying the nerve.
- **Medial:**
  - *Uses:*
    - Medial malleolar fracture, medial ankle arthrotomy, deltoid repair, and exposure of the posterior tibial tendon.
  - *Position:*
    - Supine with leg naturally externally rotated. A bump under the contralateral hip is not necessarily needed.
  - *Superficial landmarks:*
    - The medial malleolus is subcutaneous and easily palpated.
    - The soft apex of the intersection of the tibial plafond and medial malleolus denotes the anterior aspect of the medial malleolus.
    - The medial aspect of the navicular can be identified by following the course of the posterior tibial tendon and by rotation of the foot through the Chopart joint.
    - Incision: A longitudinal curvilinear incision is made over the midline of

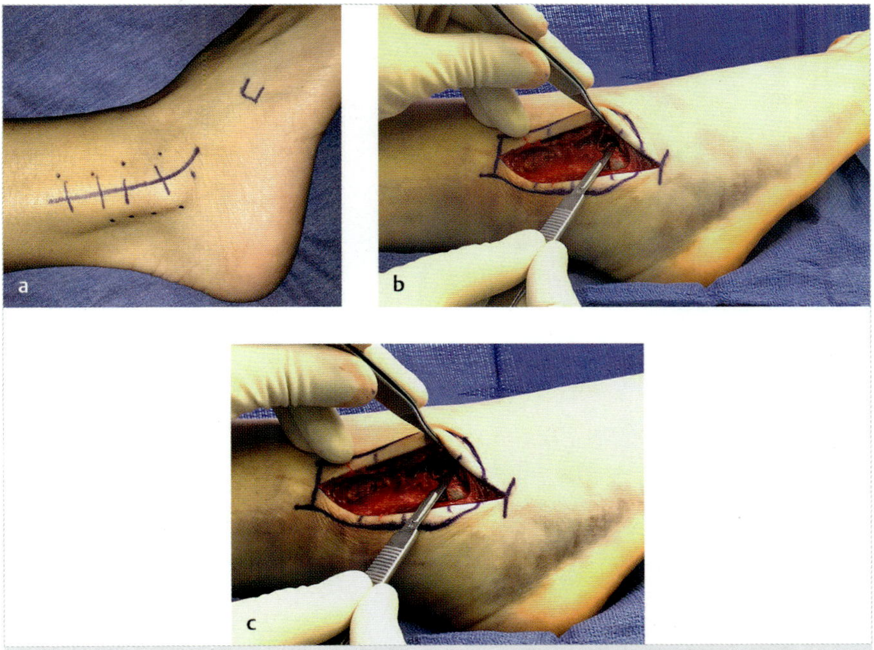

Fig. 2.3 Lateral ankle approach. **(a)** Incision centered over the midline of the fibula, then curved anteriorly over the anterior malleolus. **(b)** Superficial dissection over lateral fibula. Care is taken to protect the superficial peroneal nerve, which variably crosses from lateral to medial in the area of this incision. **(c)** Deep fascial incision with periosteal elevation.

the medial malleolus, curving anteriorly toward the navicular at the distal aspect (▶ Fig. 2.4a).

- *Superficial dissection:*
  - The skin and subcutaneous tissue are sharply divided. The long saphenous vein and saphenous nerve generally lie anterior to the incision, but may be encountered and run parallel to the incision (▶ Fig. 2.4b).
- *Deep dissection:*
  - The anterior skin flap is gently retracted to protect the saphenous nerve and vein. Posteriorly, the flexor retinaculum over the posterior tibialis tendon is palpable and can be opened to retract the tendon and expose the posterior aspect of the tibia[4] (▶ Fig. 2.4c, d).
  - To expose the anterior ankle joint, capsule is incised over the soft spot, described above, where the tibial plafond and medial malleolus intersect. This allows a read of the shoulder of the anteromedial portion of the ankle joint in the setting of a pilon or medial malleolar fracture.
  - The joint capsule is then subperiosteally elevated to expose the tibiotalar articulation.
- *Hazards:*
  - The long saphenous vein and nerve run in line with the incision anteriorly but can be immediately under the incision.
  - The posterior tibial tendon courses immediately posterior to the medial malleolus and can easily be damaged or incarcerated by hardware.
- *Technique pearls:*
  - Marking the anteromedial soft spot of the ankle should be marked prior

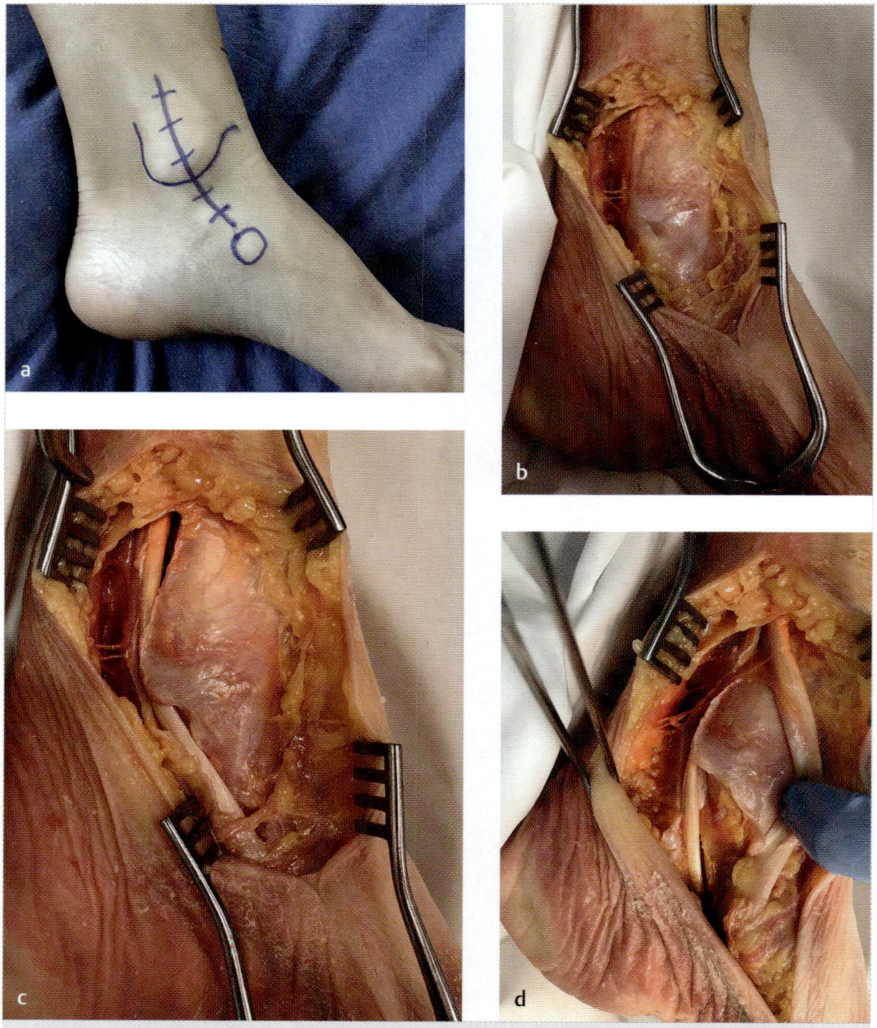

Fig. 2.4 Medial ankle approach. (a) Navicular and medial malleolus outlined and curvilinear incision marked. (b) Superficial dissection with the anterior skin flap retracted protecting the saphenous vein and nerve. (c) Flexor retinaculum split over the palpable posterior tibialis tendon. (d) Posterior tibialis tendon retracted anteriorly to expose the posterior tibia.

to placing incision as an anatomical reference.

- Preoperative planning of the incision is important to allow exposure to critical structures. If exposure of the ankle joint is important, the incision can be shifted anteriorly or the curve can be placed further anterior. Alternatively, if the posterior tibial tendon is involved, a slightly more posterior incision should be made.
- When posterior hardware is being placed, isolation and retraction of the posterior tibial tendon minimizes injury.

◦ *Anatomical reference:*
  - Apex of the ankle joint and medial malleolus.

2.2 Foot Approaches

- **Dorsal midfoot (medial):**
  - *Uses:*
    - Lisfranc ORIF, tarsometatarsal (TMT) fractures, and midfoot arthrodesis.
  - *Position:*
    - Supine with bump under ipsilateral hip.
  - *Superficial landmarks:*
    - It is difficult to palpate the proximal landmark for this approach. It is useful to use a radiopaque instrument to mark the proximal first and second TMT junction using fluoroscopy.
    - The distal endpoint of the incision is over the first webspace.
    - The specific medial to lateral placement of the incision is based on the joints that need to be accessed.
    - Incision is made longitudinally from the proximal aspect of the cuneiform to roughly the midpoint of the metatarsal shaft and taken distally (▶ Fig. 2.5a).
  - *Superficial dissection:*
    - The skin and subcutaneous tissue are sharply divided. Depending on the position of the incision, the anatomic structures encountered next will vary.
    - The extensor retinaculum is incised and the EHL and extensor hallucis brevis (EHB) should be identified.
  - *Deep dissection:*
    - The neurovascular bundle of the dorsalis pedis artery and deep peroneal nerve travels deep to the EHB. This bundle then dives into the first webspace.
    - With the EHL tendon retracted laterally and the EHB medially (with the neurovascular bundle) expose the first and second TMT articulation (▶ Fig. 2.5b).
    - The periosteum is incised and elevated exposing the TMT joints.[5] (▶ Fig. 2.5c).
  - *Hazards:*
    - Deep neurovascular bundle: The dorsalis pedis artery and the deep peroneal nerve course underneath the EHB tendon and dives into the first webspace.
  - *Technique pearls:*
    - Prior to inflating the tourniquet, the dorsalis pedis pulse should be palpated and its position noted.
    - Care should be taken to adequately mobilize and protect the

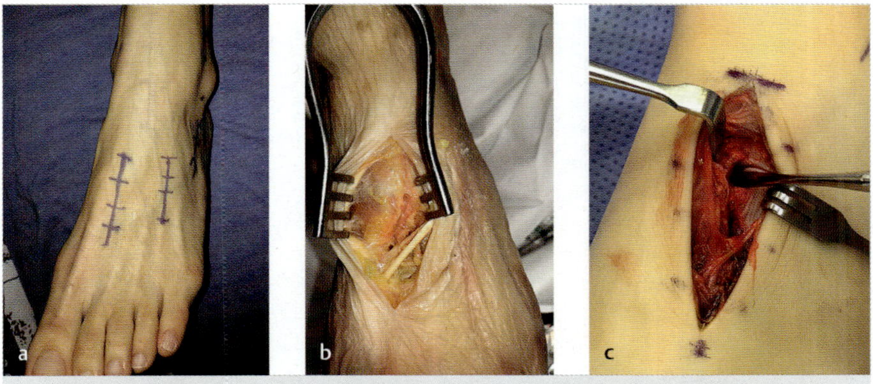

Fig. 2.5 Medial approach of the dorsal midfoot. **(a)** Planned incisions for the medial and lateral midfoot approaches (right foot). We recommend using a metallic object and fluoroscopy to identify the tarsometatarsal (TMT) joint of choice. **(b)** Extensor hallucis longus (EHL) tendon retracted laterally, extensor hallucis brevis (EHB), and neurovascular bundle retracted medially (left foot). **(c)** Deep dissection, with periosteal elevation, exposing the first and second TMT articulations.

    neurovascular bundle to allow working room underneath it. This allows a diamond or "U" type plates to be placed over the first and second TMT joints in a safe manner.
    - It is often necessary to extend the incision proximally and distally to allow adequate exposure without excessive traction on the wound. In higher energy cases, one may want to extend the incision distally to the naviculocuneiform joints to ensure that these joints are not unstable.
  - *Anatomical reference:*
    - EHB and EHL.
- **Dorsal midfoot (lateral):**
  - *Uses:*
    - TMT fractures and midfoot arthrodesis. This incision can be made in conjunction with the dorsomedial approach. Ideally, the distance between the two incisions is 3cm.
  - *Position:*
    - Supine with bump under ipsilateral hip.
  - *Superficial landmarks:*
    - It is difficult to palpate the proximal landmark for this approach. It is useful to use a radiopaque instrument to mark the proximal third and fourth TMT junction using fluoroscopy.
    - The distal endpoint of the incision is over the third webspace (▶ Fig. 2.5a).
  - *Superficial dissection:*
    - Sharply incise the skin and branches of the SPN subcutaneous tissue. The SPN lies immediately subcutaneous and is often crossing this incision in an irregular pattern. This should be mobilized and carefully retracted.
    - The extensor retinaculum is then divided.
  - *Deep dissection:*
    - Expose the extensor tendons. The third and fourth long extensor tendons are retracted exposing the extensor digitorum brevis (EDB; ▶ Fig. 2.6a, b).
    - Bluntly develop the intramuscular plane between the muscle bellies of the EDB.
    - The muscle bellies are then retracted exposing the joint capsule and periosteum.
    - Sharply incise the periosteum, and subperiosteal dissection exposes the lateral TMT articulations (▶ Fig. 2.6c).
  - *Hazards:*
    - The branches of the SPN can have varying anatomy, and careful superficial dissection is required to identify and protect the nerve.
  - *Technique pearls:*
    - The EDB originates lateral of the anterior calcaneus; therefore, the muscle and tendon units will be oriented obliquely in the wound. Blunt dissection from distal to proximal will allow greater ease in finding the intramuscular plane.
  - *Anatomical reference:*
    - EDB.
- **Sinus tarsi:**
  - *Uses:*
    - Subtalar arthrodesis, lateral talar process fractures, calcaneus ORIF, lateral column lengthening, and access to lateral talonavicular joint.
  - *Position:*
    - Lateral.
    - Supine with large bump under ipsilateral hip.
  - *Superficial landmarks:*
    - Proximal: the tip of the fibula.
    - Distal: the base of the fourth metatarsal.
    - Incision: A straight line should be drawn between the proximal and distal landmarks, which should trace over the inferior portion of the sinus tarsi, or the soft spot between the talus and calcaneus (▶ Fig. 2.7a).
  - *Superficial dissection:*
    - Sharply incise the skin and divide the subcutaneous tissue.

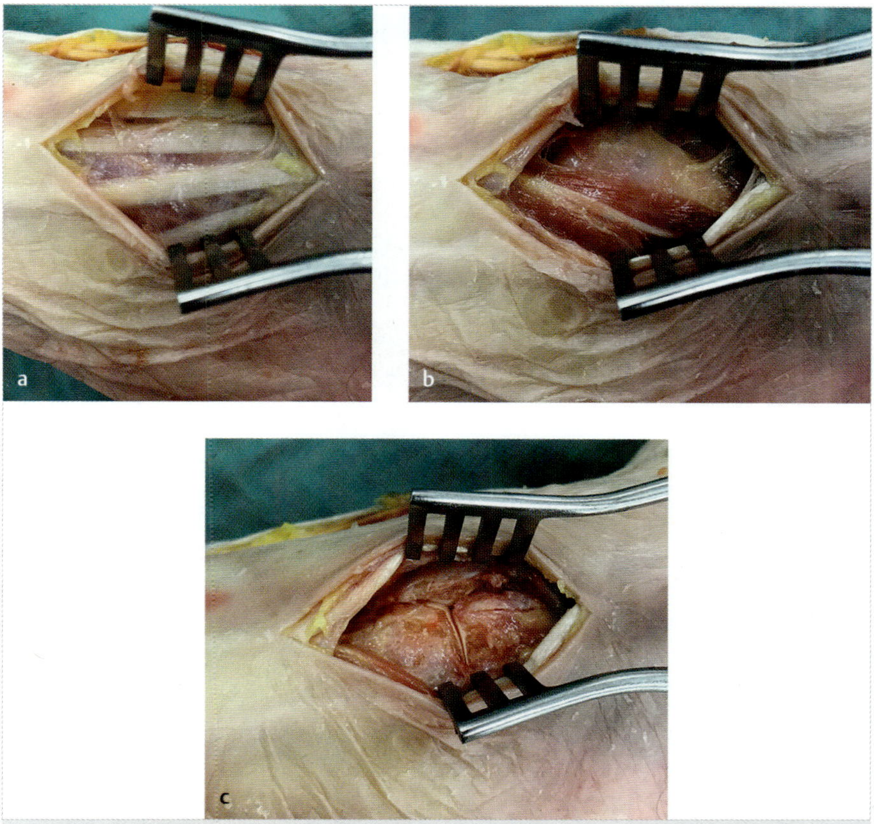

Fig. 2.6 Lateral approach to the dorsal midfoot. **(a)** Superficial dissection, the exposing extensor tendons. **(b)** Extensor digitorum longus (EDL) tendons retracted exposing extensor digitorum brevis (EDB), which can be bluntly dissected to develop intramuscular plane. **(c)** EDB muscle bellies retracted, and subperiosteal dissection exposing lateral tarsometatarsal (TMT) joints.

- The sural nerve courses plantar and parallel and plantar to this incision but is often encountered at the proximal aspect of the wound.
- The fascia is incised in line with the wound and retracted, exposing the EDB (▶ Fig. 2.7b).

◦ *Distally, Deep dissection:*

- The EDB plantar origin is sharply elevated off the calcaneus and retracted anteriorly (▶ Fig. 2.7c).
- This exposes the sinus tarsi and the subtalar joint.
- Using fluoroscopy, a blunt instrument can be inserted into the sinus tarsi to confirm its trajectory.
- If access to the calcaneocuboid joint is required, the sharp elevation of the EDB is carried toward the anterior process of the calcaneus and the joint capsule is then incised vertically. The peroneals will need to be retracted either superiorly or inferiorly.

◦ *Hazards:*

- The sural nerve courses parallel to the incision.
- Posteriorly, the peroneal tendons can be damaged.
- The artery of the sinus tarsi is at risk with dissection into the sinus tarsi.

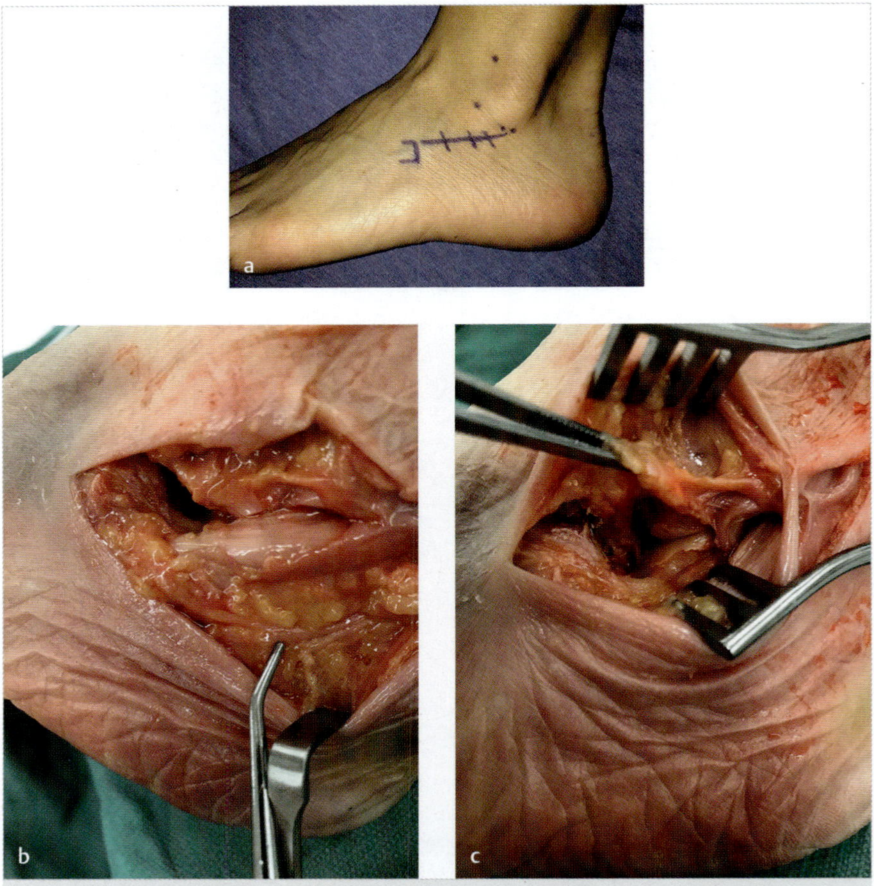

Fig. 2.7 Sinus tarsi approach. **(a)** Planned incision from the base of the fourth metatarsal and distal fibula landmarks. **(b)** Superficial dissection displaying sural nerve coursing parallel and plantar to incision, as well as extensor digitorum brevis (EDB) exposure. **(c)** Deep dissection with EDB elevated, exposing the sinus tarsi and subtalar joint.

- *Technique pearls:*
  - When performing a subtalar arthrodesis, it can be useful to elevate the EDB gently, keeping its fascia intact. This will act as a separate layer to close, preventing graft displacement and possibly better blood supply.
  - In severe valgus deformity, the ankle joint can be confused for the subtalar joint during the lateral approach. Prior to any irreversible procedural steps, fluoroscopy should be employed to confirm the appropriate joint is exposed.
  - Once identified, the sural nerve should be protected but manipulated only as absolutely necessary as it is sensitive and can often lead to postoperative neuritis or neuromas.
- *Anatomical reference:*
  - Sinus tarsi.

- **Great MTP Joint—medial:**
  - *Uses:*
    - Hallux valgus correction, akin osteotomy, medial sesamoidectomy, medial sesamoid ORIF, medial sesamoidectomy, first MTP joint fusion, and plantar plate repair.
  - *Position:*
    - Supine.
  - *Superficial landmarks:*
    - Proximally, it is centered over the medial metatarsal shaft.
    - Distally, it is centered over the proximal phalanx.
    - Incision: The connection of these lines should create an obtuse angle with the apex at the medial eminence. Often the surgeon chooses there to be a slight curve (▶ Fig. 2.8a).
  - *Superficial dissection:*
    - The skin and subcutaneous tissues are sharply divided.
    - The medial and oftentimes superior medial dorsal cutaneous nerve runs parallel to the incision. This should be identified and protected throughout the case (▶ Fig. 2.8b).
  - *Deep dissection:*
    - The capsule and periosteum are sharply incised in line with the incision from the midpoint of the proximal phalanx to proximal to the medial eminence.
    - The capsule is elevated proximally and distally using an inside-out technique exposing the MTP joint (▶ Fig. 2.8c).
    - Plantarly, the proximal extent should be limited to the metatarsal medially, avoiding deep and lateral elevation to protect the blood supply to the metatarsal head.
  - *Hazards:*
    - The medial dorsal cutaneous nerve courses parallel and generally dorsal

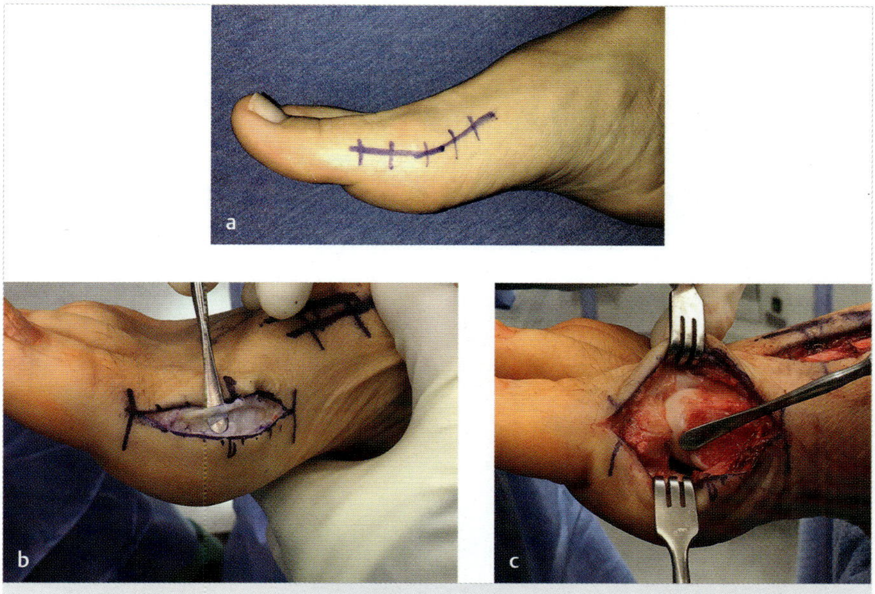

Fig. 2.8 Medial approach of the great metatarsophalangeal (MTP) joint. **(a)** Planned incision of the medial great MTP joint approach. Note the slightly curvilinear incision has apex centered over the medial eminence. **(b)** Medial great MTP dissection. Note the medial dorsal cutaneous nerve identified by the freer elevator. **(c)** Exposed great MTP joint using an inside-out approach with capsular elevation proximally and distally.

to the incision. Depending on the incision, it can be immediately in line with the incision. Care should be taken to identify this immediately and protect it. Painful incisions can occur when this is incorporated into the closure.
    - The first metatarsal plantar artery enters the plantar lateral corner of the metatarsal head. Soft-tissue dissection laterally should be avoided proximal to the metatarsal head.[6] One may release the lateral structures safely through an interval between the sesamoids and plantar metatarsal head with a lamina spreader
  - *Technique pearls:*
    - Often the proximal portion of the incision is made too plantar due to the amount of soft tissue below the metatarsal. Malposition can be mitigated by grasping the metatarsal from dorsal to plantar in the surgeon's nondominant hand and marking out the line bisecting this width.
    - Optimal joint exposure can be obtained by opening the capsule in one pass. This is done pressing the knife sharply to bone on the proximal phalanx and, without lifting off, bringing the knife across the joint to the base of the medial eminence.
    - When the capsule is kept intact, the closure and medial soft-tissue imbrication can be more robust.
- **First MTP joint: dorsal:**
  - *Uses:*
    - Dorsal cheilectomy, first MTP joint arthrodesis, first MTP joint resurfacing, and metatarsal ORIF.
  - *Position:*
    - Supine with bump under ipsilateral hip.
  - *Superficial landmarks:*
    - The hallux MTP joint is easily identified by flexion and extension. The EHL runs dorsally over the MTP joint.
    - Proximally, the center of the EHL is marked 2 to 4 cm proximal to the MTP joint.
    - Distally, the center of the interphalangeal joint can be identified by flexion and extension.
    - The incision is marked from the center of the EHL just proximal to the interphalangeal joint and taken proximally along the EHL onto the metatarsal shaft (▶ Fig. 2.9a).
  - *Superficial dissection:*
    - The skin and subcutaneous tissue are sharply divided.
    - The EHL is immediately identified and care should be taken to avoid disrupting its sheath (▶ Fig. 2.9b).
    - While still in its sheath, the EHL is isolated and mobilized. It is then retracted carefully laterally (▶ Fig. 2.9c).
    - This exposes the EHB and dorsal joint capsule.
  - *Deep dissection:*
    - The EHB is confluent with the dorsal joint capsule at the level of the MTP joint. This inserts dorsally on the proximal phalanx.
    - The EHB is sharply divided in line with the incision starting on the proximal phalanx carried proximally to the shaft of the metatarsal.
    - The capsule and periosteum are sharply elevated off the proximal phalanx and metatarsal neck, exposing the MTP joint.
    - To enhance the exposure of the metatarsal head, the collateral ligaments are elevated off the metatarsal neck (▶ Fig. 2.9d).
  - *Hazards:*
    - The EHL is directly in line with the incision. This can easily be injured or avulsed from its distal insertion if not carefully isolated and retracted.
    - When opening the first MTP joint capsule, the cartilage of the metatarsal head should be carefully

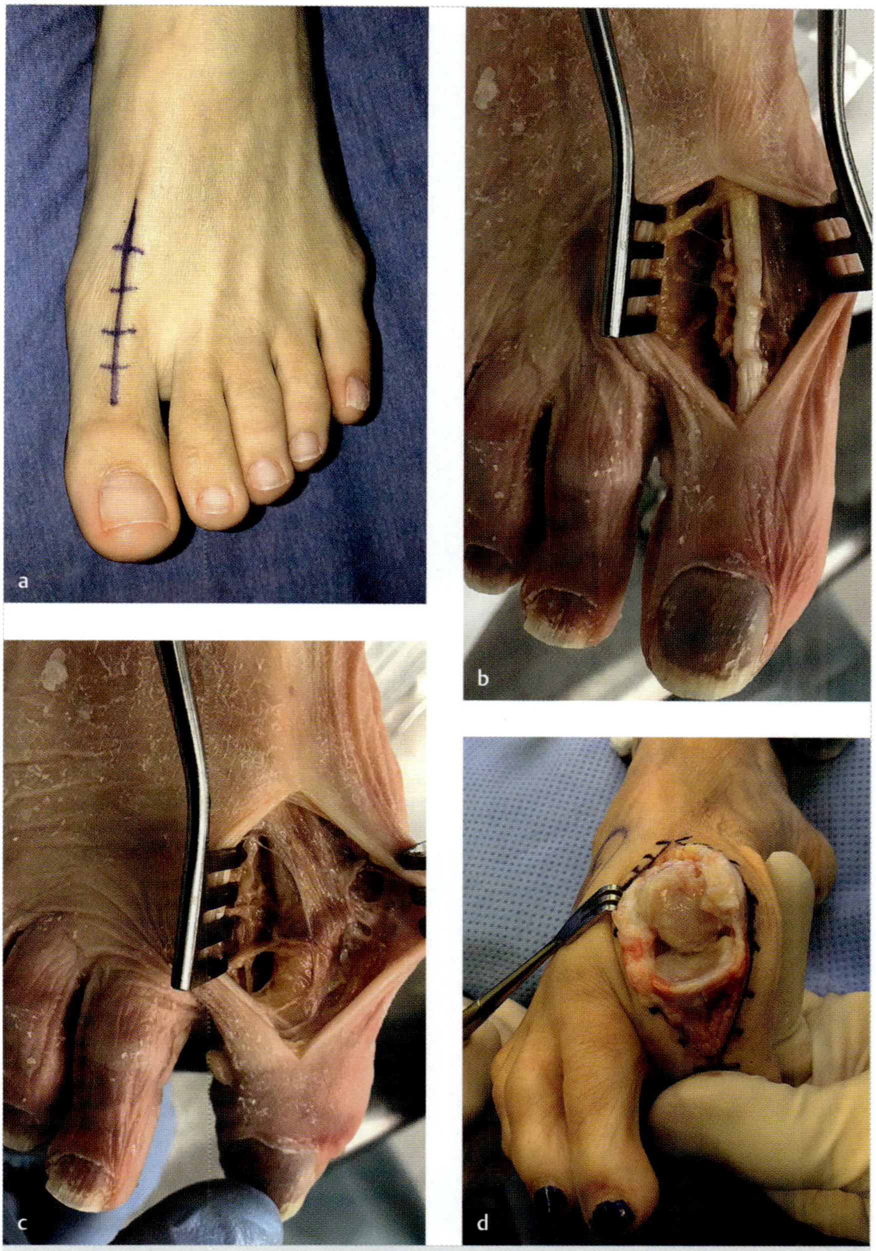

Fig. 2.9 Dorsal approach of the great metatarsophalangeal (MTP) joint. **(a)** Planned incision centered over the extensor hallucis longus (EHL) tendon. **(b)** Superficial dissection exposing the EHL tendon. **(c)** Deep dissection, with EHL tendon retracted laterally, and exposure of the extensor digitorum brevis (EDB) overlying the great MTP joint. **(d)** After capsular and periosteal elevation off the proximal phalanx and metatarsal neck, the great MTP joint is exposed. Further exposure is possible by elevating the collateral ligaments off the metatarsal neck, allowing access to the metatarsal head as seen here.

avoided as to not damage the cartilage.

- *Technique pearls:*
  - Keeping the EHL in its sheath minimizes adhesions postoperatively.
  - Incorporating the EHB when opening the MTP joint will give more robust tissue for closure.
- *Anatomical reference:*
  - MTP joint.

- **Dorsal lesser toe MTP joint:**
  - *Uses:*
    - Metatarsal shortening osteotomy, plantar plate repair, hammertoe correction, neuroma excision, and metatarsal head resection.
  - *Position:*
    - Supine with bump under the ipsilateral hip.
  - *Superficial landmarks:*
    - Proximal: the metatarsal shaft and extensor tendon.
    - Distal: the proximal phalanx is subcutaneous.
    - Incision: from the midline of the proximal phalanx carried proximally over the extensor tendon and metatarsal shaft (▶ Fig. 2.10a).
  - *Superficial dissection:*
    - The skin and subcutaneous tissue are sharply divided.
    - The deep fascia is sharply incised with care taken to avoid injury to the extensor digitorum longus (EDL; (▶ Fig. 2.10b).
    - The EDL is bluntly dissected and retracted laterally (▶ Fig. 2.10c).
  - *Deep dissection:*
    - The joint capsule is encountered next. Sharply incise and expose the joint by periosteal elevation of the proximal and distal capsule (▶ Fig. 2.10d).
    - Retractors can be placed on either side of the joint for exposure.
    - Alternatively, a McGlamry elevator can be placed plantar to the metatarsal neck to expose the metatarsal head.
    - If exposure to the digital nerve is required, blunt dissection is carried into the webspace down to the stout intermetatarsal ligament.
    - Once the intermetatarsal ligament is identified, a blunt Joker elevator is used to slide plantar to the ligament, bluntly separating and protecting the digital nerve.
    - After the elevator is in place, sharp dissection through the ligament onto the elevator is performed with care taken to ensure not to slide off the elevator.
  - *Hazards:*
    - EDL tendon: During the approach, the tendon can be inadvertently damaged, which can lead to adhesions.
    - Digital artery: Travels parallel to the metatarsal shaft, dorsal to the deep transverse metatarsal ligament and is at risk whenever dissection is directed away from the osseous ray.[7]
    - Metatarsal head cartilage: When using a McGlamry elevator, care should be taken to avoid damage to the metatarsal head cartilage during placement.
  - *Technique pearls:*
    - Planning of lesser toe incisions is critical. When consecutive metatarsals require surgery, an incision in their webspace can be utilized to avoid a narrow skin bridge.
    - When dissecting in a webspace, using a blunt instrument (i.e., handle of Adson forceps) can minimize the risk of damaging the neurovascular bundles.
    - The MTP joint capsule can be incised longitudinally for exposure; alternatively when dorsal soft-tissue contracture is part of the pathology (i.e., hammertoe), often a transverse capsulotomy is performed.
    - Careful inside-out technique is employed when performing capsulotomies or exposing joints to

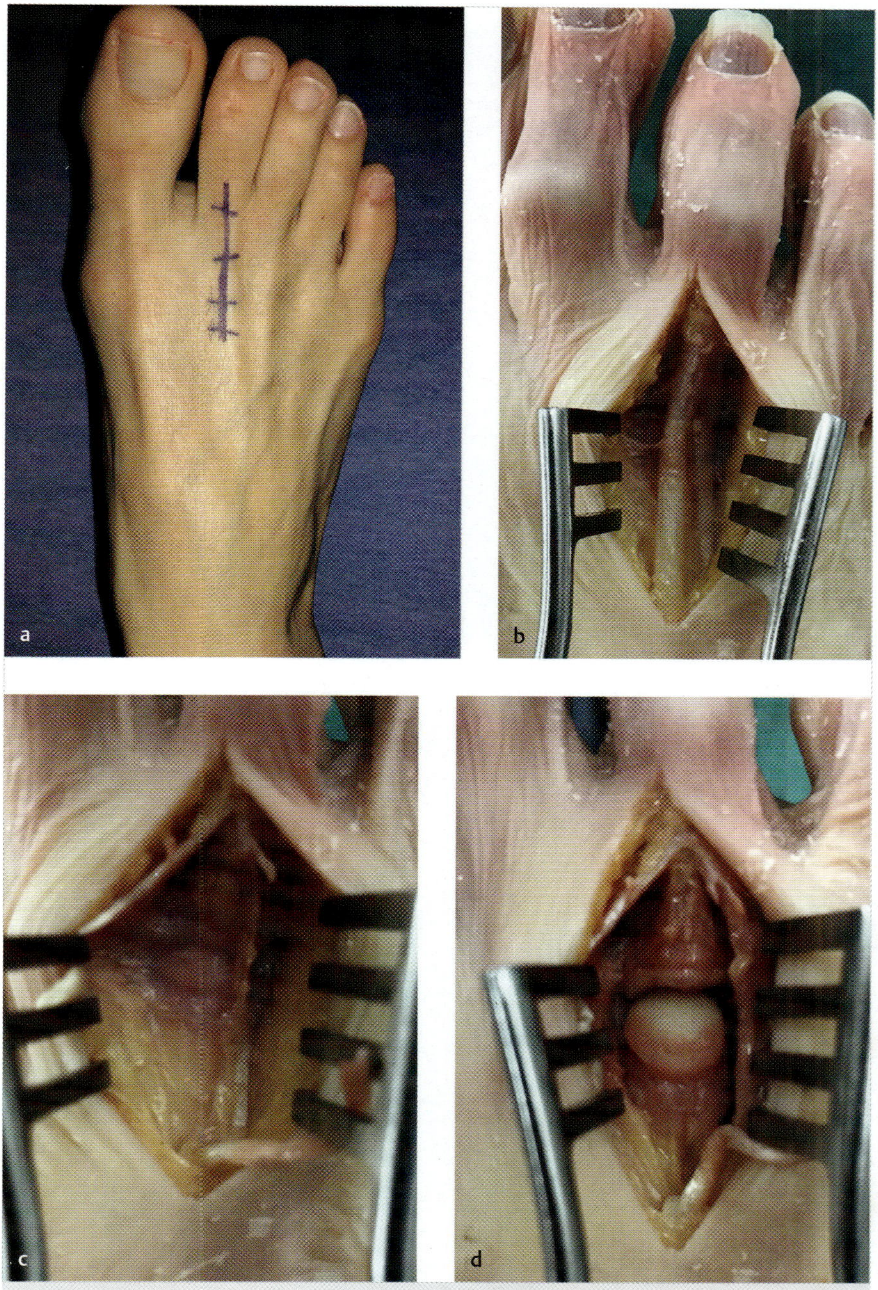

Fig. 2.10 Dorsal approach of the lesser metatarsophalangeal joint. **(a)** Lesser metatarsophalangeal joint dorsal incision centered over the proximal phalanx and the metatarsal shaft. **(b)** Superficial dissection with exposure of the extensor digitorum longus (EDL) tendon. **(c)** EDL bluntly dissected and retracted laterally. **(d)** Capsular incision and periosteal elevation gaining access to the lesser metatarsophalangeal (MTP) joint.

minimize risk to the neurovascular bundles.
  - When isolating the intermetatarsal ligament, the blunt Joker elevator can be placed, and replaced several times to ensure separation from the digital nerve.
- *Anatomical reference:*
  - Intermetatarsal ligament.

2.3 Key Testing Facts

Approach	Hazards
Anterior ankle	• Superficial peroneal nerve • Anterior tibial artery and deep peroneal nerve deep to the extensor hallucis longus tendon
Posterolateral ankle	• Sural nerve and small saphenous vein • Posterior tibial nerve and artery medial to the flexor hallucis longus tendon • Peroneal artery while elevating the flexor hallucis longus muscle body
Lateral ankle	• Superficial peroneal nerve
Medial ankle	• Long saphenous vein/nerve
Dorsal midfoot (medial)	• Dorsalis pedis artery and deep peroneal nerve under extensor hallucis brevis into the first webspace
Dorsal midfoot (lateral)	• Superficial peroneal nerve branches
Sinus tarsi	• Sural nerve • Artery of sinus tarsi
Great MTP joint (medial)	• Medial dorsal cutaneous nerve • First metatarsal plantar artery
Great MTP joint (dorsal)	• Extensor hallucis longus insertion
Dorsal lesser toe MTP joint	• Extensor digitorum longus • Digital artery

References

[1] Colonna PC, Ralston EL. Operative approaches to the ankle joint. Am J Surg. 1951; 82(1):44–54

[2] Rüedi TP, Murphy WM. AO Principles of Fracture Management. New York, NY: Thieme; 2000

[3] Duscher D, Wenny R, Entenfellner J, Weninger P, Hirtler L. Cutaneous innervation of the ankle: an anatomical study showing danger zones for ankle surgery. Clin Anat. 2014; 27(4):653–658

[4] deBoer P, Buckley R, Hoppenfeld S. Surgical Exposures in Foot & Ankle Surgery. Philadelphia, PA: Lippincott Williams & Wilkins; 2012

[5] Easley ME, Wiesel SW. Operative Techniques in Foot and Ankle Surgery. Philadelphia, PA: Lippincott Williams & Wilkins; 2016

[6] Malal JJG, Shaw-Dunn J, Kumar CS. Blood supply to the first metatarsal head and vessels at risk with a chevron osteotomy. J Bone Joint Surg Am. 2007; 89 (9):2018–2022

[7] Kelikian AS, Sarrafian SK. Sarrafian's Anatomy of the Foot and Ankle: Descriptive, Topographic, Functional. Philadelphia, PA: Wolters Kluwer Health/Lippincott Williams & Wilkins; 2011

3 Biomechanics of the Foot and Ankle

Benjamin B. Lindsey, Fred T. Finney, and Todd A. Irwin

Abstract
Understanding the biomechanics of the foot and ankle is an important first step in understanding both the normal patient and one with pathology. This chapter introduces the anatomical considerations of the foot and ankle in the context of biomechanics, in particular the motion of the foot and ankle segments (kinematics) and the forces across these segments (kinetics). The gait cycle is described in both walking and running, with correlation to the anatomy discussed. Clinical correlation is provided for some common foot and ankle pathology and gait disorders.

Keywords: biomechanics, anatomy, kinematics, kinetics, gait cycle

3.1 Introduction

- The anatomy and biomechanics of the ankle and foot are complex and often not well covered in initial anatomy instruction.
- Understanding the motion of the ankle and foot joints (kinematics) and the forces applied across these joints (kinetics) is important.
- The gait cycle in walking and running analyzes both the kinetics and kinematics of the ankle and foot.

3.2 The Ankle Joint

3.2.1 Anatomy

- The ankle joint is a hinged (ginglymus) joint incorporating the tibia, fibula, and talus.
- Stability of the ankle joint is provided by both the bony architecture and the ligamentous anatomy.[1]
- The dome of the talus is trapezoidal in shape when viewed transversely, wider anteriorly than posteriorly.
    - Due to this shape, the ankle is more stable in dorsiflexion.
- Additionally, the talus can be described as trochlear (or biconcave).
    - It has a central trochlea (sulcus) with a radius of curvature that is greater laterally than medially.
    - This creates a conical shape with the apex of the cone directed medially (▶ Fig. 3.1).
- Ligamentous stability is conferred by the anterior talofibular ligament (ATFL), posterior talofibular ligament (PTFL), and calcaneofibular ligament (CFL) laterally, and the deltoid ligament medially (please see Chapter 1 for more details).
    - The deltoid is the primary stabilizer of the ankle during stance.[2]

3.2.2 Kinematics of the Ankle Joint

- The axis of the ankle joint runs between the tips of the malleoli obliquely from plantar lateral to dorsomedial.
- This axis defines the primary motion of the ankle joint, from 20 degrees of dorsiflexion to 50 degrees of plantar flexion with significant variability between individuals.
- The obliquity of the axis permits horizontal rotation to occur in the foot or tibia as the ankle moves through plantar flexion and dorsiflexion.
- When the foot is free and not planted on the ground, the foot externally rotates (~15 degrees) with dorsiflexion and internally rotates with plantar flexion.
- When the foot is planted on the ground and thus immobilized, ankle dorsiflexion results in internal rotation of the tibia and ankle plantar flexion results in external rotation of the tibia.[3]

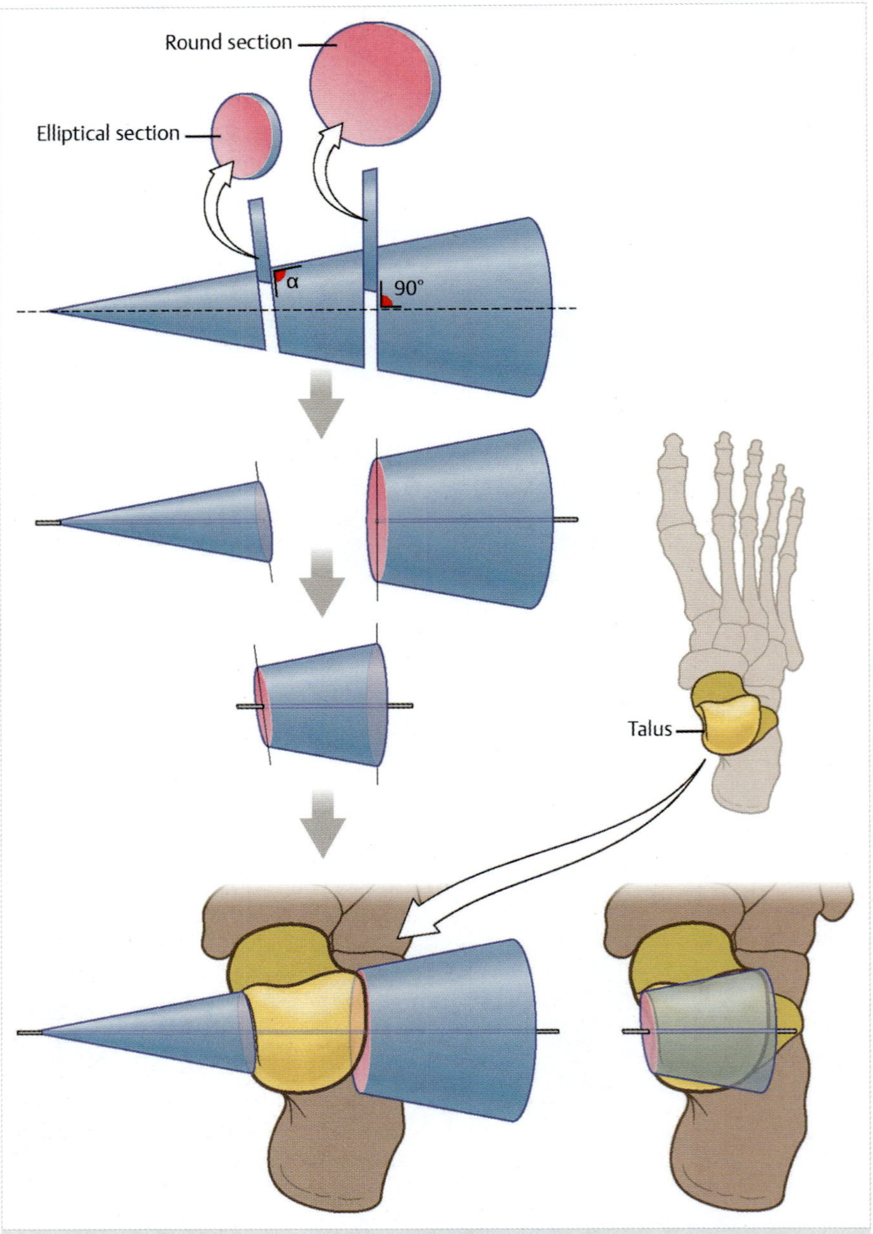

Fig. 3.1 The body of the talus resembles a conical shape with the apex of the cone directed medially along the axis of the talar body.

3.2.3 The Distal Tibiofibular Articulation (Syndesmosis)

- The syndesmosis helps control motion in the sagittal and coronal planes.
  - It allows for a small amount (~2 degrees) of fibular rotation within the incisura fibularis.
  - The fibula externally rotates and translates proximally with

dorsiflexion, and internally rotates and translates distally with plantar flexion.
  - The syndesmosis, along with the deep deltoid, helps prevent lateral talar translation.[2]
- The fibula accounts for approximately 15% of the axial load across the ankle via the tibiofibular and talofibular articulations.[4]

3.3 The Hindfoot

3.3.1 Anatomy and Kinematics

- The subtalar joint:
  - Primary motion is inversion (~30 degrees) and eversion (~15 degrees), although it is variable and difficult to measure clinically.[5]
  - The axis of the subtalar joint is an oblique axis that runs from plantar lateral to dorsomedial.
  - It is angled 42 degrees from the horizontal plane and 16 degrees from the sagittal plane (▶ Fig. 3.2).
  - The obliquity of the subtalar joint axis allows for rotation of the tibia to be converted into inversion and eversion of the subtalar joint.
    - Internal rotation of the tibia→ eversion of the subtalar joint.
    - External rotation of the tibia→ inversion of the subtalar joint.
- The transverse tarsal joint:
  - Primary motion is adduction (~20 degrees) and abduction (~10 degrees).
  - Forefoot supination and pronation also occur through the transverse tarsal joints.

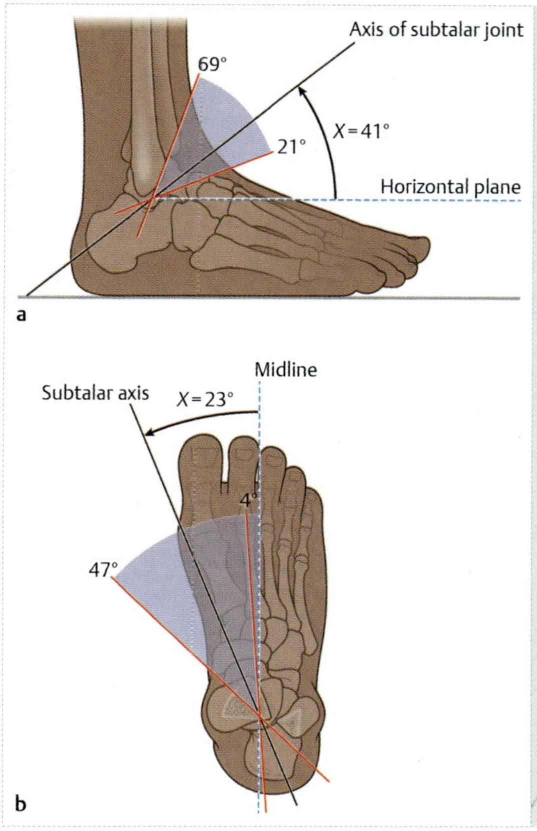

Fig. 3.2 (a,b) Axis of the subtalar joint.

- The transverse tarsal joint works in conjunction with the subtalar joint, through coupled actions, to control foot flexibility with ambulation.
- These actions work to lock and unlock the midfoot.[3,4]

3.3.2 Relationship of the Subtalar and Transverse Tarsal Joints

- With eversion of the subtalar joint, the calcaneocuboid (CC) and talonavicular (TN) joints become parallel in alignment, unlocking the joint (▶ Fig. 3.3).
  - Flexible shock absorption is then enabled through the midfoot.
  - The elasticity of the plantar fascia also contributes to shock absorption.
- With inversion of the subtalar joint, the CC and TN joints become convergent in alignment, locking the joints.
  - The midfoot becomes rigid providing a lever arm for push-off.
  - Patients with high arches (cavus) often have relative heel inversion (hindfoot varus), also called cavovarus.
    - This creates a more rigid midfoot with less ability to dissipate forces and increased stress across the midfoot and lateral column.
- The posterior tibialis tendon (PTT) functions to invert the hindfoot, thereby locking the transverse tarsal joint.
  - Patients with PTT dysfunction have difficulty with heel rise and are susceptible to progressive eversion (hindfoot valgus).[3]

3.4 The Midfoot

3.4.1 Anatomy

- The midfoot includes the naviculocuneiform (NC), intercuneiform, and tarsometatarsal (TMT) joints.
- These joints have dense dorsal and plantar ligamentous connections, which lead to limited motion and increased stability of the midfoot.
- The bony anatomy of the midfoot creates a transverse arch with the base of the second metatarsal joint serving as the keystone of this arch.[1]

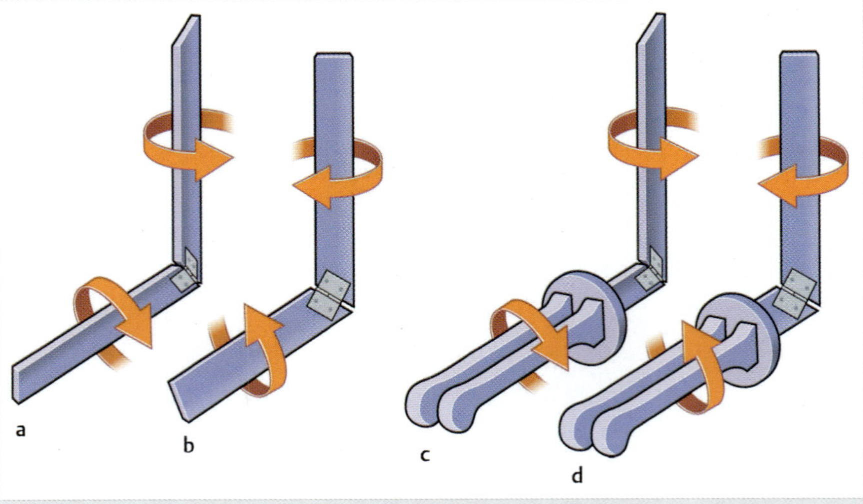

Fig. 3.3 (a–d) With eversion of the subtalar joint, the calcaneocuboid (CC) and talonavicular (TN) joints become parallel in alignment, unlocking the joint.

3.4.2 Function and Three-Column Theory

- The midfoot serves as a bridge between the hindfoot and forefoot providing both stability and flexibility for normal gait.
- The foot can be divided into three longitudinal columns (▶ Fig. 3.4).
- These columns are reflective of the difference in rigidity throughout the foot, thus delineating which portions of the foot enable push-off through a rigid lever arm and which portions of the foot are flexible for ambulation on uneven ground.
    - The medial column is composed of the first metatarsal, the medial cuneiform, and the navicular bones including the first TMT joint and the first NC joint.
        - The medial column has limited mobility and bears a significant portion of the weightbearing load during the gait cycle.
    - The intermediate (middle) column is composed of the second metatarsal, the third metatarsal, the middle cuneiform, and the lateral cuneiform including the second and third TMT joints and the second and third NC joints.
        - The intermediate column is rigid as the second TMT joint and only has approximately 1 to 2 degrees of sagittal motion.
        - This rigidity provides for a rigid lever arm during push-off.
    - The lateral column is composed of the fourth and fifth metatarsal joints and the cuboid, including the fourth and fifth TMT joints.
        - The lateral column is mobile, as the fourth and fifth TMT joints have approximately 5 to 17 degrees of sagittal motion.
        - This sagittal mobility of the lateral column allows for the flexibility necessary to ambulate on uneven terrain.[2]

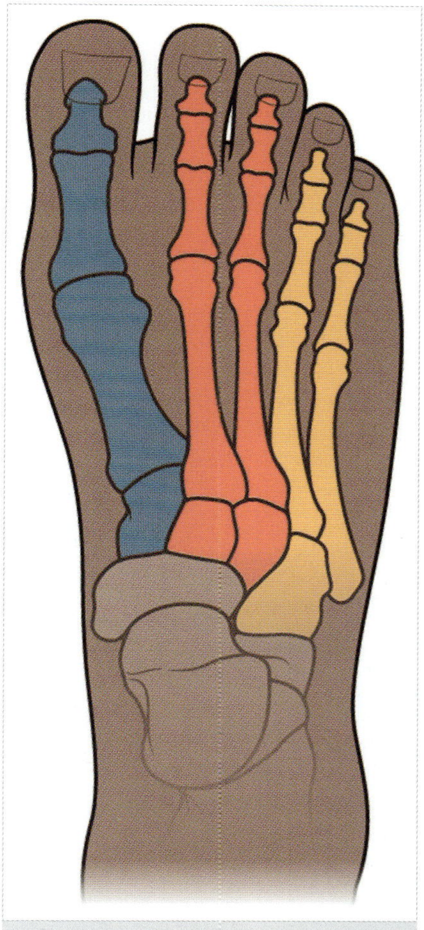

Fig. 3.4 Medial, middle, and lateral columns of the foot.

3.5 The Forefoot and Windlass Mechanism

3.5.1 Anatomy and Kinematics

- The forefoot includes the metatarsophalangeal (MTP) joints and the interphalangeal joints.
- The second through fifth MTP joints slope obliquely in a proximal direction going from medial to lateral, which is commonly referred to as the metatarsal break.

- The plantar fascia (aponeurosis) originates proximally at the medial aspect of the calcaneal tuberosity and inserts distally on the plantar plates and bases of the five proximal phalanxes, along with on the base of the fifth metatarsal.[1]
- With the foot at rest, mobility exists throughout the midfoot through a loose plantar fascia.
  - This mobility enables flexibility with ambulation over uneven surfaces.
- As dorsiflexion of the MTP joints occurs with push-off, the plantar fascia tightens, raising the longitudinal arch, inverting the heel, and decreasing the mobility of the midfoot.
  - This is termed the "windlass mechanism."
- The oblique metatarsal break contributes to lower extremity external rotation and inversion of the calcaneus as the body passes over the metatarsal heads with gait.[3,6]

3.5.2 The Foot as a Tripod

- When the subtalar joint is in neutral, the normal forefoot is positioned parallel to the ground.
- This enables the foot to function as a tripod, with pressure approximately evenly distributed between the first metatarsal head (20–25% total pressure in stance), the heads of the lesser metatarsals (25–30% total pressure in stance), and the calcaneus (45–55% total pressure in stance), with some variations depending on sex.[7]
  - As the first metatarsal bears a large load, it is the widest metatarsal.
- Understanding changes in the tripod helps us to understand some foot and ankle pathology.
  - Plantar flexion of the first ray or medial column of the foot leads to inversion of the heel and relative cavovarus foot (▶ Fig. 3.5).
  - Elevation or collapse of the first ray or medial column leads to loss of arch, hindfoot valgus, and relative flatfoot[3,4] (▶ Fig. 3.6).

3.6 The Gait Cycle

3.6.1 Definition of the Gait Cycle

- Gait cycle is the highly coordinated process by which the lower limbs are used for forward ambulation.
- One full gait cycle is defined by the period of activity between two

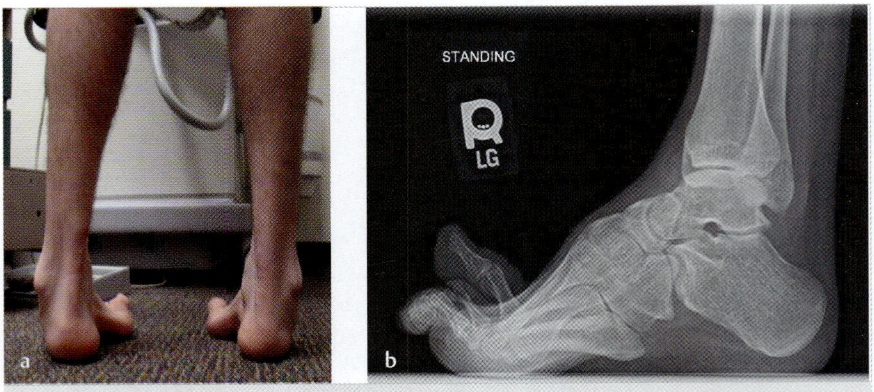

Fig. 3.5 (a) Clinical photograph and **(b)** lateral foot radiograph of a patient with plantarflexed first ray and heel inversion and resultant severe cavovarus foot deformity.

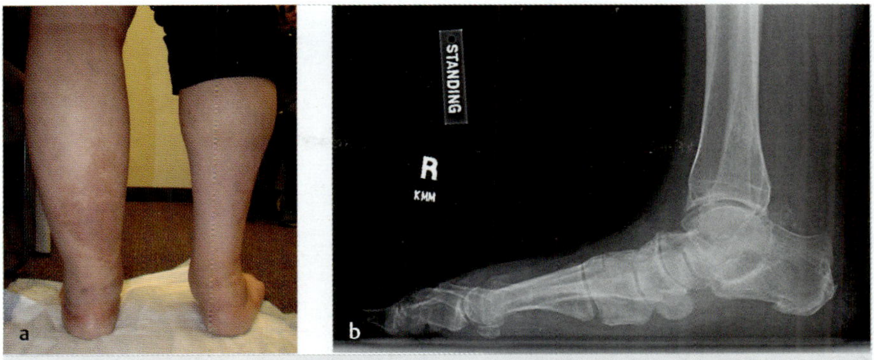

Fig. 3.6 **(a)** Clinical photograph and **(b)** lateral foot radiograph of a patient with collapse of the medial column, hindfoot valgus, and resultant significant flatfoot deformity.

consecutive heel strikes of the ipsilateral foot and is termed a "stride."[2]

- It is comprised of two major phases: stance phase and swing phase[2,3,8] (▶ Fig. 3.7).
  - The stance phase is the period between heel strike and toe-off in which the limb is loaded and in contact with the ground (62% of gait cycle).
  - The swing phase is the period between toe-off and heel strike in which the limb is moving forward and not contacting the ground (38% of gait cycle).
  - As gait speed increases, duration of the stance phase decreases.
- Walking is characterized by always having one foot in contact with the ground as well as a period of double-limb support in which both feet are contacting the ground.
  - Ground reaction forces reach approximately 1.5 times the body weight.[2]
- During running, there is a period in which neither foot is in contact with the ground, and there is no period of double-limb support.
  - Ground reaction forces reach approximately three to four times the body weight.[2]

3.6.2 Stance Phase

- The stance phase is further divided into three intervals: a period of double-limb support, a period of single-limb support, and finally a second period of double-limb support.
  - *First interval*:
    - This encompasses the first period of double-limb support and is defined as the period from heel strike to opposite foot toe-off, accounting for approximately the first 0 to 12% of gait cycle.[2,3]
    - Heel strike is characterized by the foot returning to the ground and accepting the weight of the body.
      - The hindfoot passively shifts from mildly supinated to pronated, which allows the transverse tarsal joint to unlock in order to absorb and dissipate the force of the limb returning to the ground.
    - The limb then progresses to the foot-flat position. The ankle joint plantarflexes rapidly, and the anterior muscle compartment (primarily tibialis anterior) contracts eccentrically to control the rate at which the foot returns to the ground.
      - The hindfoot remains pronated and unlocked in the foot-flat

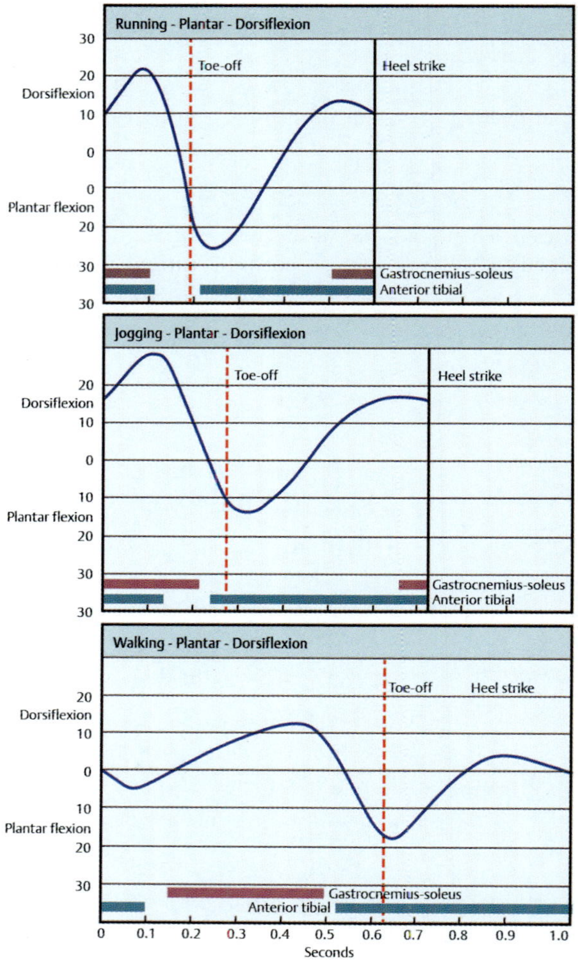

Fig. 3.7 Full gait cycle.

position for ground accommodation of uneven terrain.

* At this point, the heel of the opposite limb has lifted from the floor, but the limb remains in contact with the ground.

- *Second interval*:
  - This is defined as the period of single-limb support (from contralateral foot toe-off to contralateral foot heel strike) and occurs during 12 to 50% of the gait cycle.[2,3]
  - During this interval, the body's center of gravity advances forward over the foot as the limb progresses from foot-flat past midstance.
    * Eccentric contraction of the gastrocnemius–soleus complex as the ankle progressively dorsiflexes controls the rate at which the tibia advances over the foot, resulting in maximal load across the ankle joint.
  - As the tibia advances over the foot, progressive inversion of the hindfoot is initiated, locking the transverse tarsal joint and allowing the foot to transition from a flexible, shock-

absorbing configuration to a more rigid, load-bearing configuration.
    - Hindfoot inversion results from multiple factors:
        - The swing of the contralateral limb causes the standing limb to externally rotate, resulting in passive inversion of the subtalar joint.
        - The externally rotated orientation of the ankle joint axis and the oblique alignment of the metatarsal break contribute to hindfoot inversion.
        - With progressive dorsiflexion of the MTP joints, the windlass mechanism initiates, which tightens the plantar fascia (aponeurosis) and contributes to passive inversion of the hindfoot.
- *Third interval*:
    - This phase encompasses the second period of double-limb support and is defined as the period from contralateral heel strike to toe-off. This occurs during 50 to 62% of the gait cycle.[2,3]
        - During this time, the limb is preparing to push off the ground and begins to advance.
    - The ankle joint plantarflexes rapidly via concentric contraction of the posterior compartment musculature (primarily the gastrocnemius–soleus complex) as the limb progresses from the end of midstance to toe-off.
    - The subtalar joint continues to invert and is maximally inverted at toe-off.
        - Contraction of the posterior tibial tendon actively supinates the hindfoot.
        - This creates locking of the transverse tarsal joints and completes the transition of the foot to a rigid structure for maximal loading and push-off.

3.6.3 Swing Phase

- The swing phase makes up the final 38% of the gait cycle and is defined as the period from toe-off to heel strike during which the limb is advancing through the air.[2,3]
- As the foot leaves the ground, the ankle joint dorsiflexes through concentric contraction of the anterior compartment musculature.
    - In concert with hip and knee flexion, ankle dorsiflexion allows for clearance of the foot as the extremity advances through the air and prepares the limb for heel strike.
    - The insertion of the tibialis anterior tendon on the medial cuneiform inverts the foot such that the hindfoot is mildly supinated at heel strike.

3.6.4 Gait Changes with Running

- Running is characterized by a decreased stance phase, no period of double-limb support, and a period during which neither foot is in contact with the ground, termed the "float phase."
- As speed increases, the amount of time the foot spends on the ground decreases.
- Ground reaction forces reach approximately three to four times the body weight due to the load experienced when the foot returns to the ground following the float phase.[2]
    - The hip, knee, and ankle joints display increased motion to help dissipate and accommodate this increase.[3,8]
    - Patients with cavovarus feet absorb this increased force poorly due to heel inversion and relative locking of the transverse tarsal joints, which puts them at risk of injury such as stress fractures (e.g., the navicular and fifth metatarsal).

3.6.5 Gait Disorders

- Disorders of foot and ankle biomechanics lead to predictable and discernable changes in the gait cycle.[2,4]

- *Antalgic gait:*
  - This is a gait caused by pain and characterized by a shortened stance phase of the affected limb in order to decrease the amount of time the limb is loaded.
- *Steppage gait and slap foot gait*:
  - These result from weakness of the anterior compartment musculature.
    - A *steppage gait* results from an inability of the foot extensors to dorsiflex the ankle joint. It is marked by lifting the affected leg higher during the swing phase in order to clear the toes and forefoot from the ground.
    - In a *slap foot* gait, the affected limb is unable to control the rate at which the foot returns to the ground as the limb progresses from heel strike to foot-flat. This results in the foot "slapping" the ground.
    - The steppage and slap foot gaits are commonly seen in patients with foot drop (e.g., from injury to the common peroneal nerve) due to loss of function of the anterior compartment of the leg.
- *Calcaneal gait*:
  - This is a less common gait characterized by extended heel weight-bearing resulting from weakness of the posterior compartment musculature (inability to initiate plantar flexion and heel rise) or unbalanced spasticity of the anterior compartment as sometimes seen in traumatic brain injuries (► Fig. 3.8).

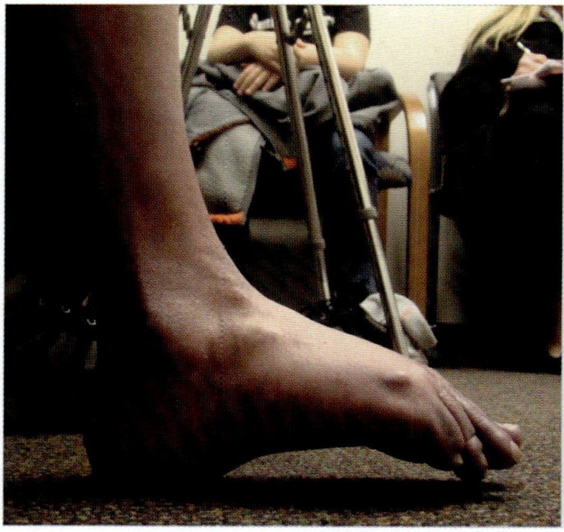

Fig. 3.8 Clinical photograph of a patient with traumatic brain injury and a calcaneal gait while standing.

3.7 Key Testing Facts

- The axis of the ankle joint runs between the tips of the malleoli obliquely from plantar lateral to dorsomedial.
- The fibula externally rotates and translates proximally with dorsiflexion, and internally rotates and translates distally with plantar flexion.
- Internal rotation of the tibia leads to eversion of the subtalar joint and external rotation of the tibia leads to inversion of the subtalar joint.
- With eversion of the subtalar joint, the CC and TN joints become parallel in alignment, which unlocks the joint, while with inversion of the subtalar joint, the CC and TN joints become convergent in alignment, which locks the joints. The midfoot then becomes rigid, providing a lever arm for push-off.
- With dorsiflexion of the MTP joints during toe-off, the plantar fascia tightens, raising the longitudinal arch, inverting the heel, and decreasing the mobility of the midfoot (termed the windlass mechanism).
- The stance phase is the period between heel strike and toe-off in which the limb is loaded and in contact with the ground (62% of gait cycle), which is then further divided into three intervals: a period of double-limb support, a period of single-limb support, and finally a second period of double-limb support.
- The swing phase is the period between toe-off and heel strike in which the limb is moving forward and not contacting the ground (38% of gait cycle).

References

[1] Thompson J. Foot/ankle. In: Thompson J, ed. Netter's Concise Orthopaedic Anatomy. 2nd ed. Philadelphia, PA: Saunders; 2010:337–383

[2] Kadakia AR, Seybold JD. Biomechanics of the foot and ankle. In: Miller MD, Thompson SR, eds. Miller's Review of Orthopaedics. 7th ed. Philadelphia, PA: Elsevier; 2016:483–488

[3] Haskell A, Mann RA. Biomechanics of the foot and ankle. In: Coughlin MJ, Saltzman CL, Anderson RB, eds. Mann's Surgery of the Foot and Ankle. 9th ed. Philadelphia, PA: Saunders; 2014:4–31

[4] Chiodo CP, Bluman EM. Biomechanics of the foot and ankle. In: Pinzur, MS, ed. Orthopaedic Knowledge Update 4: Foot and Ankle 4. Rosemont, IL: American Academy of Orthopaedic Surgeon; 2008:3–13

[5] Sammarco VJ, Taylor R. Anatomy and biomechanics of the foot and ankle. In: Boyer MI, ed. AAOS Comprehensive Orthopaedic Review 2. Rosemont, IL: American Academy of Orthopaedic Surgeons; 2014:1451–1459

[6] Hicks JH. The mechanics of the foot. II. The plantar aponeurosis and the arch. J Anat. 1954; 88(1):25–30

[7] Yamamoto T, Hoshino Y, Kanzaki N, et al. Plantar pressure sensors indicate women to have a significantly higher peak pressure on the hallux, toes, forefoot, and medial of the foot compared to men. J Foot Ankle Res. 2020; 13(1):40

[8] Czerniecki JM. Foot and ankle biomechanics in walking and running. A review. Am J Phys Med Rehabil. 1988; 67(6):246–252

4 History and Physical Examination

Adam D. Bitterman

Abstract

This chapter aims to provide a comprehensive discussion on routine and reproducible history taking as well as the necessary steps to perform a thorough physical examination. Highlighted within this text are the basic concepts behind a complete physical examination, which include look, feel, move, and test.

Keywords: history, physical examination, chief complaint, inspection, motion, provocative testing, thorough, reproducible.

4.1 History and Physical Examination

4.1.1 Introduction

- Gait evaluation is important in certain clinical situations and should be implemented as needed.
- Examination of the foot and ankle may serve as a window into systemic abnormalities involving other body systems. A low threshold should exist to refer to appropriate specialists when clinical suspicion exists regarding rheumatologic, dermatologic, and other vascular abnormalities.
- An astute clinician should be able to compile the information gathered during the history and then perform an appropriate physical examination, thus prioritizing their list of differential diagnoses, which may then be confirmed with appropriate testing.

4.1.2 History

- Accurate history taking is a crucial first step toward determining one's ailment; it is an opportunity to obtain a diagnosis by prompting the patient to provide accurate information with appropriate questioning.
- Questions pertaining to one's history should be open-ended, thus allowing the patient to provide complete responses.
- Be sure to ask questions at a level that is well within a patient's understanding based upon their age and education level.
- Initial questioning should focus on the reason for their current visit—the history of present illness.
- This is an opportunity for the patient to describe their concern in their own words. Avoid the temptation to interrupt them, but be sure to help guide them along. This will prevent tangents and keep them focused on relevant data.
- Follow-up questions allow the physician to fill in gaps regarding one's history or current complaint that may have been omitted.
- Fundamental information that must be obtained for each complaint includes the following:
    - Onset: When did the symptom(s) begin? What was happening when it started?
    - Duration: For how long have you been experiencing this problem?
    - Quality: A description of the complaint in as much detail as possible. Ask for specific characteristics of their pain (i.e., stabbing, crushing, burning, throbbing, aching, etc.).
    - Severity: Is this the worst pain ever felt? On a scale of 1 to 10, with 10 being the worst pain imaginable, how do they describe their pain?
    - Location: Where is the pain and does the pain travel to any other location?
    - Provocation: Is there a specific activity or movement that makes the symptom worse? Does anything make it better?

   - Intervention: What has been done to help the problem? Have they seen other doctors prior to you? Have they had additional procedures?
- Being on the same page as your patient with respect to their goals surrounding their problem is imperative. This enhances the physician–patient relationship and lessens the chance of any miscommunication.[1]
- Speak at a level that is understandable to each individual; never assume the patient understands medical vocabulary the way you do.
- Use this "question and answer" segment as a means to create your differential diagnosis, which will be enhanced as you trek through the physical examination and testing phase of the encounter.

4.1.3 Additional Components

- Obtaining one's prior medical diagnoses should never be missed. It may shed some light into their current complaint.
- Previous surgeries should be documented and incorporated into the overall assessment, when applicable.
- Medications may play a role in clinical symptoms, so having a complete list is imperative.
- Be sure to understand how their ailment is affecting their quality of life. This may serve as a window into a better appreciation of their treatment goals.

4.2 Physical Examination

4.2.1 Introduction

- It is important to approach this systematically in a way that is reproducible for all patient encounters, thus limiting the chances of missing vital details.
- Examiners may have the benefit of a contralateral limb, which may serve as a baseline comparison control to gauge pathologic processes.
- All examinations should incorporate a fundamental foundation that evaluates the neurologic, vascular, and integumentary system.[2]
- Be sure to perform your examination in an environment that is comfortable for the patient.
- Position yourself in a comfortable chair where you are able to visualize the leg, foot, and ankle from the front, back, and side. Furthermore, you should be able to observe their stance whether on one leg or two.
- While each examiner may personalize their approach, it is important to address each component of the physical examination. These components include inspection, palpation, movement, provocative testing, and gait evaluation.[3]
- Normal anatomic aspects of the foot and ankle are well established within a range; however, knowing the abnormal portions of one's anatomy will help ascertain the pathology and limitations to one's function.
- The goal of the physical examination is to further narrow down the list of possible diagnoses and better identify if further diagnostic testing is required.
- Subtle physical examination abnormalities may be a sign of a more systemic abnormality including peripheral vascular disease, autoimmune disorders, metabolic syndromes, or neurologic diseases.[2,3]

4.2.2 Inspection

- Be sure to have the patient in loose-fitting clothing (gown, shorts, etc.) to enable ease of motion of the joints above and below the area of concern. Both limbs should be exposed, thus enabling asymmetry to be best identified.
- Exposure of the affected limb should include the knee, leg, ankle, and foot.

- Gait can be evaluated in the examination room or as the patient moves from the waiting area to the examination room.
- Standing inspection from the anterior aspect, posterior aspect, and side should be easily attainable.
- Having the patient bear weight provides a reliable assessment of alignment, rotation, and limb shortening.

4.2.3 Standing Examination

Anterior Evaluation

- The patient stands with their feet about shoulder width apart. The examiner should be able to see the pelvis, patellae, anterior tibia, and feet.
- Rotational deformities of the limb in question may be seen at this point. Furthermore, abnormalities in the coronal plane (valgus, varus) emanating at the knee or within the tibia should be assessed.
- Arch heights can be evaluated for abnormal height or flattening, pes cavus or pes planus, respectively (▶ Fig. 4.1).
- Assessment of the midfoot and forefoot posture may occur during this phase. Evaluation of the toes, while standing, may demonstrate contractures, crossover toe, hammering, hallux valgus, or great toe pronation.

Posterior Evaluation

- Having the patient face away from you gives you full visualization of their heels and Achilles tendon.
- Alignment from behind can be assessed to determine if the hindfoot is in valgus, varus, or neutral (▶ Fig. 4.2).
- The Achilles tendon can be inspected for bulbous regions or areas void of tendon (defects) consistent with tendinosis or rupture, respectively.
- Too many toes sign, representative of posterior tibial tendon dysfunction (PTTD), can be seen.
- Having the patient attempt a single- and double-limb heel rise should be done while inspecting the patient from behind. If the posterior tibial tendon is fully functional, their hindfoot should invert as the transverse tarsal joint locks for heel lift. Any dysfunction or weakness will be easily detected. Be careful of cheating patients who may lean on a supporting examination table or those who hoist themselves up (▶ Fig. 4.3).

4.2.4 Seated Examination

General Assessment

- As the examiner, you may consider being seated as well, in a position that is lower than the patient, which allows easy access to assess the foot (▶ Fig. 4.4).

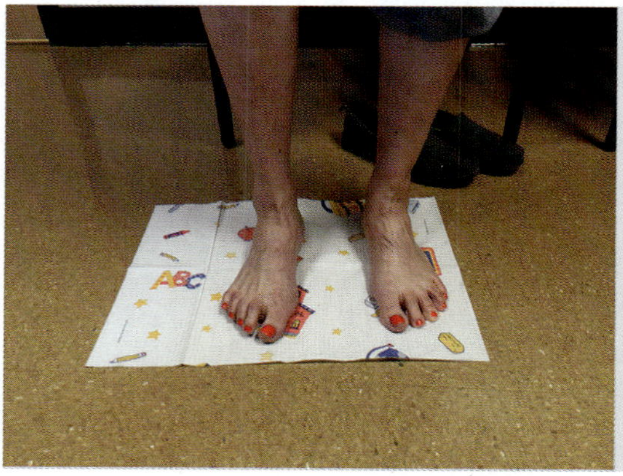

Fig. 4.1 Clinical photograph of both feet while standing.

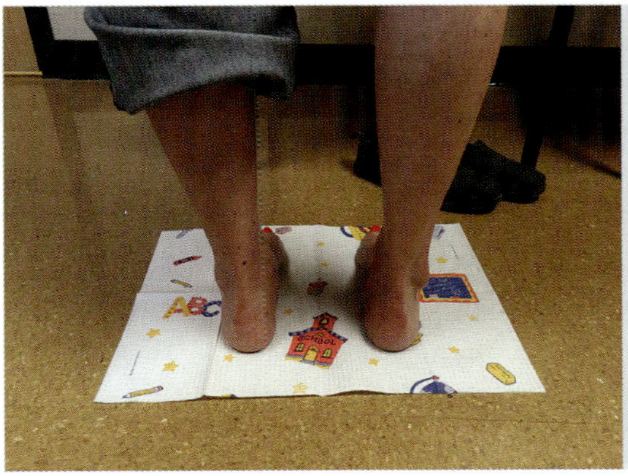

Fig. 4.2 Evaluation of the patient's stance from behind.

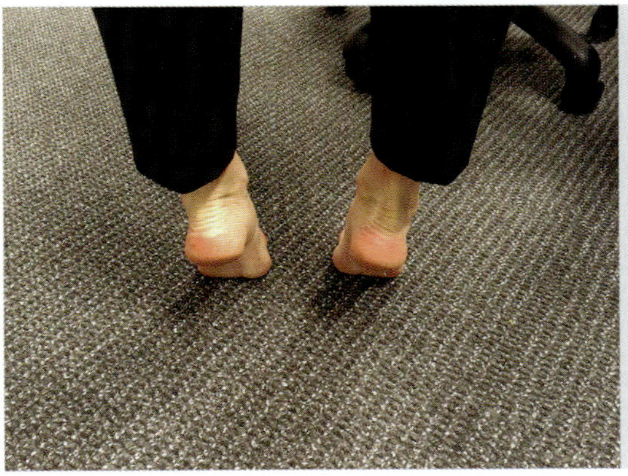

Fig. 4.3 Assessment of the patient performing a single- and double-limb heel rise. Critical focus of the hindfoot can be performed to ensure appropriate inversion during this maneuver.

- Focusing on the foot and ankle, the sequence of examination steps should include inspection of the skin for any dermatologic concerns, vascular anomalies, bony abnormalities, neurovascular evaluation, motion assessment, palpation of bony, tendon, and ligament landmarks, as well as special tests.[2]
- Assessment should include the limb's temperature, areas of erythema, ecchymosis, swelling, muscle atrophy, and hair loss. Any area of suspicion should be compared to the unaffected side.
- Skin assessment should focus on the plantar surface of the foot and the interdigital webspaces, looking for open wounds, callosities, corns, areas of impending breakdown, or evidence of foreign material.
- Previous incision sites should be appropriately recorded as should other wounds that are open or in various stages of healing.
- Care must be taken to thoroughly evaluate the skeletal anatomy, and a provider should be able to recognize any anatomical deviation within the toes and midfoot, especially when compared to the contralateral side.
- Areas of concern, as a result of tenderness upon palpation or with noticeable deformity, should be closely investigated with advanced imaging studies.

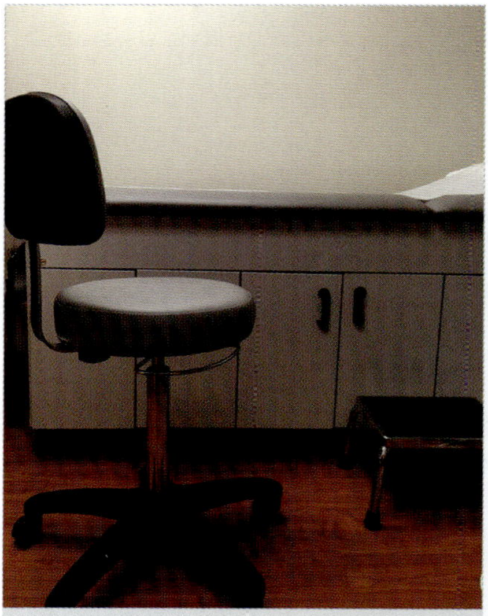

Fig. 4.4 Photograph of examination table and chair setup with the examiner being below the patient and positioned to enable easy accessibility to the foot.

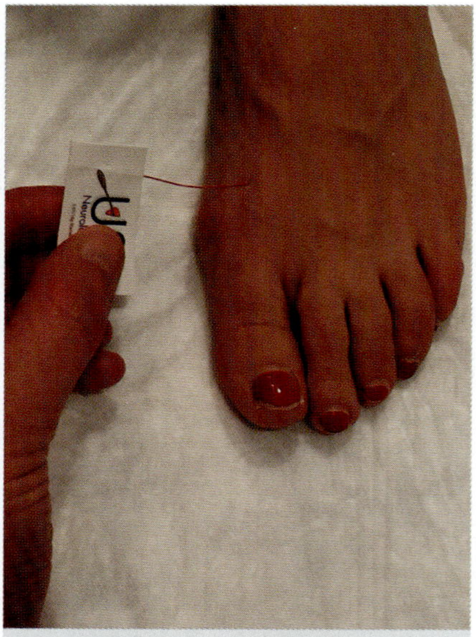

Fig. 4.5 Sensory nerve distribution being examined by a Semmes–Weinstein monofilament.

Neurovascular Examination

- Thorough assessment of the vascular perfusion and neurologic status of the foot may provide significant input on other systemic illnesses.
- Vascular status from the knee within the popliteal crease should then be followed by evaluation of the dorsalis pedis and posterior tibial artery. Capillary refill may serve as a surrogate should the pulses be too difficult to palpate.
- Any discrepancy or concern regarding circulation should be compared to the unaffected side or further investigated with non-invasive vascular studies and a referral to a vascular surgeon.
- Concern for peripheral vascular disease or other systemic illnesses should lead to additional preoperative evaluation leading to surgical optimization.
- Suspicion regarding nerve injury may arise from the patient's description while obtaining their history.
- Nerve-related pain or abnormalities may be related to local compression within specific areas of the foot or ankle, or may be a result of systemic illnesses such as diabetes.
- Care must be taken to evaluate all sensory dermatomes with a Semmes-Weinstein monofilament. Positional and vibratory sensation should be noted as well (▶ Fig. 4.5).
- Abnormalities should raise clinical suspicion for possible central nervous system involvement and lead to further clinical investigation as warranted.
- Compressive neuropathies about the foot and ankle may be further assessed via percussion and electrodiagnostic studies as indicated. Be sure to account for anatomic causes (space occupying lesions) or previous incision sites near the course of nerve structures. Scar tissue may result in nerve entrapment.
- Neurologic conditions of the forefoot may manifest as numbness or burning.

Assessment for a forefoot neuroma should include medial and lateral directed compression that may cause a palpable click (Mulder's sign) and reproduces pain within the toes.

4.2.5 Testing

- All joints of the foot and ankle should be palpated and put through their respective ranges of motion.
- Palpation of all bony landmarks and tendinous structures must occur in a regimented sequence that is reproducible among patients.
- Tendon structures and muscle bellies must be palpated to assess for defects or areas of spasm. Be sure to know the main action of each muscle when positioning the foot and ankle for specific testing.
- With joint assessment, examiners should assess for pain, blocks to motion, crepitus, and evidence of instability.
- Having a firm understanding of the biomechanics of the ankle joint, subtalar joint, syndesmosis, transverse tarsal joint, tarsometatarsal joints, and metatarsophalangeal joints will aid in the overall assessment.
- Not only should the degree of motion be assessed, but also the percent difference between the asymptomatic contralateral side should be noted.
- A great deal of variability exists within a physical examination and documented values serve as a range of norms and variability.
- Specific maneuvers may be utilized to isolate each joint and assess for pathology.

4.2.6 Ankle Joint

- Normal range of motion is based on a conical orientation of the talus within the tibial plafond.[2] Range: 15-degree dorsiflexion to 50-degree plantar flexion.
- The axis begins anteromedially and travels posterolateral through the malleoli. With a wider radius of curvature laterally, the foot will deviate medially with plantar flexion and laterally with dorsiflexion.[2]
- Anterior drawer testing involves gripping the posterior heel with the dominant hand and shifting the ankle and hindfoot anteriorly while stabilizing the anterior tibia with the opposite hand. Lack of a firm endpoint may indicate instability. Deltoid ligament assessment may occur via an external rotation moment to the anterior drawer examination.
- This test must be done with the ankle in plantarflexion and at neutral.
- Inversion talar tilt testing has the examiner invert the heel while the fingers are palpating the lateral process of the talus for gapping and instability.

4.2.7 Syndesmosis

- Gliding joint between the tibia and the fibula, roughly 15 degrees posterior to the coronal plane.
- Proximal calf squeeze may elicit pain within the syndesmosis as well as external rotation of the foot upon the tibia.

4.2.8 Subtalar Joint and Midfoot Joints

- Involve motion between the talus and the calcaneus where inversion and eversion occur with a range from 40 and 10 degrees, respectively.
- Assessment involves the patient in a seated position with one hand stabilizing the midfoot and forefoot, while the opposite hand grips the calcaneus and passively inverts and everts.
- Midfoot assessment involves gripping the hindfoot and forefoot separately and taking the distal examining hand into adduction and abduction.
- Evaluation of the tarsometatarsal joints varies depending on the ray. The medial

column can be assessed by gripping the first metatarsal in one hand and passively dorsiflexing and plantarflexing it while the hindfoot is stabilized. As one examines the lesser rays, the second ray will be fairly rigid due to its recessed nature as will the third metatarsal; however, the fourth and fifth metatarsals are mobile within the sagittal plane.

4.2.9 Metatarsophalangeal Joint

- Motion of this joint is compared to the long axis of the metatarsal. Evaluation involves passive motion and the point where pain begins.
- Drawer testing may be done to evaluate the collateral ligaments and overall stability.

4.2.10 Forefoot

- In the setting of positional deformities to the hindfoot, the forefoot may compensate to maintain a plantigrade foot.
- Best done in the seated position dangling off the examining table, assessment involves the hindfoot passively placed in neutral while the midfoot is manipulated with the other hand such that neutral talonavicular positioning is obtained.
- Inspecting through the long axis of the foot allows the metatarsal cascade to be seen superimposed about a line perpendicular to the long axis of the calcaneus. Forefoot varus and valgus may be assessed at this point (▶ Fig. 4.6).

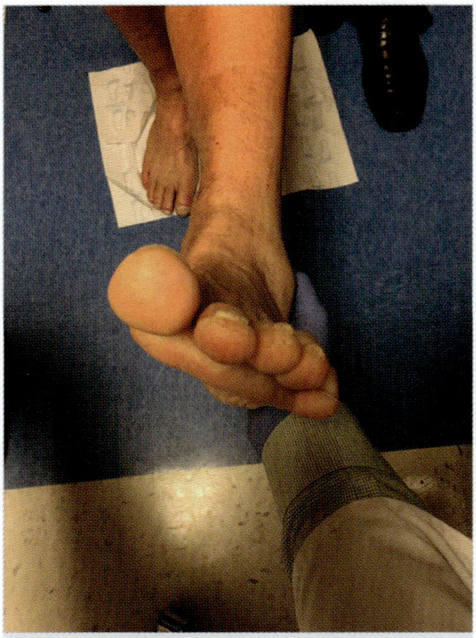

Fig. 4.6 Varus position of the forefoot with the hindfoot neutralized.

4.2.11 Tendons

- Anterior tendons include the tibialis anterior and the extensor tendons. Having the patient resist the action of the tendon in question will assess its strength while allowing an opportunity to palpate for any defect.
- Resisted eversion is mainly a result of the peroneus brevis.[2] The peroneal tendons may be evaluated in their retrofibular groove with circumduction about the ankle.
- Prone examination will allow direct visualization of the Achilles tendon and posterior ankle. Bulbous regions of the tendon may be a sign of tendinosis or previous rupture. With the knee at 90 degrees, resting plantar flexion tension of approximately 15 degrees about the ankle can be assessed and compared to the uninjured side. Loss of tendon continuity may result in a hyperdorsiflexed position (▶ Fig. 4.7).
- A Thompson test may be done when the calf is squeezed while the foot is off the bed, thus allowing passive plantar flexion when the tendon is intact.

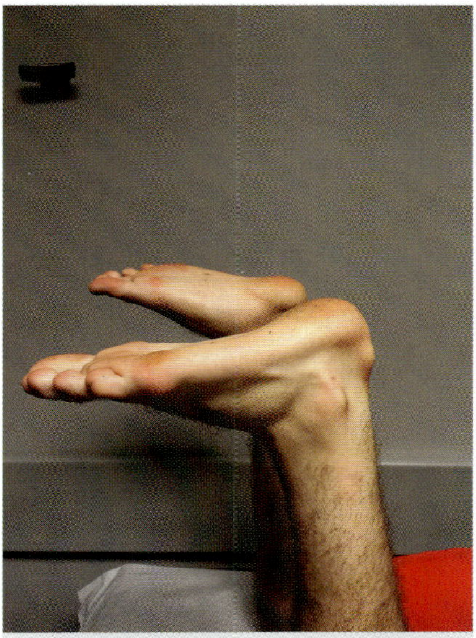

Fig. 4.7 Clinical photography of the Matles sign with loss of normal resting plantar flexion tension of the right ankle.

4.2.12 Gait Evaluation

- A firm understanding of the gait cycle is critical to assess pathology during ambulation.
- Gait assessment may provide further insight into postural abnormalities of the foot and ankle.
- Patient's ambulation should be viewed from the front, back, and side, and it should occur at varying speeds.[3]
- Specific attention should focus on the hindfoot and how it accommodates the ground and whether the foot is favoring one specific side. The examiner must watch the longitudinal arch and assess for collapse.
- Pathologic gait patterns may be a result of musculoskeletal disorders of the muscles, tendons, and joints of the leg and foot, or may be due to a neurologic disorder. Such neurologic disorders may be caused by systemic illnesses that affect the visual, vestibular, or proprioceptive systems.[3]

4.2.13 Shoe and Orthotic Evaluation

- External examination of the patient's shoe wear is vital to assessing pressure points during gait. Seeing how the shoe preferentially loses cushioning will lend some insight into their foot posture and pathology.[4]
- Evaluating one's inserts will allow the clinician to assess for areas of stress that may require offloading.
- Have the patient stand on their orthotics to see if they are corrective or accommodative and correlate with their examination.
- Understanding the means by which the orthotic was used will allow the clinician to make appropriate recommendations to improve prognosis.

4.3 Key Testing Facts

- The history and physical examination provide the clinician with information pertinent to the patient's complaint, ultimately leading to a diagnosis and appropriate therapeutic modalities.
- Obtaining a thorough yet focused history requires communication that a patient understands. The clinical provider must be able to elicit appropriate responses that will yield insight into one's ailment. It should not be expected that the patient will volunteer information. Thus, one must question in an open-ended format that will have the highest yield for valuable information.
- Results of the history and physical examination should catapult the provider to arrive at a presumptive diagnosis, which can then be confirmed with appropriate testing, when applicable.

References

[1] Hampton JR, Harrison MJ, Mitchell JR, Prichard JS, Seymour C. Relative contributions of history-taking, physical examination, and laboratory investigation to diagnosis and management of medical outpatients. BMJ. 1975; 2(5969):486–489

[2] Irwin T, Anderson RB, Davis WH. Principles of the physical examination of the foot and ankle. In: Coughlin MJ, Saltzman CL, Anderson RB, eds. Mann's Surgery of the Foot and Ankle. Amsterdam: Elsevier Saunders; 2014:37–60

[3] Papaliodis DN, Vanushkina MA, Richardson NG, DiPreta JA. The foot and ankle examination. Med Clin North Am. 2014; 98(2):181–204

[4] Boulton AJ, Armstrong DG, Albert SF, et al. American Diabetes Association, American Association of Clinical Endocrinologists. Comprehensive foot examination and risk assessment: a report of the task force of the foot care interest group of the American Diabetes Association, with endorsement by the American Association of Clinical Endocrinologists. Diabetes Care. 2008; 31(8):1679–1685

5 Imaging

Craig Chike Akoh and Phinit Phisitkul

Abstract

The foot and ankle are complex biomechanical structures that allow for locomotion. The intricate anatomy between different tendons and ligaments requires a variety of imaging modalities to determine the appropriate diagnosis for pathologic conditions. Plain radiographs are the most widely used imaging modality for foot and ankle. Radiographs are commonly used in trauma, infection, arthritis, and lower limb deformity. Weight-bearing plain films such as the Saltzman view or tripod index allow for the visualization of bony articulations under physiologic loading. Ultrasound is an excellent imaging modality for assessing superficial soft-tissue structures such as nerves, tendons, and ligaments of the foot and ankle. Computer tomography (CT) scan is the best imaging modality for complex bony anatomy. Magnetic resonance imaging (MRI) is a highly sensitive modality that allows for high quality imaging of soft-tissue injuries without ionizing radiation. Lastly, nuclear medicine imaging utilizes radioisotopes to delineate bioactivity in the setting of infection and implant loosening. Utilizing a combination of these imaging modalities allows for the accurate diagnosis of complex ankle conditions.

Keywords: foot and ankle, plain radiographs, ultrasound, MDCT, magnetic resonance imaging, tripod index, Saltzman's view, EOS, nuclear medicine scan

5.1 Purpose of Imaging

- The foot and ankle contain a complex region of closely located anatomic structures.
- The complex biomechanics of the foot and ankle increase the difficulty of obtaining an accurate diagnosis.
- Advanced imaging modalities improve the capability of accurately diagnosing and treating foot and ankle pathologies.

5.1.1 Indications

- *Diagnosis:* fractures, soft-tissue injuries, tarsal coalition, arthritis, and tumors.
- *Treatment planning:* articular involvement, three-dimensional (3D) reconstruction, and fracture fixation.
- *Posttreatment follow-up:* Fracture reduction, articular congruity, and bony union.

5.2 Plain Radiographs

5.2.1 Basic Principles

- *Plain radiographs* are the most widely used imaging modality in the foot and ankle. It is commonly used to assess trauma, infection, arthritis, and lower limb deformity. Plain radiographs utilize ionizing radiation to visualize calcium deposition in organic bony structures.
- **Advantages:**
  - Plain radiography allows for the visualization of osseous integrity, joint surface contour, osteophyte formation, and periosteal reaction.
  - The affordability and efficiency of plain radiography allow this to be the most commonly used modality for initial diagnosis and follow-up.
- **Disadvantages:**
  - Low-dose ionizing radiation (50–60 kV) is required for proper penetrance of bone.[1]
  - Plain radiographs lack 3D visualization and soft-tissue assessment of ligamentous and tendon pathologies.

5.2.2 Standard Imaging Protocol

- **Ankle composite (anteroposterior [AP], lateral, and mortise):**
  - Proper imaging of the foot and ankle requires the limb to be weightbearing and at least two orthogonal views to clearly visualize the complex bony anatomy of the foot and ankle. Utilizing three views, although more costly, increases the detection of ankle injuries.[2]
  - Mortise view: Measurements include the incisura fibularis, medial clear space, medial malleolus, lateral malleolus, and plafond.
- **Foot composite (AP, lateral, oblique).**
- **Sesamoid view** (▶ Fig. 5.1):
  - Holly's method—taken with the patient supine. Use a towel or strap to passively dorsiflex the toes. Aim the X-ray beam downward vertically toward the posterior aspect of the first metatarsophalangeal (MTP) joint.
  - Lewis' method—taken with the patient in the prone position. The patient dorsiflexes the foot so that it is 15 to 20 degrees from the vertical. With the cassette under the great toe, dorsiflex the first ray with the beam aimed downward in the vertical plane. This may be difficult for painful conditions.

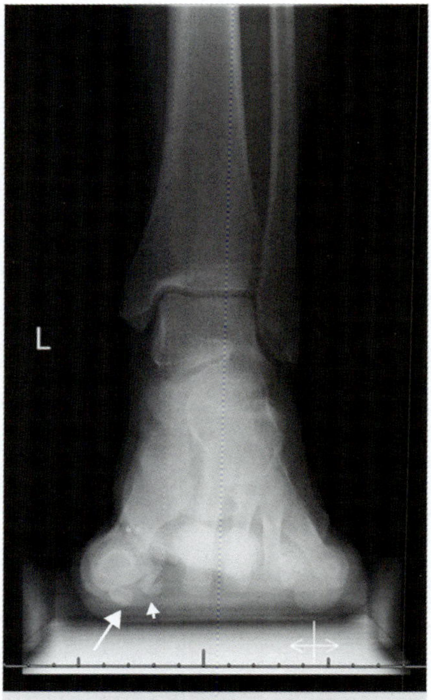

Fig. 5.1 Sesamoid view. Tibial sesamoid (*arrow*) and fibular sesamoid (*arrowhead*).

5.2.3 Weight-Bearing Films

- Weight-bearing films allow for the visualization of bony articulations under physiologic loading. Bilateral imaging on the same cassette is obtained to compare differences in alignment and joint space narrowing in the malalignment and arthritic population.
- **Ankle:**
  - *Bilateral AP*:
    - Weight-bearing films are obtained by placing both feet on a cassette with 50% of one's body weight placed on the affected limb.
    - Studies have shown that there is significant variability in the percentage of body weight being placed during imaging, potentially affecting its utility.[3]
  - *Saltzman's hindfoot view*:
    - The Saltzman view is obtained by having the patient stand with both feet on a radiolucent platform with equal weight distributed between them. The cassette is placed anterior to the patient's feet and angled 20 degrees from the vertical line. The X-ray tube is aimed 20 degrees from the horizontal so that it is perpendicular to the cassette (▶ Fig. 5.2).[4]
  - *Long leg alignment*:
    - Long leg alignment views allow for more accurate assessment of coronal alignment when compared to limited AP radiographs (▶ Fig. 5.3).[5]

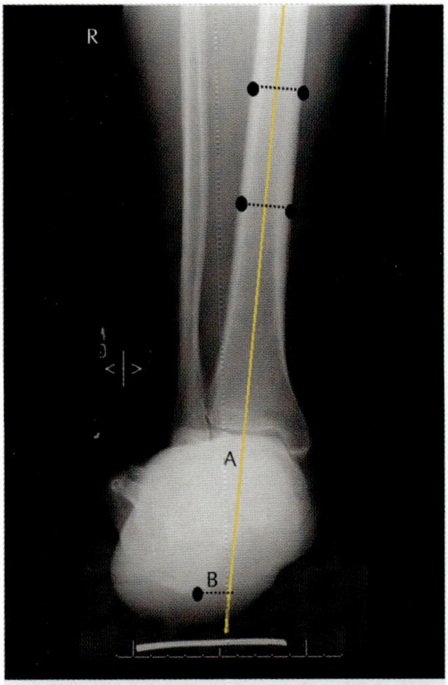

Fig. 5.2 Saltzman's view. *Line A* is the anatomic axis of the tibia. *Point B* is the inferior-most aspect of the calcaneus. The perpendicular distance from *line A* to *point B* measures the amount of hindfoot coronal malalignment. This radiograph shows mild valgus hindfoot alignment.

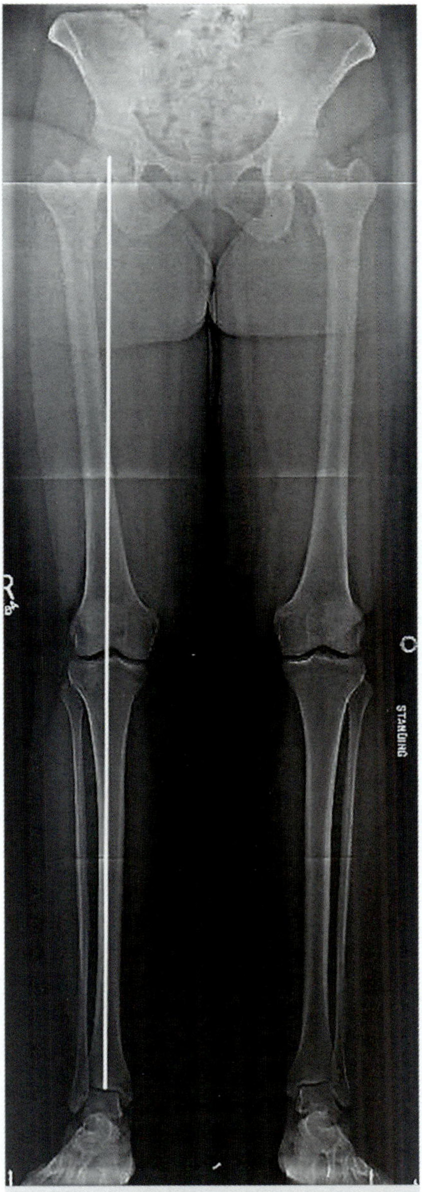

Fig. 5.3 Long leg alignment view. The *solid line* shows the mechanical axis of the right lower extremity, measured from the center of the femoral head to the center tibial plafond.

- Biplanar imaging (EOS; ▶ Fig. 5.4):
  - Digital imaging system that allows for the simultaneous acquisition of two orthogonal AP and lateral radiographs during weight bearing.
  - Utilizes multiple beams and linear scanning to generate images instead of utilizing a projection from a single X-ray beam.
  - Can obtain long leg images with less radiation and artifact.
  - Radiographic measurements using EOS are comparable to conventional radiographs, with the exception of the staggered hindfoot view.[6]
- Foot:
  - *Tripod index*:
    - The tripod index is measured from the weight-bearing AP foot view to assess aggregate coronal malalignment (▶ Fig. 5.5).[7]

 - It has been shown to be an accurate measurement for cavovarus and planovalgus deformities.[8]
 - A tripod index values greater than 26% and less than −39% were used as the cutoff values for radiographic diagnosis of pes planus and cavovarus feet, respectively.

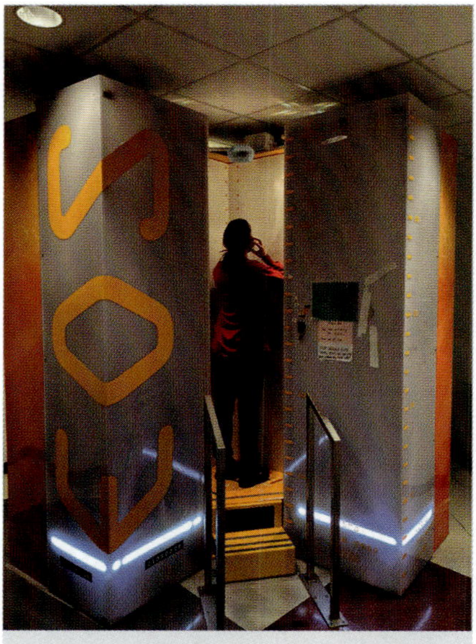

Fig. 5.4 EOS device. The patient stands while simultaneous anteroposterior (AP) and lateral images of the lower limbs and the entire body are obtained.

- *Lateral*:
 - Lateral weight-bearing foot images allow for the dynamic evaluation of foot deformity cases including cavovarus and pes planovalgus deformities (▶ Fig. 5.6).
 - Meary's angle is the angle between the long axis of the first metatarsal and the talus. Normal is −4 to 4 degrees.[9]
 - The calcaneal pitch angle is measured between the line along the calcaneus plantar surface and the floor. Normal value is 30 degrees.[9]
 - Hibbs' angle is the angle between a line through the long axis of the calcaneus and the long axis of the first metatarsal. Normal is less than 45 degrees.[9]
 - The medial cuneiform–fifth metatarsal distance is the distance from the plantar aspect of the fifth metatarsal to the plantar surface of the medial cuneiform.
 - The medial cuneiform–fifth metatarsal distance and calcaneal pitch are the most reliable measurements for planovalgus deformity.[10]

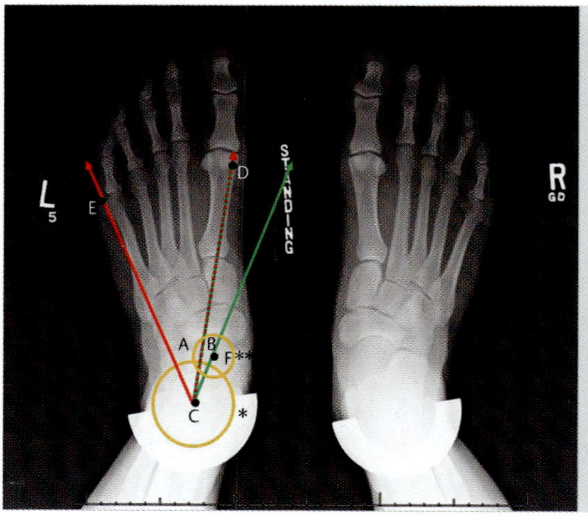

Fig. 5.5 Tripod index (TI). A perfect circle is drawn with the hemispheric marker as the center (*). Lines are drawn from the first perfect circle to the medial sesamoid (green dashed), the lateral border of the fifth metatarsal (red), and through the central talus axis (solid green) that bisects the perfect circle at the talar neck (**). Angle A is the angle between lines CE and CD. Angle B is the angle between CD and CF. The TI = (angle B/A) × 100.

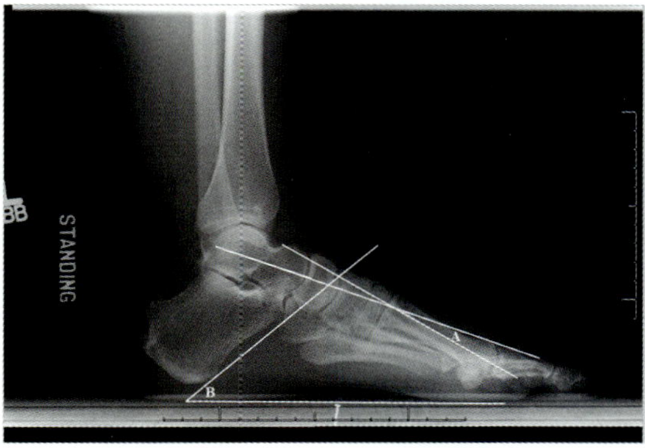

Fig. 5.6 Radiographic angles for lateral weight-bearing films: Meary's angle (A) and calcaneal pitch angle (B).

5.2.4 Stress Radiographs

- **Gravity stress**:
  - An AP radiograph of the ankle is obtained with the leg parallel to the floor and hanging free from the end of a table.
- **External rotation view**:
  - There are conflicting data if the medial ankle clear space widening is influenced by the ankle position (varus and plantarflexion) during the external rotation stress examination.[11,12,13,14]
  - Additionally, there is debate as to whether medial clear space widening correlates with magnetic resonance imaging (MRI) confirmed injury to the deep deltoid ligament.[15]
- **Comparing stress views**:
  - Studies have shown that detection of medial clear space widening is comparable for gravity and external rotation stress examinations.[16]

5.3 Ultrasound

5.3.1 Basic Principles

- Ultrasound is an excellent imaging modality for assessing superficial soft-tissue structures such as nerves, tendons, and ligaments of the foot and ankle.[17]
- Small high-frequency transducers of at least 7.5 MHz allows for visualization of the superficial tendon and ligament structures of the foot and ankle.[1]
- Optimizing ultrasound imaging includes placing the transducer perpendicular to the structure of interest and minimizing the depth.
- Advantages: Ultrasound allows for easy contralateral comparison, dynamic evaluation of soft-tissue structures, Achilles tendon rupture,[18] peroneal tendon subluxation,[19] flexor hallucis longus (FHL) stenosing tenosynovitis, plantar fasciitis, Morton's neuromas, nerve entrapment syndromes, superficial masses, and therapeutic injections.[17]
- Disadvantages: Effective use of ultrasound requires a steep learning curve, and its accuracy is extremely dependent on the skill level of the operator.

5.3.2 Dynamic Evaluation

- Peroneal tendon subluxation is evaluated at the retromalleolar space. Instability of the peroneal tendons is usually due to an avulsion injury of the superior extensor retinaculum. In order to visualize peroneal tendon instability, one must actively dorsiflex and evert the affected foot (▶ Fig. 5.7 and ▶ Fig. 5.8).

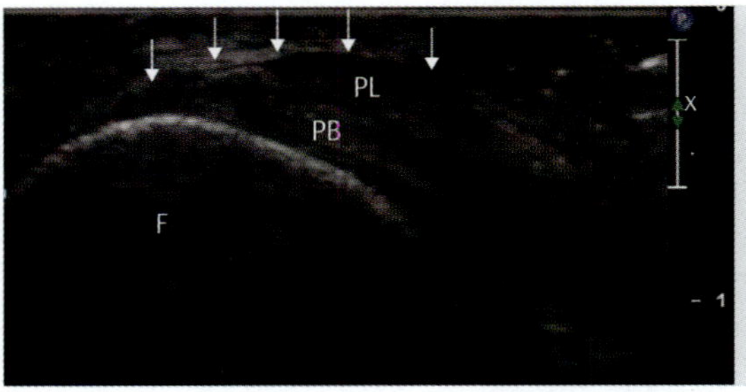

Fig. 5.7 Ultrasound peroneal tendon anatomy. Short axis view at the retromalleolar groove with the peroneal tendons located in their normal position at rest. F, fibula; PB, peroneal brevis; PL, peroneal longus. *Arrows* indicate the fibular retinaculum. Posterior to the right.

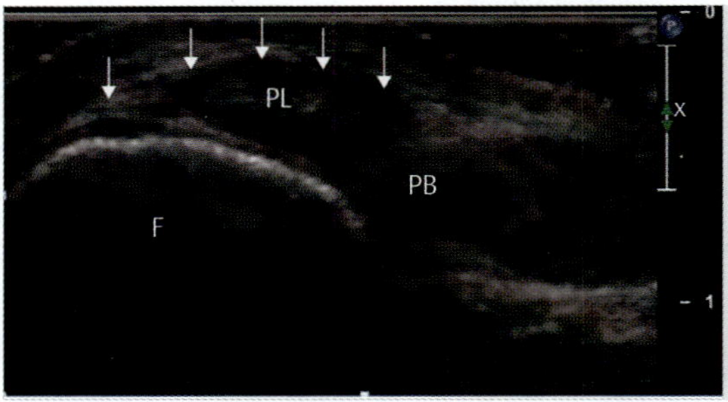

Fig. 5.8 Dynamic ultrasound peroneal tendon subluxation. Short axis view at the retromalleolar groove during active resisted ankle dorsiflexion and eversion showing dynamic instability with active ankle eversion. F, fibula; PB, peroneal brevis; PL, peroneal longus. *Arrows* indicate the fibular retinaculum. Posterior to the right.

5.3.3 Achilles Tendon Rupture

- Ultrasound evaluation can be used to assess tendon apposition and guide management of acute Achilles tendon injuries. Significant gapping greater than 5 mm may require surgical intervention.[20]
- Additionally, real-time Achilles ultrasound Thompson (RAUT) improves the accuracy of diagnosing acute Achilles tendon injuries.[18]

5.3.4 Therapeutic Injections

- Ultrasound-guided injections improved the accuracy of perineural and small joint injections.[21,22]

5.4 Computer Tomography Scan

5.4.1 Basic Principles

- Utilization of computed tomography (CT) scans has rapidly increased over the past 10 to 15 years, especially in the polytraumatized patient. CT imaging utilizes ionizing radiation to produce axial, coronal, and sagittal images.
- **Advantages:**
  - CT scan is the best imaging modality for complex bony anatomy.
  - It allows for improved characterization of intra-articular fractures, cortical erosion, soft-tissue calcification, and coalitions for surgical planning.
- **Radiation safety**:
  - Although there are reports of high-dose CT scan–associated cancers, extremity multidetector CT (MDCT) scans utilize low effective radiation dose (0.001 mSv) when compared to conventional CT imaging (0.07 mSv) by allowing for 3D reformatting without requiring imaging in multiple planes.[23,24]

5.4.2 Innovations

- **MDCT scan**:
  - In contrast to conventional CT, MDCT allows for higher resolution, quicker

image acquisition time, and 3D image reformating.[23]
  - Reducing pitch and increasing current allows for improved imaging quality.
- **Cone beam CT (CBCT) scan:**
  - CBCT is a newer technology that utilizes pulsed X-ray radiation onto a silicon flat-panel detector. Over 300 images are obtained within 18 seconds. Small platform sizes allow for specific field of view imaging for the lower extremity.[25]
  - Weight-bearing images with rotatable platforms allow for dynamic assessment of bony alignment.[25]
  - One retrospective comparison study showed that pediatric patients undergoing CBCT have shown significantly lower mean effective radiation dose than MDCT.[26]

5.4.3 Weight-Bearing Computed Tomography

- **Tibiotalar arthritis:**
  - Weight-bearing CT scan has shown an increased incidence of talus internal rotation in varus tibiotalar joint arthritis.[27]
- **Syndesmosis evaluation:**
  - Weight-bearing CT can be used to detect subtle instability of the syndesmosis. Arthroscopic diastasis highly correlates with greater than 2 mm of the anterior syndesmosis widening at the joint line during CT imaging.[28]
- **Subfibular impingement:**
  - ► Fig. 5.9 shows a weight-bearing CT scan of a patient with an accessory lateral talus causing subfibular impingement.

5.5 Magnetic Resonance Imaging

5.5.1 Basic Principles

- MRI is a highly utilized imaging modality that allows for high-quality imaging of soft-tissue injuries.
- When a magnetic field is placed onto one's body, hydrogen particles in a given tissue will align in a steady state of equilibrium.

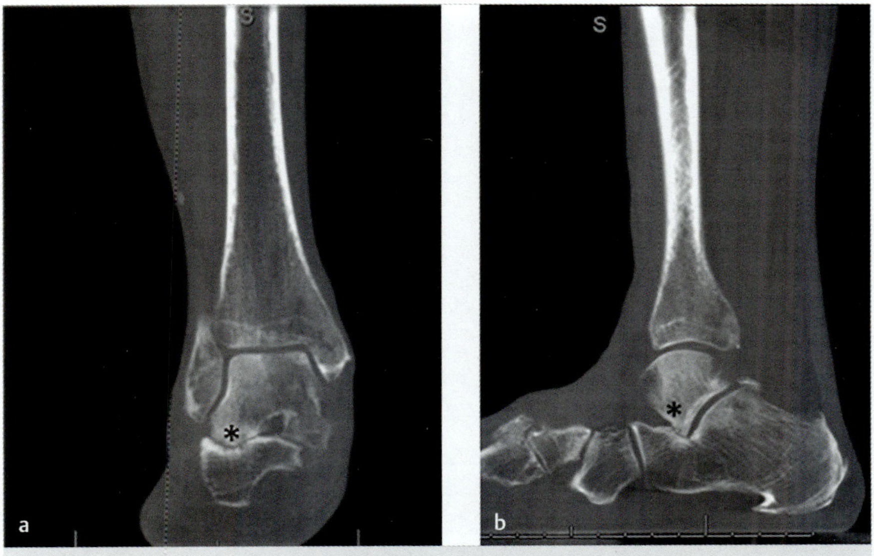

Fig. 5.9 Weight-bearing ankle computed tomography (CT). **(a)** Anteroposterior (AP) and **(b)** lateral weight-bearing CT of the ankle shows a patient with an accessory lateral talus process (*asterisk*), causing subfibular impingement and pain. This patient underwent an arthroscopic ostectomy.

- Radiofrequency pulse is applied to this magnetic field, and high-quality images are obtained by processing the radiofrequency emitted by excited protons with a receiver coil.[29]
- Advancements in MRI include the utilization of high-field scanners with magnetic fields greater than 1.5 T in order to shorten scanning time and allow for thinner image slices.
- Having a small field of view less than 16 cm^2 can improve the image resolution.
- **Advantages:**
  - MRI allows for high-quality multiplane images without the high-dose radiation used in plain radiographs and CT scans.
- **Disadvantages**:
  - Too much sensitivity. When tendons and ligaments are aligned at the magic angle (55 degrees) in relation to the magnetic field, a signal artifact is produced falsely mimicking pathology.[30]
  - Additionally, the use of MRI is contraindicated in patients with cardiac pacemakers, internal hearing aids, metallic foreign bodies, intravascular stents placed within 6 weeks, and first-trimester pregnancy. Additionally, although most orthopaedic implants are MRI compatible, significant metal artifact can obscure soft-tissue anatomy.

5.5.2 Tissue-Specific Imaging

Tissue-specific images were obtained at different times during proton relaxation back to their steady state.

- **T1-weighted imaging** (▶ Fig. 5.10):
  - T1-weighted imaging is best for delineating anatomic structures and has a high signal-to-noise ratio. The time to repetition values is less than 1,000 milliseconds.[31] Fat appears hyperintense during T1-weighted imaging.
- **T2-weighted imaging** (▶ Fig. 5.11):
  - T2-weighted imaging is best for contrasting normal and abnormal anatomy. The time to repetition values is greater than 1,000 milliseconds.[31] Water appears to be hyperintense during T2-weighted images.
  - Structures with little fat or water are hypointense on both MRI sequences,

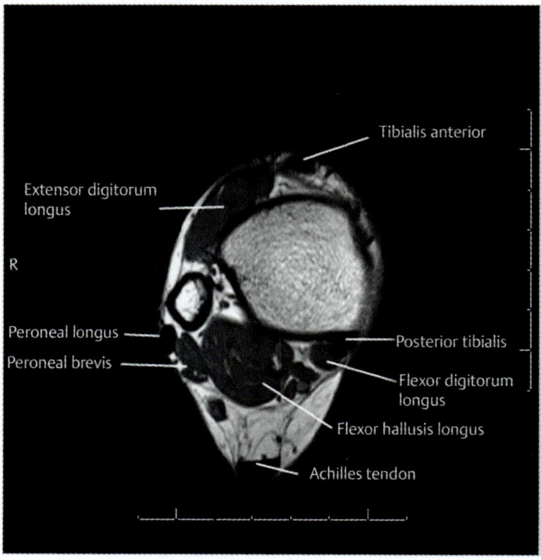

Fig. 5.10 T1-weighted ankle magnetic resonance imaging (MRI) showing a T1-weighted axial image at the level of the distal tibia and fibula.

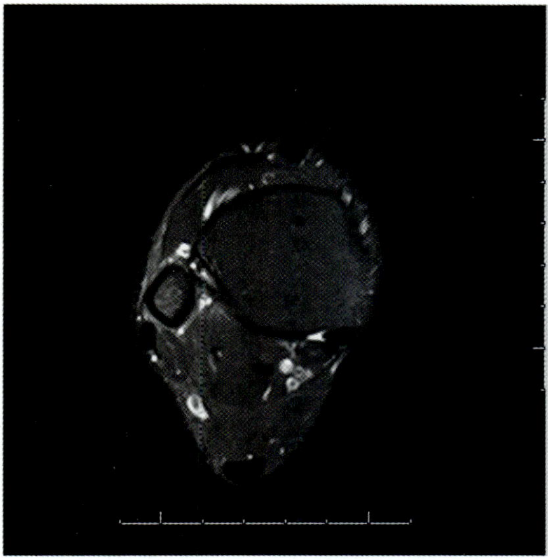

Fig. 5.11 T2-weighted ankle magnetic resonance imaging (MRI) showing a T2-weighted axial image at the level of the distal tibia and fibula.

such as cartilage, ligaments, fibrous tissue, and high-flow arterial blood flow.[31]

- **Other sequences**:
- Contrast enhancement can be utilized to detect and differentiate infection from a benign fluid collection.
- Fat suppression (short tau inversion recovery [STIR], T2 fat suppression).

5.6 Nuclear Medicine Scanning

5.6.1 Technetium-99 Bone Scan

- **Basic principles** (▶ Fig. 5.12):
  - It utilizes technetium-99 m phosphate binds to osteoblasts and hydroxyapatite crystal formation.
- **Indications**:
  - Osseous tumors, osteomyelitis, periprosthetic joint infection, aseptic loosening, stress fractures, and complex regional pain syndrome.
- **Disadvantages**:
  - It lacks anatomic localization.
  - It binds nonspecifically during bone formation and may not be a very specific test.
- **Phase studies**:
  - First phase:
    - Immediate blood flow phase through arterial system.
  - Second phase:
    - Blood pool phase at which there is tracer accumulation through intravascular volume at 30 minutes.
  - Third phase:
    - Delayed tracer accumulation at 4 hours (▶ Fig. 5.12).

5.6.2 Single-Photon Emission CT Scan

- The addition of positron emission improves the anatomic localization of osteoblastic activity (▶ Fig. 5.13).
- It can be used in patients with chronic periprosthetic ankle pain concerning for aseptic loosening (▶ Fig. 5.13).[32]

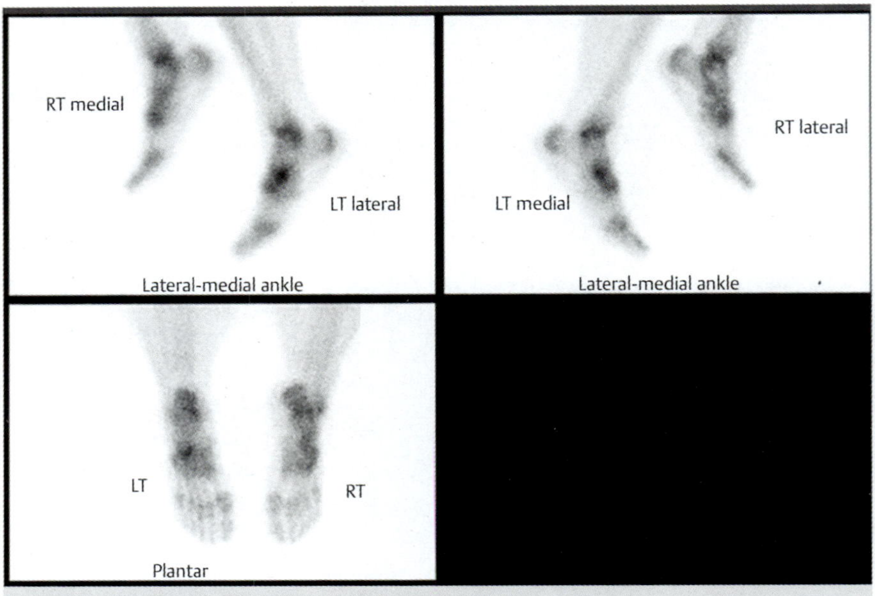

Fig. 5.12 Technetium-99 bone scan. Blood pool phase of the left foot reveals increased signal at the lateral midfoot, consistent with lateral cuneiform-cuboid osteoarthritis.

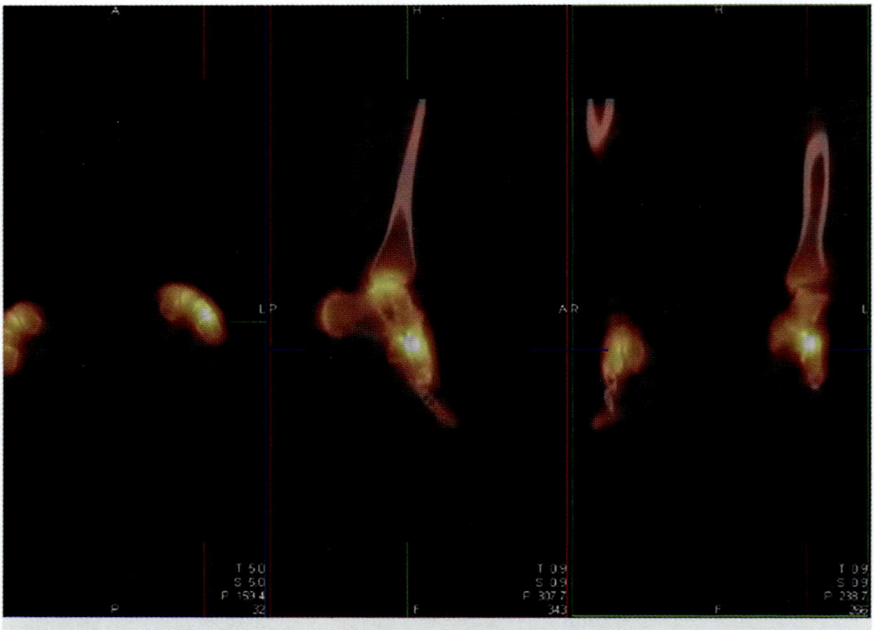

Fig. 5.13 Single-photon emission computed tomography (SPECT)/CT. The image illustrates increased osteoblastic activity at the lateral midfoot, consistent with lateral cuneiform-cuboid osteoarthritis.

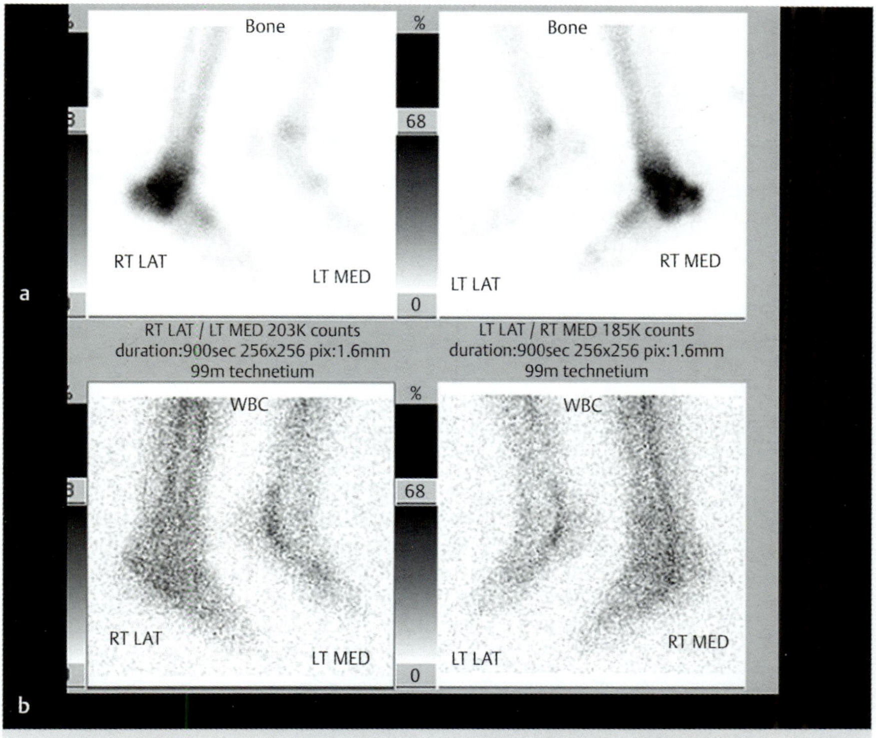

Fig. 5.14 Tagged white blood cell (WBC) I-111 scan. **(a)** Pool phase: Tc-99 bone scan of the right ankle in a patient with a painful foot 4 months after a revision subtalar fusion. **(b)** A tagged WBC I-111 bone scan that did not have increased signal at the ankle. There was no concern for osteomyelitis and the patient was diagnosed with a nonunion.

5.6.3 Tagged White Blood Cell Scan

- **Gallium-67 isotope**:
  - Localization to sites of inflammation, infection, or tumor involvement.
- **Indium-111 isotope** (▶ Fig. 5.14):
  - Localization to sites of infection.

5.7 Key Testing Facts

- The foot and ankle are a complex anatomic structure that requires multiple imaging modalities for the diagnosis of various conditions.
- Plain radiographs provide static assessment of the osseous structures.
- Stress views and standing plain radiographs provide dynamic assessment of bony alignment.
- Ultrasound imaging provides an affordable modality for the dynamic assessment of soft-tissue structures.
- Advanced imaging, such as CT imaging and MRI, provides detailed assessment of bony structures and soft-tissue structures, respectively.
- Nuclear medicine imaging allows for the assessment of infection and biologic bone activity.

References

[1] Doherty BTMW. General imaging principles. In: Pope T, Bloem HL, Beltran JB, Morrison WB, Wilson DJ, eds. Musculoskeletal Imaging. 2nd ed. Philadelphia, PA: Elsevier; 2015:1–12

[2] Brandser EA, Berbaum KS, Dorfman DD, et al. Contribution of individual projections alone and in combination for radiographic detection of ankle fractures. AJR Am J Roentgenol. 2000; 174(6): 1691–1697

[3] Miller CP, Ghorbanhoseini M, Ehrlichman LK, Walley KC, Ghaheri A, Kwon JY. High variability of observed weight bearing during standing foot and ankle radiographs. Foot Ankle Int. 2017; 38(6): 690–693

[4] Saltzman CL, el-Khoury GY. The hindfoot alignment view. Foot Ankle Int. 1995; 16(9):572–576

[5] Zampogna B, Vasta S, Amendola A, et al. Assessing lower limb alignment: comparison of standard knee Xray vs long leg view. Iowa Orthop J. 2015; 35:49–54

[6] Rungprai C, Goetz JE, Arunakul M, et al. Validation and reproducibility of a biplanar imaging system versus conventional radiography of foot and ankle radiographic parameters. Foot Ankle Int. 2014; 35 (11):1166–1175

[7] Arunakul M, Amendola A, Gao Y, Goetz JE, Femino JE, Phisitkul P. Tripod index: a new radiographic parameter assessing foot alignment. Foot Ankle Int. 2013; 34(10):1411–1420

[8] Arunakul M, Amendola A, Gao Y, Goetz JE, Femino JE, Phisitkul P. Tripod index: diagnostic accuracy in symptomatic flatfoot and cavovarus foot: part 2. Iowa Orthop J. 2013; 33:47–53

[9] Schwend RM, Drennan JC. Cavus foot deformity in children. J Am Acad Orthop Surg. 2003; 11(3): 201–211

[10] Sensiba PR, Coffey MJ, Williams NE, Mariscalco M, Laughlin RT. Inter- and intraobserver reliability in the radiographic evaluation of adult flatfoot deformity. Foot Ankle Int. 2010; 31(2):141–145

[11] Ashraf A, Murphree J, Wait E, et al. Gravity stress radiographs and the effect of ankle position on deltoid ligament integrity and medial clear space measurements. J Orthop Trauma. 2017; 31(5): 270–274

[12] Baumfeld D, Baumfeld T, Cangussu J, et al. Does foot position and location of measurement influence ankle medial clear space? Foot Ankle Spec. 2018; 11(1):32–36

[13] Park SS, Kubiak EN, Egol KA, Kummer F, Koval KJ. Stress radiographs after ankle fracture: the effect of ankle position and deltoid ligament status on medial clear space measurements. J Orthop Trauma. 2006; 20(1):11–18

[14] Femino JE, Vaseenon T, Phisitkul P, Tochigi Y, Anderson DD, Amendola A. Varus external rotation stress test for radiographic detection of deep deltoid ligament disruption with and without syndesmotic disruption: a cadaveric study. Foot Ankle Int. 2013; 34(2):251–260

[15] Koval KJ, Egol KA, Cheung Y, Goodwin DW, Spratt KF. Does a positive ankle stress test indicate the need for operative treatment after lateral malleolus fracture? A preliminary report. J Orthop Trauma. 2007; 21(7):449–455

[16] Gill JB, Risko T, Raducan V, Grimes JS, Schutt RC, Jr. Comparison of manual and gravity stress radiographs for the evaluation of supination-external rotation fibular fractures. J Bone Joint Surg Am. 2007; 89(5):994–999

[17] Girish G, Finlay K, Landry D, et al. Musculoskeletal disorders of the lower limb: ultrasound and magnetic resonance imaging correlation. Can Assoc Radiol J. 2007; 58(3):152–166

[18] Griffin MJ, Olson K, Heckmann N, Charlton TP. Realtime Achilles Ultrasound Thompson (RAUT) test for the evaluation and diagnosis of acute Achilles tendon ruptures. Foot Ankle Int. 2017; 38(1):36–40

[19] Pesquer L, Guillo S, Poussange N, Pele E, Meyer P, Dallaudière B. Dynamic ultrasound of peroneal tendon instability. Br J Radiol. 2016; 89(1063): 20150958

[20] Kotnis R, David S, Handley R, Willett K, Ostlere S. Dynamic ultrasound as a selection tool for reducing Achilles tendon reruptures. Am J Sports Med. 2006; 34(9):1395–1400

[21] Walter WR, Burke CJ, Adler RS. Ultrasound-guided therapeutic injections for neural pathology about the foot and ankle: a 4 year retrospective review. Skeletal Radiol. 2017; 46(6):795–803

[22] Khosla S, Thiele R, Baumhauer JF. Ultrasound guidance for intra-articular injections of the foot and ankle. Foot Ankle Int. 2009; 30(9):886–890

[23] Fayad LM, Bluemke DA, Fishman EK. Musculoskeletal imaging with computed tomography and magnetic resonance imaging: when is computed tomography the study of choice? Curr Probl Diagn Radiol. 2005; 34(6):220–237

[24] Biswas D, Bible JE, Bohan M, Simpson AK, Whang PG, Grauer JN. Radiation exposure from musculoskeletal computerized tomographic scans. J Bone Joint Surg Am. 2009; 91(8):1882–1889

[25] Tuominen EK, Kankare J, Koskinen SK, Mattila KT. Weight-bearing CT imaging of the lower extremity. AJR Am J Roentgenol. 2013; 200(1):146–148

[26] Pugmire BS, Shailam R, Sagar P, et al. Initial clinical experience with extremity cone-beam CT of the foot and ankle in pediatric patients. AJR Am J Roentgenol. 2016; 206(2):431–435

[27] Kim JB, Yi Y, Kim JY, et al. Weight-bearing computed tomography findings in varus ankle osteoarthritis: abnormal internal rotation of the talus in the axial plane. Skeletal Radiol. 2017; 46 (8):1071–1080

[28] Ahn TK, Choi SM, Kim JY, Lee WC. Isolated syndesmosis diastasis: computed tomography scan assessment with arthroscopic correlation. Arthroscopy. 2017; 33(4):828–834

[29] White D. Magnetic resonance imaging in orthopaedics. In: Azar F, ed. Campbell's Operative Orthopaedics. 13th ed. Philadelphia, PA: Elsevier; 2017:134–164

[30] Erickson SJ, Prost RW, Timins ME. The "magic angle" effect: background physics and clinical relevance. Radiology. 1993; 188(1):23–25

[31] Miller MDTS, Hart JA. Imaging and Special Studies. Review of Orthopaedics. 6th ed. Philadelphia, PA: Elsevier Saunders; 2012:113–118

[32] Mason LW, Wyatt J, Butcher C, Wieshmann H, Molloy AP. Single-photon-emission computed tomography in painful total ankle replacements. Foot Ankle Int. 2015; 36(6):635–640

6 Disorders of the First Ray

Phillip T. Kirn, Samuel AbuMoussa, and Christopher E. Gross

Abstract

This chapter comprehensively covers disorders affecting the first ray of the foot, focusing primarily on hallux valgus, hallux varus, hallux rigidus, sesamoid pain, and turf toe. Each condition is explored in detail, starting with etiology and pathophysiology, progressing through symptoms, diagnostic methods, classification, and culminating in both conservative and surgical treatment options. For hallux valgus, the chapter emphasizes the importance of determining the chief complaint and appropriate surgical planning based on joint congruence and severity of deformity. Hallux varus is highlighted as frequently iatrogenic, requiring careful assessment. Hallux rigidus is discussed with a focus on its degenerative nature and the necessity for surgical intervention in advanced stages. Sesamoid pain and turf toe are also examined, with emphasis on their impact on athletic performance and specific surgical techniques for refractory cases. The chapter aims to provide a thorough understanding of these conditions to guide effective treatment strategies.

Keywords: Hallux Valgus, Hallux Varus, Hallux Rigidus, Sesamoid Pain, Turf Toe

6.1 Hallux Valgus

Hallux valgus is medial deviation of the first metatarsal and lateral deviation of the great toe.

6.1.1 Etiology

- ***Intrinsic***: genetics, ligamentous laxity, pes planus, rheumatoid arthritis (RA), cerebral palsy.
- ***Extrinsic***: certain shoes (narrow toe box, high heels).

6.1.2 Pathophysiology

- Attenuation of medial metatarsophalangeal (MTP) joint capsule.
- The first proximal phalanx begins to deviate laterally.
- As the abductor hallucis migrates medially, it begins to act as a plantar flexor and pronates the great toe.
- The first metatarsal drifts medially.
- Secondary contracture of the lateral MTP joint capsule and adductor hallucis.

6.1.3 Symptoms

- Pain over medial eminence.
- Cosmesis: not a reason to perform surgery.
- Transfer metatarsalgia.
- Second toe deformity.
- Difficulty wearing shoes due to medial eminence.
- **Important to determine what exactly is the patient's chief complaint.**

6.1.4 Diagnostics

Physical Examination

- With the patient standing, observe hindfoot alignment and forefoot changes.
- Observe the position of the great toe in relation to the lesser toes.
- Evaluate the first MTP joint motion; limited dorsiflexion suggests that full motion will not be achievable after surgery.
- Evaluate the second toe for MTP joint instability (Lachman) and presence of hammertoe.
- Assess stability of the first tarsometatarsal (TMT) joint:
  - About 10% of patients with severe hallux valgus will have instability at this joint.[1]

  - Important to recognize for surgical planning as a Lapidus procedure may be necessary.

Radiographs

- Weight-bearing anteroposterior (AP), lateral, and oblique foot views.
- Evaluate the following:
  - Hallux valgus angle (HVA): Angle between line drawn along the shaft of the first metatarsal and proximal phalanx (normal < 15 degrees).
  - Intermetatarsal angle (IMA): Angle between long axis of the first and second metatarsal (normal < 9 degrees).
  - Distal metatarsal articular angle (DMAA): Angle between the articular surface and the long axis of the first metatarsal (normal < 10 degrees).
  - Hallux valgus interphalangeus: Angle between the first proximal and distal phalanx (normal < 10 degrees of valgus).
  - First TMT joint: More than 15 degrees of varus may indicate instability.
  - First MTP joint arthritis.
  - First MTP joint incongruence: Proximal phalanx joint surface is not parallel to the distal metatarsal joint surface. DMAA > 10 degrees also indicates incongruent joint.

6.1.5 Classification

Classification of the hallux valgus is used to guide the surgical plan:

- Is the first MTP joint stiff or arthritic? If yes, then perform first MTP arthrodesis.
- Is the first MTP joint congruent?
  - Most important factor when determining the best surgical intervention.
  - If the joint is incongruent, then procedure should restore congruency.
- Is the metatarsocuneiform joint unstable or arthritic? If yes, then perform a 1st tarsometatarsal fusion.
- Severity of deformity based on HVA and IMA.
  - *Mild:* HVA < 30 degrees and IMA < 13 degrees→ chevron osteotomy or other distally-based osteotomy.
  - *Moderate:* HVA < 40 degrees and IMA > 13 degrees→ Proximal osteotomy
  - *Severe:* HVA > 40 degrees and IMA > 20 degrees→ first MTP arthrodesis or TMT fusion.

6.1.6 Conservative Management

- For the most part, all hallux valgus deformities can and should initially be treated conservatively.
- *Modify shoe wear:* wide and deep toe box to accommodate deformity.

6.1.7 Surgical Intervention

- Over 130 surgical procedures have been described.
- Should NEVER be performed for cosmetic reasons.
- Most appropriate surgical intervention is determined by both clinical findings and imaging.

6.1.8 Akin Procedure (Proximal Phalanx Osteotomy)

Indications

- Hallux valgus interphalangeus.

Contraindications

- Incongruent joint or DMAA > 15 degrees. Results in worsening of deformity.

Technical Considerations

- Make osteotomy distal to concavity of joint to avoid inadvertent arthrotomy.

Key Testing Facts

- Usually performed as a secondary procedure to correct hallux valgus interphalangeus after a metatarsal osteotomy or distal soft-tissue procedure.
- Can be performed in isolation if hallux valgus interphalangeus is the only deformity present.

6.1.9 Chevron Procedure (Distal Metatarsal Osteotomy)

Indications

- Mild deformity.

Contraindications

- HVA > 35 degrees and IMA > 15 degrees.

Technical Considerations

- Medial approach to avoid dorsal medial cutaneous nerve.
- Minimize soft-tissue stripping and avoid medial capsulotomy, which may compromise blood flow to metatarsal head and result in avascular necrosis.
- If DMAA > 10 degrees, then perform additional medial closing wedge osteotomy (biplanar chevron osteotomy; ▶ Fig. 6.1).

Key Testing Facts

- Excellent procedure for mild deformity.

Modified McBride Procedure (Distal Soft-Tissue Procedure)

Indications

- Very mild deformity.

Contraindications

- HVA > 35 degrees and IMA > 15 degrees.
- DMAA > 15 degrees.

Technical Considerations

- Procedure includes release of adductor hallucis, lateral capsulotomy, and medial capsule imbrication.
- *Original McBride Procedure*: fibular sesamoid removal. Resulted in hallux varus
- *Modified McBride's procedure*: does not resect the fibular sesamoid.
- *Make two incisions*: one along medial side of the joint and the other in the first webspace.
- Resect medial eminence in line with the medial border of the foot (Silver osteotomy).

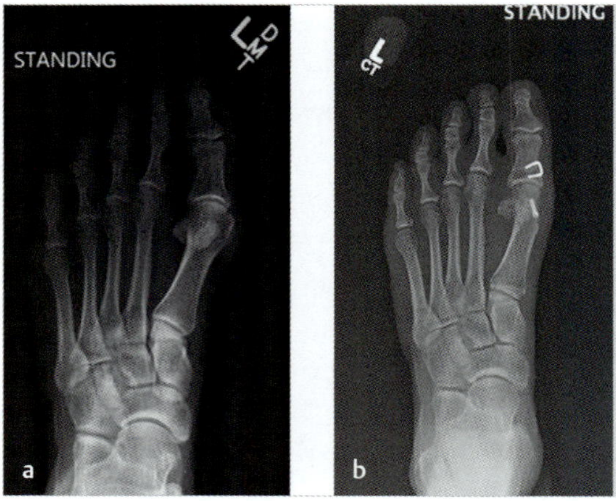

Fig. 6.1 (a,b) Chevron + Akin procedure for hallux valgus.

- Completely release the soft tissue along the lateral aspect of the joint.
- Use postoperative dressing to maintain correction for 8 weeks.

Key Testing Facts

- Rarely indicated as the primary procedure.
- Usually performed with metatarsal osteotomy or first TMT fusion.

Proximal Metatarsal Osteotomy + Distal Soft-Tissue Procedure

Indications

- Moderate to severe deformity.

Contraindications

- Presence of arthrosis.

Technical Considerations

- There is a variety of proximal metatarsal osteotomy options including crescentic osteotomy, broomstick osteotomy, Ludloff's osteotomy, and scarf osteotomy.
- The goal is to correct IMA while avoiding shortening and excessive lateral displacement of metatarsal head.

Key Testing Facts

- Can be used for most hallux valgus deformities.

Lapidus Procedure (First TMT Fusion + Distal Soft-Tissue Procedure)

Indications

- Unstable or arthritic first TMT joint with moderate hallux valgus deformity.
- Severe hallux valgus deformity.

Contraindications

- Active, young patients.
- Normal metatarsocuneiform stability.

Technical Considerations

- Technically difficult.
- Joint should be fused plantarward and laterally.

Key Testing Facts

- Results in increased stiffness of the foot and should be avoided in a young, active patient.

First MTP Joint Fusion

Indications

- Stiff or painful first MTP joint (RA, osteoarthritis [OA], gout).
- Spasticity (stroke, cerebral palsy).
- Severe deformity.
- Salvage procedure.

Technical Considerations

- Alignment is critical.
- Fifteen-degree dorsiflexion, 15-degree valgus, and neutral rotation.

Key Testing Facts

- Excellent long-term results but should be avoided in less severe deformities when there are other options.
- Salvage procedure.

Keller's Procedure (First Proximal Phalanx Resection Arthroplasty)

Indications

- Severe deformity or MTP arthrosis in elderly, inactive patients.

Contraindications

- Active patients.

Technical Considerations

- Destabilizes the first MTP joint.
- Stabilizes the joint with a pin for 3 to 4 weeks.

> **Key Testing Facts**
>
> - Do not use in active patients.
> - Rarely indicated and rarely performed.

6.1.10 Postoperative Care

- Use dressing to help maintain corrected alignment.
- Noncompliant patients who bear weight too early are at risk of recurrence.

6.2 Hallux Varus

- Medial deviation of the great toe.

6.2.1 Etiology

- Most commonly an iatrogenic deformity resulting from a surgical procedure to correct a hallux valgus deformity.[2]
- RA: loss of capsular restraint.

6.2.2 Pathophysiology

Soft-Tissue Factors

- Over-resection of medial eminence.
- Incompetent lateral capsule (i.e., excessive release).
- Tight medial capsule (i.e., over-plication).
- Medial displacement of the tibial sesamoid.
- Overpull of the abductor hallucis muscle.

6.2.3 Symptoms

- Main complaint is often cosmetic or difficulty wearing shoes. Usually not painful.

6.2.4 Diagnostics

Physical Examination

- Determine if deformity is fixed or flexible.
- Flexibility of deformity is important for surgical planning.

Imaging

Radiographs

- Obtain weight-bearing views.
- IMA < 0 degrees.
- Determine the presence of MTP or interphalangeal joint arthritis.

6.2.5 Conservative Management

- *Modify shoe wear*: Wide toe box to accommodate deformity.
- Taping/splinting to correct deformities that occur after a hallux valgus surgery.

6.2.6 Surgical Intervention

Joint-Preserving Procedures

- *Lateral closing wedge osteotomy:* Indicated when varus deformity is the result of overcorrection from previous metatarsal or proximal phalangeal osteotomy.
- *Tendon transfer and medial capsule release:* Indicated for flexible MTP joint deformity in a young patient.

Joint-Sacrificing Procedures

- *First MTP arthrodesis:* Indicated for fixed MTP joint deformity or when painful MTP joint arthritis is also present.

Key Testing Facts

- Usually an iatrogenic deformity following a hallux valgus corrective surgery.
- If deformity is flexible, perform a joint-preserving procedure.
- If deformity is fixed, perform arthrodesis.

6.3 Hallux Rigidus

- Painful first MTP joint arthrosis with limited dorsiflexion.

6.3.1 Etiology

- Not well understood.

6.3.2 Pathophysiology

- Degenerative OA of the first MTP joint.
- Dorsal aspect of the joint affected first.
- Cartilage loss begins to occur in plantar half of the joint as disease progresses.

6.3.3 Symptoms

- Main complaint is often pain that is worse during extremes of motion.
- Main source of pain is dorsal impingement from osteophytes.

6.3.4 Diagnostics

Physical Examination

- Evaluate range of motion (i.e., loss of dorsiflexion).
- Initially, pain occurs at extremes of motion, especially plantar flexion.
- Pain during midrange of motion suggests more extensive MTP joint arthritis.
    - These patients often need arthrodesis.

Imaging

Radiographs

- Obtain weight-bearing AP, lateral, and oblique views.
- Evaluate dorsal osteophytes on lateral view.
- Joint space narrowing best evaluated on oblique view.

6.3.5 Classification

Classification of hallux rigidus based on severity is presented in detail in ▶ Table 6.1.

6.3.6 Conservative Management

- Should be attempted before considering surgical intervention.

Table 6.1 Classification of hallux rigidus based on severity[3]

Grade	Dorsiflexion (degrees)	Radiographs	Examination
0	40–60	Normal	No pain
1	30–40	Dorsal osteophyte Minimal joint space narrowing	Mild pain at extremes of motion
2	10–30	Dorsal, lateral ± medial osteophytes < 50% joint space narrowing	Moderate pain just before extremes of motion
3	≤ 10	Dorsal, lateral ± medial osteophytes > 50% joint space narrowing	Severe pain but not at the midrange of motion
4	≤ 10	Dorsal, lateral ± medial osteophytes > 50% joint space narrowing	Pain at the midrange of motion

- *Modify shoe wear:* Wide toe box, rigid rocker sole, or Morton's extension to decrease motion at the first MTP joint.
- Activity modification, nonsteroidal anti-inflammatory drugs (NSAIDs) ± corticosteroid injections.

6.3.7 Surgical Intervention

Cheilectomy

Indications

- Pain with mild to moderate limitations in dorsiflexion exists.

Technical Aspects

- Make dorsal incision over the MTP joint, open capsule, and perform synovectomy. Remove the medial and lateral osteophytes.
- Remove the dorsal osteophytes and approximately 30% of the dorsal articular surface of the metatarsal head until approximately 65 degrees of dorsiflexion is obtainable.[4]
- May also perform proximal phalanx dorsal closing wedge osteotomy (i.e., Moberg's procedure) to improve dorsiflexion (▶ Fig. 6.2 and ▶ Fig. 6.3).

Postoperative Care

- Post-op shoe until wound has healed, then encourage active motion.
- May take several months for maximal improvement.

Keller's Resection Arthroplasty

Indications

- Consider in sedentary patients older than 80 years.

Technical Aspects

- Remove the base of the proximal phalanx.
- Results in MTP joint instability, which can lead to transfer metatarsalgia, toe-off weakness, and hallux cockup deformity.

MTP Joint Arthrodesis

Indications

- Standard of care for severe arthritis (i.e., grades 3 and 4).

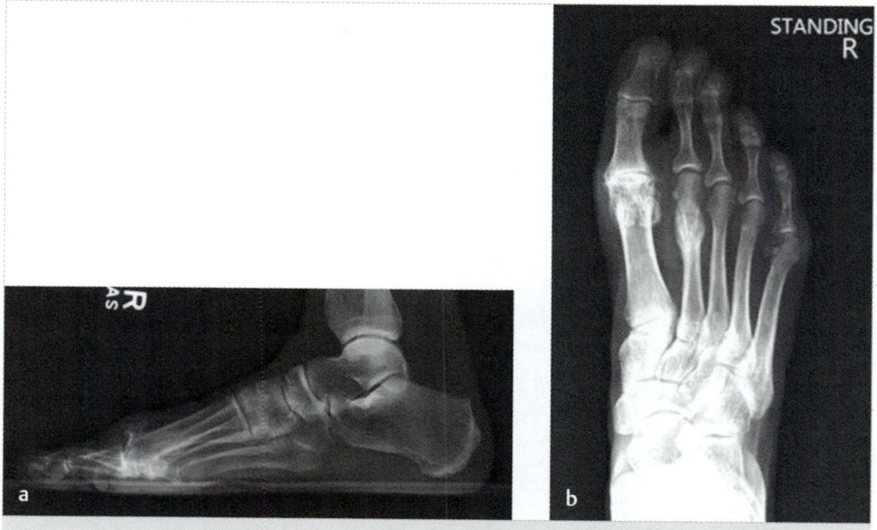

Fig. 6.2 (a,b) A 63-year-old woman with hallux rigidus.

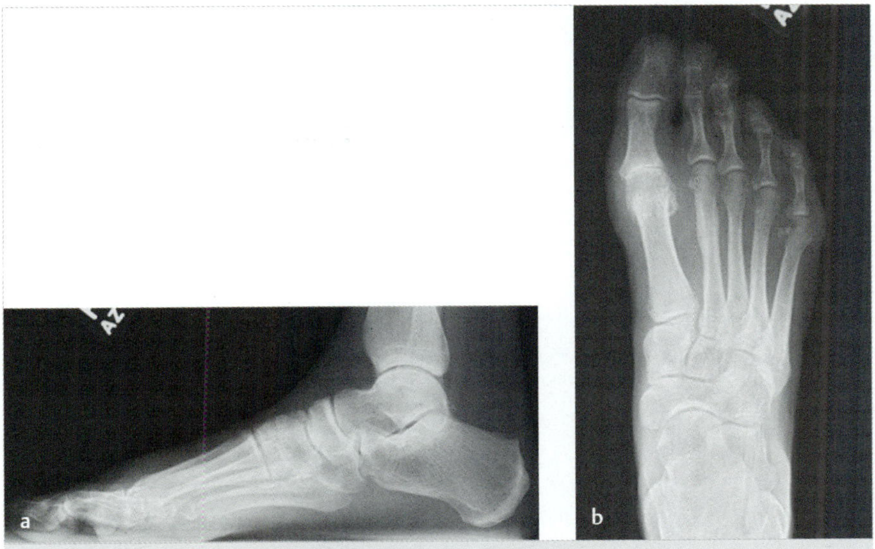

Fig. 6.3 (a,b) The patient in ▶ Fig. 6.2 underwent a cheilectomy.

Technical Aspects

- Several fixation methods to choose from: K-wires, staples, plates, and/or screws.
- Fuse the great toe in 10- to 15-degree dorsiflexion and 10 to 15 degrees of valgus (▶ Fig. 6.4 and ▶ Fig. 6.5).

Implant Arthroplasty

- Includes total joint arthroplasty, metatarsal hemiarthroplasty, and proximal phalanx hemiarthroplasty.
- Fusions have better outcomes.
- **Implant arthroplasty is not recommended.**

Cartiva Synthetic Joint Implant

Indications

- Focal cartilage defects associated with joint pain and decreased motion.
- Severe first MTP arthritis: 96% implant survivorship and high patient satisfaction with significantly improved function at 5 years.[5,6]

Technical Aspects

- Expose the MTP joint and remove the osteophytes.
- A cavity is drilled into the metatarsal head and the cylindrical implant is inserted.

Postoperative Care

- Weight bearing as tolerated in stiff sole shoe. Begin range of motion exercises immediately.

6.4 Sesamoid Pain

6.4.1 Etiology

- Sesamoid fracture.
- *Sesamoiditis:* Occurs in young patients after repetitive trauma:
  - Bilateral sesamoiditis associated with inflammatory conditions.
- *Other causes:* Infection, osteochondritis, and turf toe.

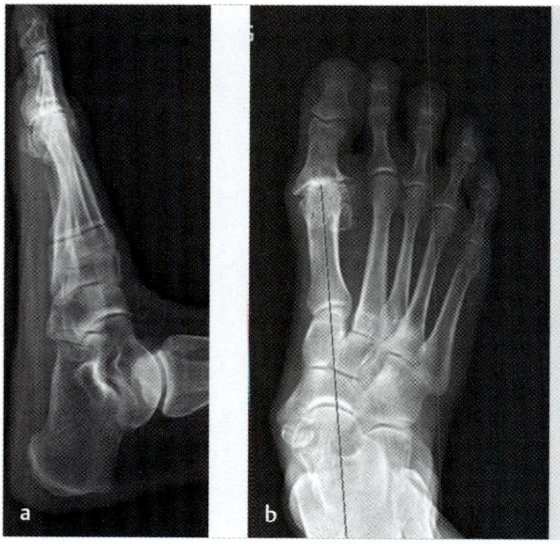

Fig. 6.4 (a,b) A 57-year-old woman with hallux rigidus.

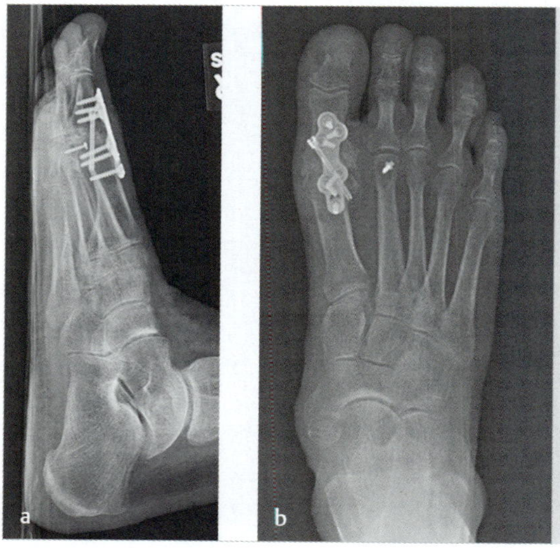

Fig. 6.5 (a,b) The patient in ▶ Fig. 6.5 underwent an arthrodesis of the first metatarsophalangeal (MTP) joint.

6.4.2 Pathophysiology

- Often injured during forced dorsiflexion of the first MTP.
- Sesamoids reside in the flexor hallucis brevis (FHB) and act as a fulcrum to increase the MTP flexion strength.
- Tibial sesamoid is larger and bears more weight than the fibular sesamoid.
  - Higher incidence of traumatic injuries to the tibial sesamoid.

6.4.3 Symptoms

- Main complaint: generalized great toe pain, especially plantarly.
- Pain often occurs during the terminal part of the stance phase when the hallux extends.

6.4.4 Diagnostics

Physical Examination

- Often tender over the sesamoid.
- Inspect for cavus deformity with plantarflexed first toe.

Radiographs

- Obtain AP, lateral oblique, and medial oblique views:
  - Medial oblique to evaluate tibial sesamoid.
  - Lateral oblique to evaluate fibular sesamoid.
- Axial sesamoid view:
  - If you see a sesamoid that appears fractured, be careful as it may be a bipartite sesamoid.
    - Bipartite sesamoid can be found in 10% of population.[7]
    - Obtaining radiographs of the other foot may be useful because 25% of patients with this condition will have it in both feet.

Bone Scan

- Can help differentiate a fracture from a bipartite sesamoid.
- A fracture will have increased uptake compared to the uninjured side.

Magnetic Resonance Imaging

- Helpful if avascular necrosis is suspected.

6.4.5 Conservative Management

Sesamoid Fracture

- Molded orthosis with metatarsal pad.
- If orthosis fails, then short-leg walking cast with toe plate for 6 weeks.

Sesamoid Stress Fracture

- Non-weight-bearing in a cast/controlled ankle motion (CAM) boot for 6 to 8 weeks.
- If symptoms persist, then consider surgical intervention.

Sesamoiditis

- Shoe modifications, activity modification, orthosis (Dancer's pad, Morton's extension orthotic), casting.
- Managed conservatively for an extensive period before considering excision.

6.4.6 Surgical Intervention

- Consider only after exhaustive trial of nonoperative measures.

Complete or Partial Sesamoidectomy

Indications

- Fail to improve after more than 3 months of nonoperative management.

Technical Aspects

- Make dorsal incision in the first intermetatarsal space or plantar incision in the first webspace to remove the fibular sesamoid.
- Make a medial plantar incision to remove the tibial sesamoid and protect the medial branch of the plantar digital nerve during approach.
- Try to avoid excising both sesamoids to avoid cockup deformity and recalcitrant pain.
- Repair FHB after sesamoid excision.

6.5 Turf Toe

- Hyperextension injury of the first MTP joint.

6.5.1 Etiology

- Common in contact sports played on hard surfaces (i.e., football players on turf).

6.5.2 Pathophysiology

- Hyperextension of the first MTP joint when the ankle is in plantar flexion and axial load is applied to the heel → tearing of plantar capsuloligamentous structures.
- Football players frequently have their foot in this position with significant loading that accounts for the high prevalence of turf toe in these athletes.
- Results in joint instability.

6.5.3 Symptoms

- Main complaint is acute MTP joint pain and swelling following an identifiable inciting event.
- Decreased push-off strength.

6.5.4 Diagnostics

Physical Examination

- Assess the first MTP joint stability.
- Evaluate the hallux flexion strength.

Imaging

Radiographs

- Obtain AP and lateral views.
- Look for sesamoid fracture.
- Proximal migration of the sesamoids may occur with disruption of the plantar capsule.

Magnetic Resonance Imaging

- Provides conclusive information with regard to the integrity of the plantar capsular structures and joint surface.

6.5.5 Classification

Classification of turf toe severity is shown in ▶ Table 6.2.

6.5.6 Conservative Management

- ***Grade I:*** taping and early rehabilitation with return to play as tolerated.
- ***Grade II:*** taping and rehabilitation with return to play in approximately 2 weeks.
  - Walking boot, turf toe plate, or carbon fiber orthosis (Morton's extension).
- ***Grade III:*** immobilize the first MTP joint in plantar flexion. Return to play in approximately 12 weeks.
  - May do better with surgical intervention.

6.5.7 Surgical Intervention

Direct Primary Repair

- Indicated after complete disruption of the plantar capsule (grade III injury).
- May take 6 to 12 months for an athlete to return to full competition.

6.5.8 Rehabilitation

- Timing depends on severity of injury.
- Focus on the first MTP joint's range of motion and plantar flexion strength.

Table 6.2 Classification of turf toe severity[8]

Grade	Plantar capsule	Swelling/ecchymosis	Motion/strength
I	Attenuated	Minimal	Normal
II	Partial tear	Moderate	Limited motion due to pain
III	Complete tear	Significant	Metatarsophalangeal (MTP) joint instability and weakness

References

[1] Coughlin MJ, Smith BW. Hallux valgus and first ray mobility. Surgical technique. J Bone Joint Surg Am. 2008; 90 Suppl 2, Pt 2:153–170

[2] Hawkins FB. Acquired hallux varus: cause, prevention and correction. Clin Orthop Relat Res. 1971; 76(76):169–176

[3] Coughlin MJ, Shurnas PS. Hallux rigidus. Grading and long-term results of operative treatment. J Bone Joint Surg Am. 2003; 85(11):2072–2088

[4] Deland JT, Williams BR. Surgical management of hallux rigidus. J Am Acad Orthop Surg. 2012; 20 (6):347–358

[5] Daniels TR, Younger AS, Penner MJ, et al. midterm outcomes of polyvinyl alcohol hydrogel hemiarthroplasty of the first metatarsophalangeal joint in advanced hallux rigidus. Foot Ankle Int. 2017; 38(3):243–247

[6] Baumhauer JF, Singh D, Glazebrook M, et al. for and on behalf of the CARTIVA Motion Study Group. Prospective, randomized, multi-centered clinical trial assessing safety and efficacy of a synthetic cartilage implant versus first metatarsophalangeal arthrodesis in advanced hallux rigidus. Foot Ankle Int. 2016; 37(5):457–469

[7] Richardson EG. Hallucal sesamoid pain: causes and surgical treatment. J Am Acad Orthop Surg. 1999; 7 (4):270–278

[8] Anderson RB, Hunt KJ, McCormick JJ. Management of common sports-related injuries about the foot and ankle. J Am Acad Orthop Surg. 2010; 18(9): 546–556

7 Lesser Toe Deformities

Justin Tsai and Steven M. Raikin

Abstract
Lesser toe deformities include mallet/hammer/claw deformities, bunionettes, and Freiberg's infarction. Mallet/hammer/claw toe deformities develop as a result of imbalance between flexor and extensor mechanisms, and mostly occur secondary to extrinsic causes such as tight shoe wear and/or trauma. A bunionette is a deformity of the fifth metatarsal resulting in a prominent fifth metatarsal head. Freiberg's infarction describes osteonecrosis of the second metatarsal head. Nonoperative treatment options for lesser toe deformities include wearing wider shoes, shaving of callosities, and activity modification. Operative treatment is dependent on the type of deformity/pathology present, the flexibility of the deformity, and the location of pathology.

Keywords: deformity, hammer toe, mallet toe, claw toe, Freiberg's, bunionette

7.1 Anatomy

- The extensor digitorum longus (EDL) divides into three slips over the proximal phalanx (▶ Fig. 7.1):
  - The central slip inserts onto the middle phalanx.
  - The lateral slips diverge and merge again at the distal phalanx.
- The extensor hood attaches at the plantar aspect of the metatarsophalangeal joint (MTPJ), which centralizes and contains the extensor tendon.
- The main function is to extend at the MTPJ (dorsiflex the proximal phalanx).
- The extensor mechanism has no direct attachment onto the proximal phalanx, and thus its extension ability at the MTPJ is through the indirect action of the extensor hood.

7.1.1 Flexor Mechanism

- The flexor digitorum longus (FDL) inserts onto the plantar aspect of the distal phalanx.
- The flexor digitorum brevis (FDB) inserts onto the plantar aspect of the middle phalanx.
- Their action is antagonized by the EDL.
- With persistent extension at the MTPJ that occurs with wearing fashionable shoe wear, the extrinsic extensors cannot extend at the proximal interphalangeal joint (PIPJ) and distal interphalangeal joint (DIPJ), and the flexors are the only extrinsic forces acting, leading to persistent PIP and DIP flexion. They easily overpower the intrinsic muscles, which normally contribute to PIP and DIP extension.

7.1.2 Intrinsic Muscles

- Both the tendons of the lumbricals and interossei are plantar to the MTPJ center of rotation and dorsal to the PIPJ and DIPJ center of rotation (▶ Fig. 7.2).
- As a result, they flex at the MTPJ and extend at the PIPJ and DIPJ.
- Interossei are dorsal to intermetatarsal ligament, while lumbricals are plantar.
- Lumbricals attach to the medial aspect of the extensor hood.
- Interossei attach to the proximal phalanx.

7.1.3 Plantar Plate

- Strong fibrous structure that attaches thinly to the metatarsal metaphysis proximally, and more robustly into the proximal phalanx adjacent to the articular surface.
- *Other contributions:* distal fibers of the plantar fascia, accessory collateral

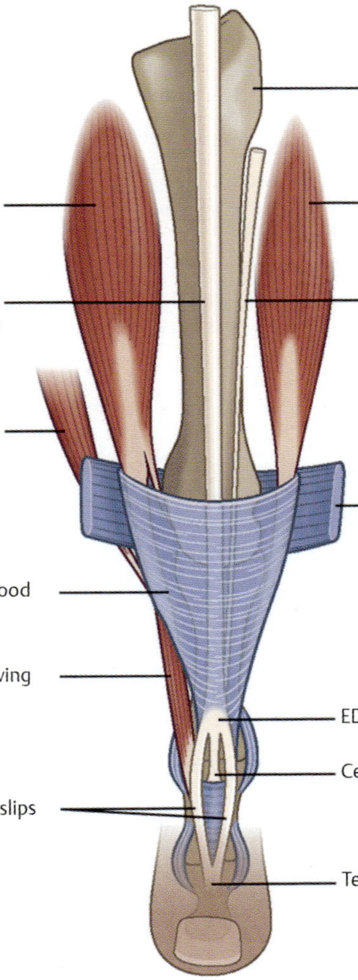

Fig. 7.1 Dorsal view of the lesser toe extensor mechanism.

ligaments, transverse metatarsal ligament, interosseous tendons, and fibrous sheath of the flexor tendon.[1]

- It is the most important stabilizer of the MTPJ.[2]
- Also acts to cushion compressive force, support the windlass mechanism, and contribute to medial/lateral instability with its broad insertion onto the base of the proximal phalanx.

7.1.4 Collateral Ligaments

- Made up of two components:
  - Proper collateral ligament—inserts onto the proximal phalanx.

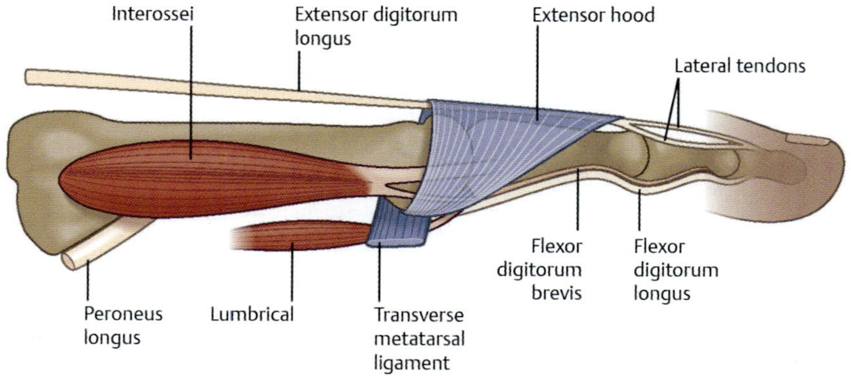

Fig. 7.2 Intrinsics passing plantar to the metatarsophalangeal joint (MTPJ) and dorsal to the proximal interphalangeal joint (PIPJ) and distal interphalangeal joint (DIPJ).

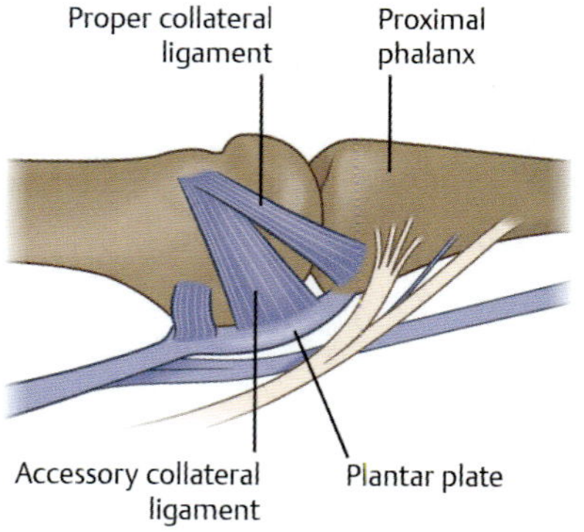

Fig. 7.3 The collateral ligaments act as secondary stabilizers of the metatarsophalangeal joint.

- ◦ Accessory collateral ligament—inserts onto plantar plate (▶ Fig. 7.3).
- Act as secondary stabilizers of the MTPJs.

7.2 Mallet Toe

- Mallet deformity is defined as a flexion deformity at the DIPJ in isolation, and further classified as being flexible or rigid.

7.2.1 Etiology and Pathophysiology

- The incidence of mallet toe is less common that other deformities, accounting for only 5% of lesser toe deformities.[3]
- Various causes have been implicated:
  - Increased relative length of toe, constricting shoe wear, and hyperflexion injuries resulting in avulsion of the distal extensor tendon are all commonly described mechanisms.[4,5]

7.2.2 Symptoms/Physical Examination

- Present with pain related to the flexion deformity at the DIPJ.
- Inability to demonstrate active extension at the DIPJ.
- If related to trauma, a dorsal laceration or signs of blunt trauma may be present.
- In chronic mallet toes, a callus may be present at the dorsal aspect of the DIPJ or

distal pulp. Nail abnormalities may be present secondary to constant pressure.

- The examiner should assess for flexibility of the deformity. Test the patient standing and siting down, and with and without ankle plantar flexion.

7.2.3 Diagnostics and Classification

- See ▶ Table 7.1 for comparison of deformities present in the mallet, hammer, and claw toes.
- The diagnosis is made clinically; advanced imaging is rarely of additional value.

7.2.4 Nonoperative Management

- Flexible deformities: passive stretching of flexor tendons.
- Shoe wear modification to shoes with wide tow boxes and wider low heels and soft insoles.
- Shaving of callosities.
- Padding over symptomatic areas.
- Trauma: extension splinting for 6 to 10 weeks.
- Unlike mallet finger, do not fare as well without operative treatment.[6]

7.2.5 Operative Management

Options include flexor tenotomy, condylectomy, resection arthroplasty/arthrodesis, and distal phalanx amputation.[3]

Flexor Tenotomy

- Used primarily for flexible deformities.
- If dorsal osteophytes at the DIPJ are present, they need to be debrided as they may be blocking correction of the deformity.
- Technique:
    - Transverse or longitudinal incision over distal flexor crease.
    - Transect FDL tendon, taking care to avoid neurovascular bundle.
    - K-wire to maintain correction. Extension taping can also be used.
        - The wire is typically removed at 3 to 4 weeks.

Condylectomy

- Goal is to establish fibrous union.
- Results not as predictable as when used for hammer toe.
- Technique:
    - Elliptical incision over the DIPJ and dorsal extensor hood.
    - Release collaterals.
    - Isolate the distal aspect of the middle phalanx and resect with a bone cutter or microsagittal saw.
    - K-wire to maintain correction; typically removed at 4 weeks.

Resection Arthroplasty/Fusion

- The goal is to establish a bony union through the excision of the distal aspect of the middle phalanx at the supracondylar region and the articular surface of the distal phalanx.
- Reliable in regard to fusion rates, patient satisfaction, and pain relief.[5]
- Technique:
    - Elliptical incision over the DIPJ and dorsal extensor hood.
    - Release collaterals.
    - Deliver the head of the middle phalanx into incision.
    - Resect the distal aspect of the middle phalanx at the supracondylar level, taking care that the plane of resection is perpendicular to the long axis of bone.
    - Remove articular cartilage from the distal phalanx, with either curette or another perpendicular bone cut just distal to the articular surface.
    - Drive K-wire antegrade through the base of the distal phalanx out through

the tip of the toe, just underneath the nail bed.
  - Position the DIPJ in neutral, then drive the K-wire retrograde through the joint, ensuring there is enough of the wire proximal to the joint to maintain correction.
    - Remove wire at 4 to 6 weeks.

Distal Phalanx Amputation

- Reserved for low-demand elderly patients or those with infection of the distal phalanx.
- Technique:
  - "Fishmouth" incision to provide long plantar flap.
  - Disarticulate at the DIPJ.

7.3 Hammer and Claw Toes

- A hammertoe is flexion at the PIPJ, with or without extension at the MTPJ.
- Clawing involves extension at the MTP, with flexion of the PIP and DIP.
  - Also frequently associated with neuromuscular conditions.
  - Usually involves multiple toes bilaterally.

7.3.1 Etiology and Pathophysiology

- At each joint, the potential exists for strong extrinsics to overpower weak intrinsics (▶ Fig. 7.4):
  - *MTP:* Strong EDL extension overpowers weak intrinsic flexors.
  - *PIP and DIP:* Strong FDL flexors overpower weak intrinsic extensors.
- Persistent extension of the proximal phalanx leads to plantar plate attenuation/inefficiency and eventual dorsal subluxation of the proximal phalanx on the metatarsal head.
  - With the MTPJ in an extended position, the EDL is effectively shortened, limiting its ability to extend at the PIPJ and DIPJ.
- The lumbrical and interossei force vectors change and cannot effectively flex at the MTP and extend at the PIP and DIP.
- Additionally, extension at the MTPJ also tensions the FDL and FDB through the tenodesis effect.
  - The strong extrinsic flexors become dominant with the MTP persistently extended causing flexion at the PIP and DIP.
- Other causes include trauma (compartment syndrome) and inflammatory arthritides.

7.3.2 Symptoms/Physical Examination

- Pain overlying calluses at the dorsal aspect of the PIPJ.
- Greater deformity causes metatarsalgia, as a result of hyperextension at the MTP.
  - The plantar plate and plantar fascia get pulled distally and no longer cushion/protect the metatarsal heads.
  - Painful callosities can develop overlying the plantar aspect of the metatarsal head.

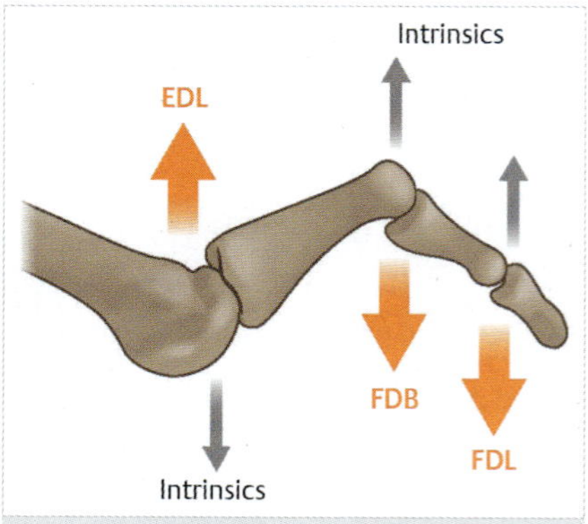

Fig. 7.4 Extrinsics overpowering the intrinsics in a claw toe deformity.

- The examiner should determine whether the deformity is flexible or rigid.
  - *Flexible:* Will correct with manipulation. Important to note ankle position during the examination, as ankle plantar flexion reduces tension on the FDL through the tenodesis effect.
- Note the position of other surrounding toes: have to account for space after re-alignment, for example, the hallux valgus may have to be corrected at the same time.

7.3.3 Diagnostics and Classification

- Mallet, hammer, and claw toes are summarized in regard to joint positions in ▶ Table 7.1.
- Diagnosis is made clinically; advanced imaging is rarely of additional value.

7.3.4 Nonoperative Management

- Similar to treatment of the mallet toe—stretching, shoe wear modification, and shaving of callosities.
- Orthotics such as a cushioned toe sleeve and a Budin splint can help relieve symptoms but do nothing to change the course of disease.

7.3.5 Operative Management

- Treatment strategies for flexible versus fixed deformities differ.
- For a flexible deformity, a flexor to extensor transfer (Girdlestone–Taylor procedure) can be performed.[7]

Flexor to Extensor Transfer

- First described by Girdlestone[8] and Taylor[9] for neurogenic claw toes.
- Technique:
  - Make a transverse incision at the plantar level of the PIPJ.
  - Access the flexor tendons with a longitudinal incision through the flexor sheath, and identify the FDL.
  - Make transverse stab incision at the DIP and release the FDL off the distal phalanx.

Table 7.1 Position of the MTPJ, PIPJ, and DIPJ in mallet, hammer, and claw toe deformities, with associated clinical pictures

DEFORMITY	MTP	PIP	DIP	Clinical image
Mallet toe	Neutral	Neutral	Flexed	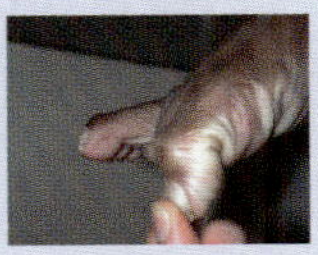
Hammer toe	Extended or neutral	Flexed	Extended, neutral, or flexed	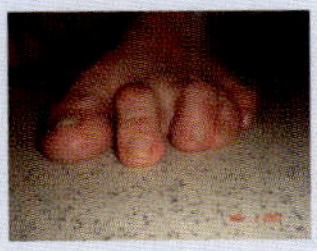
Claw toe	Extended	Flexed	Flexed	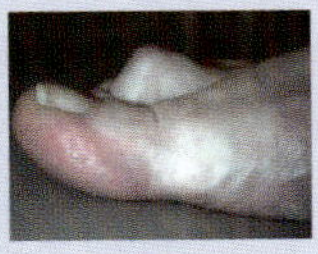

Abbreviations: DIPJ, distal interphalangeal joint; MTPJ, metatarsophalangeal joint; PIPJ, proximal interphalangeal joint.

 - Pull the FDL into proximal incision and divide the tendon longitudinally along its median raphe.
 - Make a dorsal midline longitudinal incision from the MTPJ to the PIPJ.
 - Use curved hemostat passed dorsally to proximally to retrieve the two limbs of the FDL, taking care not to entrap the neurovascular bundle.
 - Position the MTPJ in 20 degrees of plantar flexion and secure the knotted FDL to the extensor hood.

Resection Arthroplasty/ Arthrodesis

- Reserved for rigid deformities.
- Technique:
  - An elliptical incision is made over the PIPJ to avoid skin redundancy after correction of deformity.
  - Remove the extensor hood and release collaterals, and deliver the head of the proximal phalanx into wound.
  - Removal the distal aspect of the proximal phalanx with saw or bone cutter with a cut perpendicular to its long axis. If performing an arthrodesis, prepare the cartilage of the proximal aspect of the middle phalanx as well.
  - Drive a K-wire antegrade through base of middle phalanx out through the tip of the toe, just underneath the nail bed. Position the PIPJ in neutral, then drive the K-wire retrograde through the joint, ensuring there is enough of the wire proximal to the joint to maintain correction.
  - Can perform FDL tenotomy as needed, which can be done through the incision or through a separate plantar incision.
  - Intramedullary devices have also been shown to be effective clinically and radiographically in maintaining correction in mid-term follow-up.[10]

7.4 Lesser Joint MTP Instability/Plantar Plate

7.4.1 Etiology and Pathophysiology

- More common in females with age of onset in the sixth decade of life.
- The second ray is most likely to be involved because the second metatarsal is the longest.
- Mostly caused by overload/chronic inflammation of the MTPJ.
- Mechanical causes:
  - Long second metatarsal.
  - Hallux valgus.
  - Pes planus.
  - Long-term use of high-fashion footwear.
- Biologic causes:
  - Rheumatoid arthritis.
  - Other connective tissue disorders.
- As with hammer and claw toes, with hyperextension at the MTPJ, the extrinsic flexors take over at the PIPJ and DIPJ.
- The interossei becomes dorsal to axis and no longer acts as efficient flexors. Lumbrical tendons become tethered under the intermetatarsal ligament.
- With time and persistent inflammation can lose all restraints, including collaterals—leading to coronal plane deformity and a "crossover toe."

7.4.2 Symptoms/Physical Examination

- Patients may complain of "walking on a marble" or "bunched up socks."
- Swelling at first, followed by progressive deformity in the sagittal plane, and eventually in the coronal plane, manifesting in "crossover" toe.
- *Drawer test* (▶ Fig. 7.5): Even if frank subluxation/dislocation is not noted, the test is indicative of intra-articular or periarticular abnormality if the maneuver causes pain.

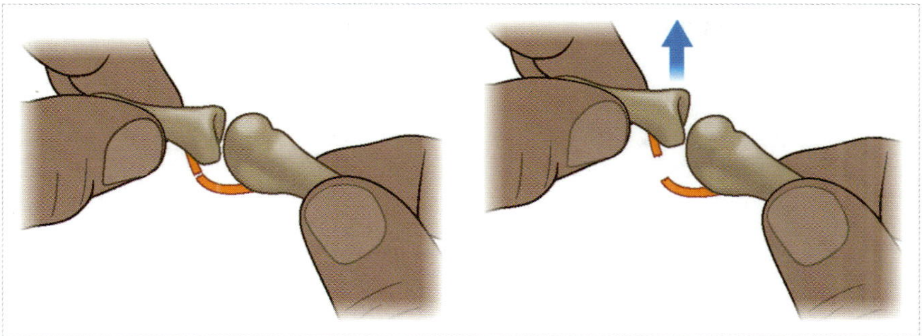

Fig. 7.5 Drawer test for MTP instability. Both ends of the joint are grasped and stabilized by the examiner (left). A dorsally directed forced is then applied to the proximal phalanx (right)

7.4.3 Diagnostics and Classification

- Magnetic resonance imaging (MRI), along with physical examination, can help differentiate between early stage synovitis/instability and other cause of pain, which include metatarsalgia, Freiberg's infraction, Morton's neuroma, stress fracture, and synovial cyst formation.

Plantar plate tears can be classified based on the orientation of the tear.[11] (▶ Table 7.2)

Table 7.2 Classification of Plantar Plate Tears

Grade	Clinical features
1	Horizontal tear with < 50% involvement off the base of the proximal phalanx
2	Horizontal tear with > 50% involvement
3	Tear with longitudinal component, in addition to a horizontal tear
4	Extensive and complex tear pattern

7.4.4 Nonoperative Management

- Carbon fiber inserts or rocker bottom soles can be used to lessen MTPJ dorsiflexion forces.[12]
- Metatarsal pads placed just proximal to the symptomatic metatarsal head help offload the joint.
- Taping and/or a Budin splint can secure the toe in a neutral position to prevent capsular contraction.[11]
- Anti-inflammatory medication.
- Intra-articular corticosteroid injections can lead to plantar plate attenuation and subsequent frank dislocation and should be avoided, especially in the second MTPJ.[13]

7.4.5 Operative Management

- Treatment options include the following:
  - Osteotomies, which shorten the metatarsal, thus decompressing the joint and reducing the magnitude of the extrinsic forces acting across the joint.
  - Direct plantar plate repair—which is often combined with a shortening osteotomy.

Weil Osteotomy

- Most commonly described osteotomy for this purpose: an intra-articular shortening osteotomy that achieves longitudinal decompression through shortening.[14]

- Technique:
  - A 2- to 3-cm dorsal incision over the symptomatic MTPJ. If adjacent, symptomatic MTPJs can make incision between the metatarsals involved.
  - Joint capsule is incised longitudinally.
  - Release the collateral ligaments off the proximal phalanx and use a McGlamry retractor to release the plantar plate off the plantar surface of the metatarsal neck.
  - Starting 2 mm from the dorsal aspect of the articular surface, perform an oblique osteotomy from distal dorsal to proximal plantar. The saw blade should be parallel to the plantar surface of the foot. A second parallel cut can be made just plantar to the first cut, or stacked saw blades utilized to prevent plantar movement of the capital fragment.
  - Translate the capital fragment to the desired amount proximally. Fixation to the shaft can be achieved in the form of commercially available twist-off screws. Ensure proper rotation, cortical contact, and length relative to the other metatarsal heads prior to closure.

Plantar Plate Repair

- Both plantar and dorsal approaches have been described.[11] The dorsal technique is outlined below.
- Dorsal technique:
  - Same approach as that for Weil's osteotomy.
  - The Weil osteotomy is performed, and the capital fragment translated as far proximally as possible and held in place using a K-wire. The K wire should not penetrate too far plantarly as this may tether the plantar plate and prevent mobilization and advancement.
  - Another K-wire driven from dorsal to plantar in the proximal phalanx, and a joint distractor passed over these two K-wires is used to open the joint.
  - The remainder of the plantar plate is released off the proximal phalanx and mobilized, taking care to avoid damage to the long flexor, which lies directly plantar.
  - Two sutures are passed through mobilized plantar plate in a horizontal mattress manner using the suture passing technique of choice.
  - Use a K-wire to drill two holes in the proximal aspect of the proximal phalanx (just distal to the proximal articular surface from dorsal to plantar.
  - Pass the plantar plate sutures through the drilled holes from plantar to dorsal.
  - Release distraction and secure osteotomy with the fixation method of choice.
  - With the toe in neutral or slight plantar flexion, tie the sutures down over the bony bridge.

7.5 Bunionette

7.5.1 Etiology and Pathophysiology

- Commonly seen in both adolescents and adults, more frequently in females.
- Causes:
  - A prominent fifth metatarsal head in thin individuals.
  - Conditions leading to friction/pressure between the shoe and the metatarsal head such as tight shoe or chronic positioning of the foot with the lateral aspect of the fifth metatarsal head contacting the ground.
  - Incomplete development of transverse metatarsal ligament.
  - Congenital dumbbell-shaped fifth metatarsal.
  - *Pes planus:* With hindfoot eversion, the fifth metatarsal rotates to a more lateral location, which can lead to increased prominence of the lateral condyle.

7.5.2 Symptoms/Physical Examination

- Present with painful deformity to the lateral aspect of the forefoot.
- Inflammation, callus, and ulceration may all be present.

7.5.3 Diagnostics and Classification

- Normal 4 to 5 intermetatarsal angle (IMA): < 6.5 to 8 degrees.
- Average is 6.5 in normal feet and 9.6 in patients with a bunionette.[15]
- Bunionettes can broadly be classified into three types (▶ Fig. 7.6):
  - Type 1: lateral prominence of the metatarsal head.
  - Type 2: lateral bowing of the fifth metatarsal.
  - Type 3: widening of the 4 to 5 IMA.

7.5.4 Nonoperative Treatment

- Shoe with a wider toe box.
- Gel or silicone pads for inflamed soft tissues/bursa.
- Shaving of hyperkeratotic areas.
- Topical or oral anti-inflammatory medication.

7.5.5 Operative Management

- Surgical options are broadly classified into one of two categories: (1) exostectomy or (2) fifth metatarsal osteotomies. Osteotomies can be further described in regard to location and type. One of these osteotomies will be discussed below.

Lateral Exostectomy

- Reserved for cases in which there is isolated dorsolateral enlargement of the fifth metatarsal head (i.e., type I deformities).[16]
- If plantar keratosis is present, lateral exostectomy alone will not be effective in isolation in reducing plantar pressure and pain.
- Technique:
  - A 2- to 3-cm incision centered over the lateral aspect of the fifth metatarsal head condyle.

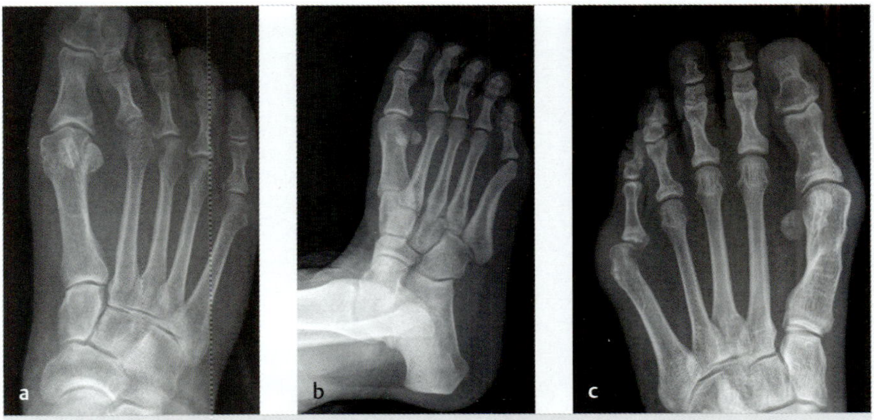

Fig. 7.6 The three different types of bunionettes: Type I (left), type 2 (middle), and type 3 (right).

- Identify and protect the lateral dorsal cutaneous nerve.
- Expose the metatarsal head using an L-shaped capsulotomy, keeping the stronger plantar and distal limbs attached.
  - Remove the lateral condylar process in line with the lateral border of the foot.
  - A medial capsular release can then be performed through the MTPJ with adequate traction.
  - Ensure an adequate capsular closure to prevent recurrence of the deformity.

S.E.R.I. (Simple, Effective, Rapid, Inexpensive) Minimally Invasive Fifth Metatarsal Osteotomy

- Indicated for symptomatic type 2 or 3 bunionettes.[17]
- Technique:
  - A 1-cm incision just proximal to the lateral prominence of the fifth metatarsal head.
  - Dissect to expose the lateral aspect of the fifth metatarsal neck.
  - Use a microsagittal saw at this level to osteotomize the metatarsal head.
  - This cut should be perpendicular to the fourth ray if length is to be maintained. For the cases in which shortening of the fifth metatarsal is desired to decompress the joint, a slight distal to proximal angulation can be utilized.
  - The saw blade can also be inclined to guide desired dorsal or plantar translation.
  - Mobilize the fifth metatarsal head with an osteotome.
  - Insert a 1.6-mm K-wire proximally to distally in the lateral soft tissue adjacent to the bone. The wire should emerge in the lateral aspect of the tip of the toe, 5 mm from the lateral edge of the nail.
  - Pull back the wire in a retrograde fashion so that the proximal tip is visualized just adjacent to the level of the osteotomy.
  - Guide the fifth metatarsal head medially and in the direction of other desired correction and advance the K-wire down the fifth metatarsal intramedullary canal from distal to proximal, stopping at the base of the fifth metatarsal.
  - Remove any remaining lateral prominence.
  - The patient can be heel weight bearing in a post-op shoe. At 4 weeks, the K-wire is removed and the transition is made to normal shoe wear.

7.6 Freiberg's Infraction

7.6.1 Etiology and Pathophysiology

- Freiberg's infraction is an osteochondrosis of the second metatarsal head.
  - Osteochondroses are a family of disorders resulting from disruption of epiphysis resulting in joint incongruity.
- Freiberg's infraction is the only osteochondrosis more common in females: a 5:1 preponderance.[18]
- It is unlikely to involve the other foot. It is bilateral in 10% of cases.
- Peak age of onset is at 11 to 17 years of age.
- The etiology is likely multifactorial, secondary to either trauma or vascular disruption.
  - *Trauma:* The second metatarsal is the longest and least mobile, which predisposes it to sustain greater stresses during normal gait.
  - *Vascular:* Anatomical variants resulting in decreased blood flow or compression of vessels due to a joint effusion or soft-tissue swelling.

7.6.2 Symptoms/Physical Examination

- Pain localized to the second metatarsal head.
- Exacerbated with walking, particularly barefoot.
- Fullness of the MTPJ; fusiform swelling of the affected toe.
- Coronal or sagittal plane deformities later in disease, with instability.
- Range of motion decreased with increase in arthrosis.

7.6.3 Diagnostics and Classification

Radiographs

- *Early disease:* Joint space widening within 3 to 6 weeks following symptoms.
- *Progression:* Sclerosis of subchondral bone and flattening of the metatarsal head.
- *Later:* Joint space narrowing, loose bodies, rarefaction, and sclerosis (▶ Fig. 7.7).
  - Thickening of the metatarsal shaft can be seen in late disease—likely representing a response to abnormal stress.[19]

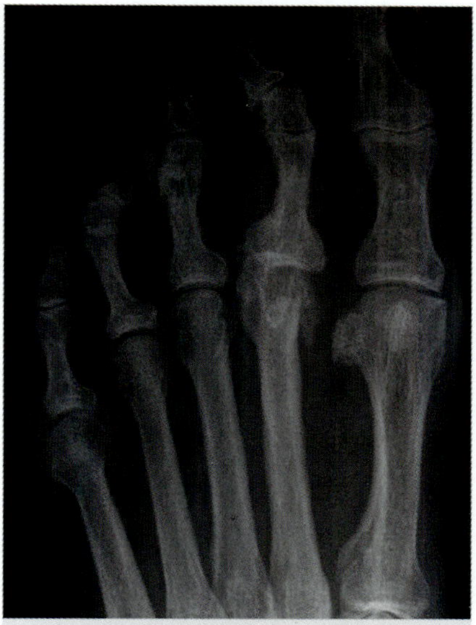

Fig. 7.7 Late stage Freiberg's disease, demonstrating joint space narrowing, loose bodies, rarefaction and sclerosis.

Advanced Imaging

- MRI is useful for early detection: Hypointense T1 and hyperintense T2. Flattening on sagittal views.
- Useful to distinguish from other diagnoses such as Morton's neuroma and a metatarsal stress fracture.
- Smillie outlined the macroscopic progression of the disease into five stages[20]:
  - *Stage 1:* Narrow fissure fracture develops in ischemic epiphysis.
  - *Stage 2:* Central collapse of the subchondral bone and overlying cartilage, secondary to absorption of cancellous bone. The plantar cartilage remains intact.
  - *Stage 3:* Further absorption of cancellous bone, with more pronounced central collapse. Plantar cartilage remains intact.
  - *Stage 4:* Further collapse leads to fracture of the plantar hinge.
    - This is when central and peripheral projections fracture, producing irreparable damage. In stages 1 to 3, the blood supply remains intact, and restoration is possible.
  - *Stage 5:* Arthrosis with marked flattening of the articular cartilage present (▶ Fig. 7.8).

7.6.4 Nonoperative Management

- The goal of nonoperative treatment is both pain relief and to offload the second metatarsal head.[21]
- Early stage treatment:
  - Activity modification—partial or non-weight-bearing.

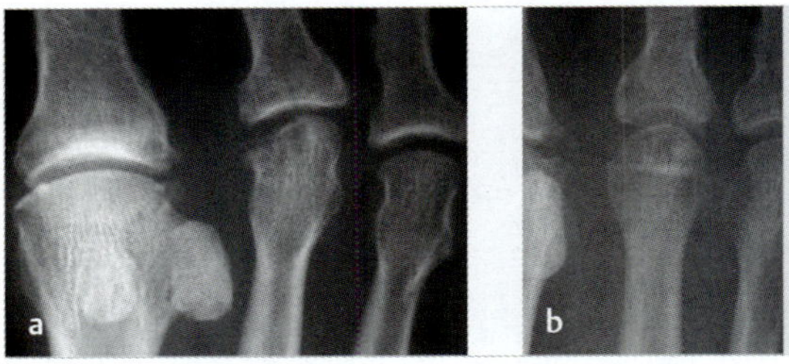

Fig. 7.8 (a,b) Radiographs of Freiberg's infarction before and after dorsiflexion closing wedge osteotomy.

- *Protected weight bearing:* stiff soled shoe, fracture boot, or short leg cast.
- Rocker bottom soles or orthotics with metatarsal bars can offload the metatarsal head.
- Only appropriate for Smillie stage I to III disease, when the blood supply remains intact and revascularization is possible.

7.6.5 Operative Management

- Two broad categories:
  - Those that aim to alter the biomechanics and/or pathophysiology.
  - Those that address the sequalae of the disease process.[18]

Biomechanics/Pathophysiology Altering

Core Decompression

- Similar to analogous situation in early stages of hip avascular necrosis. It acts to alleviate pain by reducing the intraosseous pressure in the metatarsal head.

Perichondral Grafting

- Smillie described utilizing a slot cut in the dorsal aspect of the metatarsal shaft, drilling across the epiphyseal plate to the subchondral bone.[20]
- Depressed subchondral bone is then elevated and supported with back-filled bone graft.
- The aim is to reestablish blood flow to the epiphysis across the epiphyseal plate.

Metatarsal Osteotomies

- Two main types of osteotomies:
  - Shortening osteotomies that decompress the joint.
  - Dorsal closing wedge osteotomies that redirect healthy plantar cartilage to articulate with the proximal phalanx.
- Multiple studies demonstrate fair evidence for the use of dorsal closing wedge osteotomy in providing clinical benefit to the patient.[22,23,24,25]
- ▶ Fig. 7.9 demonstrates radiographs of Freiberg's disease before and after dorsiflexion closing wedge osteotomy.

Those that Address the Sequelae of the Disease Process

Joint Debridement

- Can be performed in conjunction with other procedures or in isolation.
- Involves excision of thickened synovium, removal of loose bodies, and resection of peripheral osteophytes.

Excisional/Interpositional Arthroplasty

- Since Freiberg's disease occurs in isolation, resection of the metatarsal head and proximal aspect of the proximal phalanx can lead to transfer metatarsalgia and is generally not recommended.

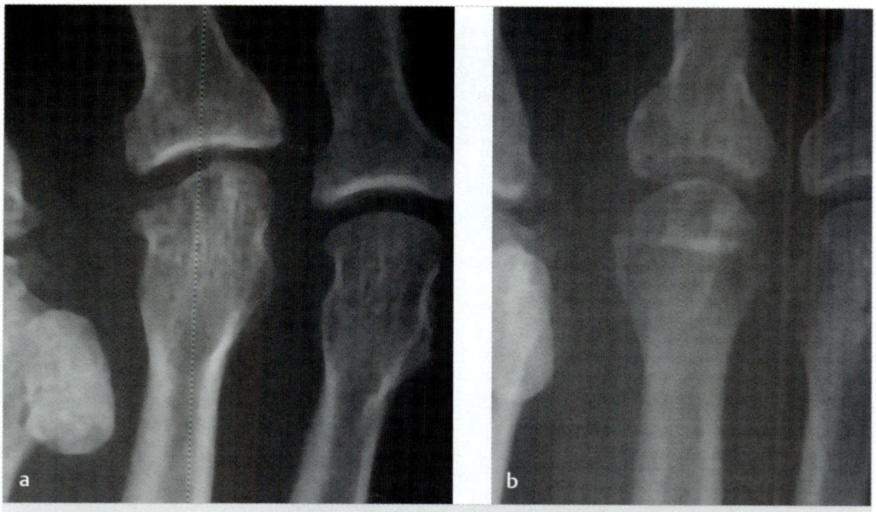

Fig. 7.9 (a,b) Radiographs of Freiberg's infarction before and after dorsiflexion closing wedge osteotomy.

- Interposition of the dorsal capsule, EDL and brevis, and the FDL has been described with limited success.[26]

Replacement Arthroplasty

- Replacement options include silicone spacers, titanium hemiarthroplasty of the proximal phalanx with debridement of the metatarsal head, and a total ceramic arthroplasty.
- Silicone spacers are not recommended for use in Freiberg's disease and evidence for metallic and spacer materials is incomplete.[18]

7.7 Key Testing Facts

- Lesser toe conditions include mallet toes, hammer toes, claw toes, MTPJ instability, bunionettes, and Freiberg's disease
- Fashionable shoe wear is largely contributory the development of many lesser toe conditions and the related symptoms
- Advanced imaging can be useful in distinguishing between different causes of pain around the second MTPJ—including Morton's neuroma, metatarsalgia, plantar plate tears, stress fracture, and Freiberg's disease
- Options for initial nonoperative management include passive stretching, orthotic inserts, taping, shoe wear modification, and anti-inflammatory medication
- The choice of operative procedure is tailored to the specific deformity present, how rigid it is, and how advanced the disease process is

Position of the MTP, PIP, and DIP joints in mallet, hammer, and claw toe deformities, with associated clinical pictures

References

[1] Deland JT, Lee KT, Sobel M, DiCarlo EF. Anatomy of the plantar plate and its attachments in the lesser metatarsal phalangeal joint. Foot Ankle Int. 1995; 16(8):480–486

[2] Suero EM, Meyers KN, Bohne WHO. Stability of the metatarsophalangeal joint of the lesser toes: a cadaveric study. J Orthop Res. 2012; 30(12): 1995–1998

[3] Molloy A, Shariff R. Mallet toe deformity. Foot Ankle Clin. 2011; 16(4):537–546

[4] Coughlin MJ. Mallet toes, hammer toes, claw toes, and corns. Causes and treatment of lesser-toe deformities. Postgrad Med. 1984; 75(5):191–198

[5] Coughlin MJ. Operative repair of the mallet toe deformity. Foot Ankle Int. 1995; 16(3):109–116

[6] Lancaster SC, Sizensky JA, Young CC. Acute mallet toe. Clin J Sport Med. 2008; 18(3):298–299

[7] Kwon JY, De Asla RJ. The use of flexor to extensor transfers for the correction of the flexible hammer toe deformity. Foot Ankle Clin. 2011; 16(4):573–582

[8] Girdlestone GR. Physiotherapy for hand and foot. Physiotherapy. 1947; 32(11):167–169

[9] Taylor RG. The treatment of claw toes by multiple transfers of flexor into extensor tendons. J Bone Joint Surg Br. 1951; 33-B(4):539–542

[10] Ellington JK, Anderson RB, Davis WH, Cohen BE, Jones CP. Radiographic analysis of proximal interphalangeal joint arthrodesis with an intramedullary fusion device for lesser toe deformities. Foot Ankle Int. 2010; 31(5):372–376

[11] Doty JF, Coughlin MJ. Metatarsophalangeal joint instability of the lesser toes and plantar plate deficiency. J Am Acad Orthop Surg. 2014; 22(4): 235–245

[12] Coughlin MJ, Baumfeld DS, Nery C. Second MTP joint instability: grading of the deformity and description of surgical repair of capsular insufficiency. Phys Sportsmed. 2011; 39(3):132–141

[13] Coughlin MJ. Subluxation and dislocation of the second metatarsophalangeal joint. Orthop Clin North Am. 1989; 20(4):535–551

[14] Espinosa N, Brodsky JW, Maceira E. Metatarsalgia. J Am Acad Orthop Surg. 2010; 18(8):474–485

[15] Fallat LM, Buckholz J. An analysis of the tailor's bunion by radiographic and anatomical display. J Am Podiatry Assoc. 1980; 70(12):597–603

[16] Bertrand T, Parekh SG. Bunionette deformity: etiology, nonsurgical management, and lateral exostectomy. Foot Ankle Clin. 2011; 16(4):679–688

[17] Giannini S, Faldini C, Vannini F, Digennaro V, Bevoni R, Luciani D. The minimally invasive osteotomy "S.E.R.I." (simple, effective, rapid, inexpensive) for correction of bunionette deformity. Foot Ankle Int. 2008; 29(3):282–286

[18] Carmont MR, Rees RJ, Blundell CM. Current concepts review: Freiberg's disease. Foot Ankle Int. 2009; 30(2):167–176

[19] Katcherian DA. Treatment of Freiberg's disease. Orthop Clin North Am. 1994; 25(1):69–81

[20] Smillie IS. Treatment of Freiberg's infraction. Proc R Soc Med. 1967; 60(1):29–31

[21] Cerrato RA. Freiberg's disease. Foot Ankle Clin. 2011; 16(4):647–658

[22] Chao KH, Lee CH, Lin LC. Surgery for symptomatic Freiberg's disease: extraarticular dorsal closing-wedge osteotomy in 13 patients followed for 2–4 years. Acta Orthop Scand. 1999; 70(5):483–486

[23] Gauthier G, Elbaz R. Freiberg's infraction: a subchondral bone fatigue fracture. A new surgical treatment. Clin Orthop Relat Res. 1979(142):93–95

[24] Kinnard P, Lirette R. Freiberg's disease and dorsiflexion osteotomy. J Bone Joint Surg Br. 1991; 73(5):864–865

[25] Lee SK, Chung MS, Baek GH, Oh JH, Lee YH, Gong HS. Treatment of Freiberg disease with intra-articular dorsal wedge osteotomy and absorbable pin fixation. Foot Ankle Int. 2007; 28(1):43–48

[26] el-Tayeby HM. Freiberg's infraction: a new surgical procedure. J Foot Ankle Surg. 1998; 37(1):23–27, discussion 79

8 Sesamoids and Accessory Bones of the Foot

Katherine Gavin and Adam D. Bitterman

Abstract

This chapter aims to briefly yet thoroughly discuss the most commonly encountered sesamoids and accessory bones of the foot. A discussion is introduced regarding form, function, pathologic conditions, treatment options, and surgical interventions.

Keywords: sesamoid, accessory bone, ossicle, metatarsophalangeal joint, os, accessory navicular

8.1 Sesamoids

8.1.1 Anatomy and Function

- The term sesamoid derived due to their resemblance to sesame seeds.[1]
- Sesamoids develop through enchondral ossification at multiple ossification centers, beginning around 6 to 8 years of age.
- They can remain cartilaginous or fibrocartilaginous, which may explain their high variability of incidence.[2]
- Hallucal sesamoids under the first metatarsophalangeal joint are considered constant.[3,4] Inconstant sesamoids include the hallucal interphalangeal sesamoid (overall prevalence of about 22%) and those of the second through fifth metatarsals (prevalence ranging from 1 to 13%).[5,6]

Anatomy

- The hallucal sesamoids are located on the plantar aspect of the first metatarsophalangeal joint (▶ Fig. 8.1).
- The dorsal surface is cartilaginous and articulates with the first metatarsal head.
- The plantar surface is in the slip of the flexor hallucis brevis (FHB) tendon.
- It is connected to the proximal phalanx via the plantar plate, which consists of FHB tendons, the phalangeal–sesamoid ligament, the collateral ligaments, and the plantar aponeurosis.[7]
- The intersesamoid ridge on the metatarsal head and the intersesamoid ligament provide intrinsic stability to the complex.
- The medial tibial sesamoid is consistently slightly larger than the lateral fibular sesamoid.[8]
- The abductor and adductor hallucis tendons also have attachments to the medial and lateral sesamoid bones, respectively. The deep aspect of the intermetatarsal ligament also has an attachment to the lateral sesamoid.
- The flexor hallucis longus (FHL) tendon travels between the sesamoids.
- Blood supply:
  - It comes proximally from the plantar arch *and* the medial plantar artery.
  - More infrequently, it is sourced from either the plantar arch *or* the medial plantar artery.
  - The distal aspect of the sesamoids has a tenuous blood supply. This may explain a high incidence of avascular necrosis and nonunion of the sesamoids.[9,10]

Function

- *Primary function*: increase the moment arm across the first metatarsophalangeal joint resulting in an improved mechanical advantage to flexion and push-off power.[11]
- *Secondary function*: cushion the metatarsophalangeal (MTP) joint by dispersing stress and protecting the FHL tendon.

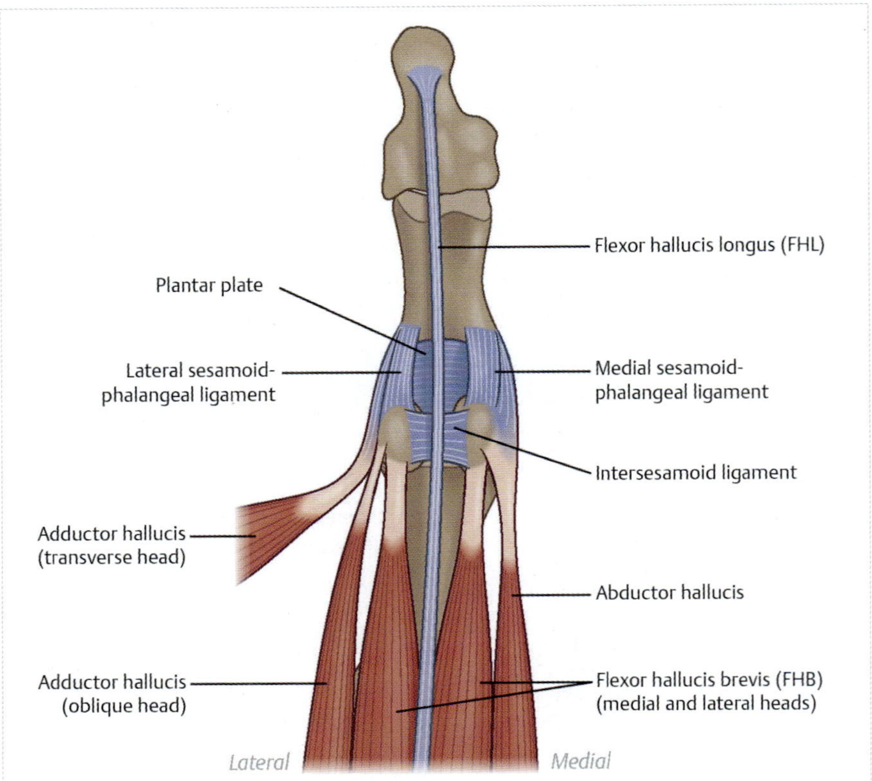

Fig. 8.1 Illustration of the sesamoid complex.

8.1.2 Clinical Examination

- History of pain on the plantar aspect of the foot, particularly with toe-off. It is important to get an idea of acuity/chronicity and prior interventions.
- A detailed motor, sensory, and vascular examination is key.
- *Possible key findings:* tenderness under the first MTP joint, intractable keratotic lesion, synovitis, and swelling at the first MTP joint. Painful or decreased range of motion, plantarflexed first ray, hallux valgus, or hallux varus.

8.1.3 Imaging

- Best viewed with a medial and lateral oblique radiograph.[11] The X-ray beam is directed 15 degrees cephalad from the lateral position.
- Axial sesamoid view shows them in an anatomic, rotated, or translated position with varying grading systems reported in the literature[12] (▶ Fig. 8.2).
- Computed tomography (CT), magnetic resonance imaging (MRI), and technetium-99 bone scan are useful in specific situations.

8.1.4 Pathologic Conditions, Including Treatment and Surgical Approaches

Bipartite Sesamoids

- Incidence of bipartite hallucal sesamoids is 12%, with the large majority (90%) of these occurring with the tibial sesamoid. Forty-two percent of all partitions were bilateral.[6]

- Most are due to incomplete ossification.
- Partitioned sesamoids fracture through the synchondrosis and become symptomatic with less force and trauma compared to nonpartitioned sesamoids due to decreased ability to resist shear and compressive forces.

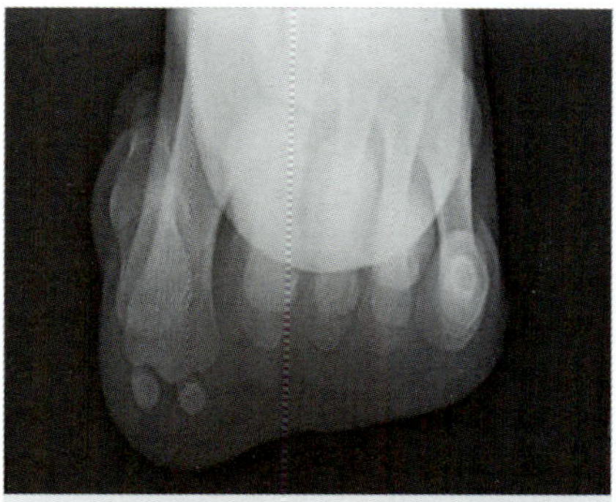

Fig. 8.2 Axial view of the hallucal sesamoids.

- It is difficult to differentiate between a symptomatic bipartite and a fractured sesamoid, although pathology specimens will show hyaline cartilage present between two ossific foci in a truly bipartite sesamoid.[13]
- Previous or contralateral foot radiographs will provide more information with bipartite sesamoids, usually showing smooth edges and a standard gap distance.[14]
- MRI or bone scan helps provide definitive diagnosis and differentiation.

Fractures

- The most common mechanism is a large forefoot plantar force with hyperextension of the MTP joint or a crush injury.
- The tibial sesamoid is more commonly fractured than the lateral sesamoid, due to increase loads through it.[15]
- Usually fractures are midsubstance and transverse on an anteroposterior (AP) or oblique radiograph (▶ Fig. 8.3).

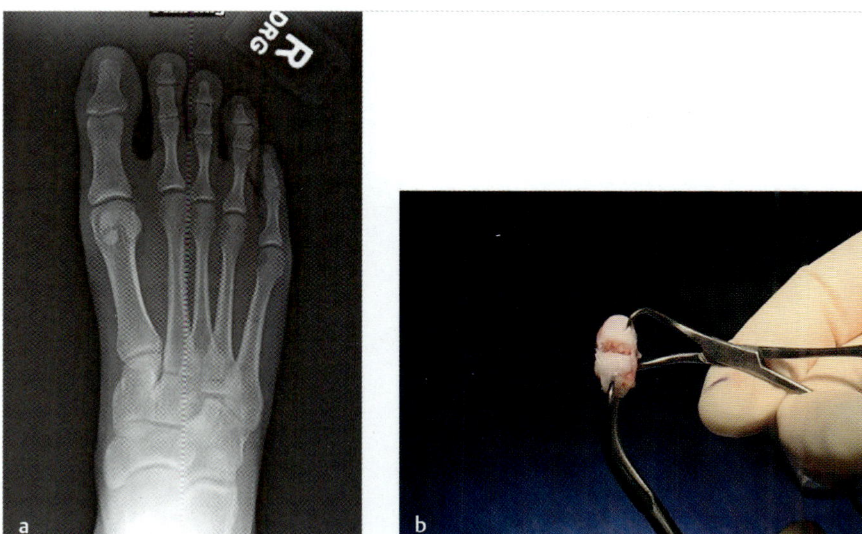

Fig. 8.3 **(a)** Anteroposterior (AP) radiograph of a tibial sesamoid fracture with persistent pain despite nonoperative measures in a high-level volleyball player. **(b)** Excised tibial sesamoid showing sharp edges at the fracture site and visible bone, helping differentiate this from a bipartite sesamoid.

- Pain is localized to the affected sesamoid and worsened with ambulation.
- Stress fractures can have an insidious onset and normal radiographs.
- It can go on to develop nonunion or avascular necrosis, usually of the distal fragment.

Congenital Absence

- It tends to be asymptomatic and is likely more common than reported in the literature.
- Tibial sesamoid absence is more commonly reported than lateral sesamoid absence and having both congenitally absent is very rare.[16]
- Symptomatic patients might have metatarsalgia, claw-toe deformity, hallux valgus, or hallux varus.

Intractable Plantar Keratoses

- Osseous abnormalities of the tibial sesamoid such as trauma, congenital deformity, exostoses, or fragmentation, as well as a cavus foot deformity, a plantarflexed first ray, or rotational deformity of the metatarsal can all lead to a plantarly directed hypertrophy resulting in painful keratoses of the foot.[17]
- Persistent pain with ambulation is commonly reported (▶ Fig. 8.4).

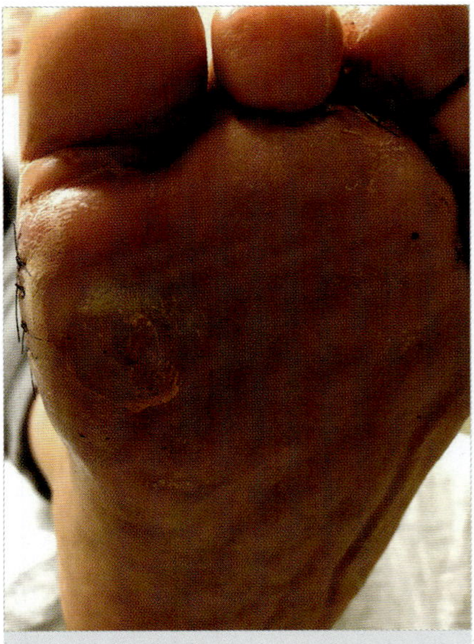

Fig. 8.4 Intractable plantar keratosis as a result of a hypertrophic tibial sesamoid, which was excised after failure of nonoperative treatment.

Nerve Compression

- Impingement of either the medial or lateral digital nerve to the hallux can occur due to close proximity of each nerve to the sesamoids. This impingement can be worsened with different sesamoid pathology, including hypertrophy, subluxation or dislocation, fracture, etc.
- It can present as aching pain or nerve pain, numbness, and possibly a positive Tinel's sign along the digital nerve.[18]
- If the nerve is not protected during surgery, a painful neuroma can develop.

Arthritis

- Arthritis is usually a result of some other pathology that causes altered mechanics across the articular surface.
- It is seen with hallux valgus, hallux rigidus, and systemic arthritides such as rheumatoid or psoriatic arthritis and diffuse idiopathic skeletal hyperostosis (DISH).[19]

Osteochondritis

- It falls within the spectrum containing osteonecrosis.
- Causal theories include severe trauma, stress fracture, and threatened sesamoid blood supply.
- Pain with passive distal push of the involved sesamoid.
- Ischemic necrosis is not visible on radiographs. Coronal T1-weighted MRI shows low signal intensity.

- After excision, macroscopic examination shows fragmented and irregular shape with necrotic bone.[20]

Sesamoiditis

- It is defined as pain at the sesamoid complex without radiographic changes.
- It is described as inflammation of the peritendinous structures involving the sesamoids or as chondromalacia with obvious articular cartilage degeneration.[21,22]
- Diagnosis of exclusion and likely falls on a spectrum depending on time of patient presentation.
- More specific examination finding is pain with dorsiflexion due to diffuse synovitis.

Treatment

General

- Address the underlying pathology.
- Conservative care of padding the metatarsal, dancers pads, taping in slight plantar flexion, stiff insoles, and custom orthotics that unload the first metatarsal head and sesamoid complex work the best.
- Activity modification including avoiding high-impact activity and a period of non-weight-bearing and casting is also effective.
- Nonsteroidal anti-inflammatory drugs (NSAIDs).
- *Corticosteroid injection:* use infrequently and not in the setting of fracture or osteonecrosis.
- Ultimately, sesamoidectomy is an option for most pathology, although removing both is not recommended.

Fracture

- Non-weight-bearing in a cast with a toe plate for 6 weeks, followed by walking boot for 4 to 6 more weeks.
- Open reduction and internal fixation is controversial, but has been done with some success using a single compression screw or cerclage wire with or without bone graft.

Intractable Plantar Keratoses

- Avoid progression to ulceration or osteomyelitis.
- A bursectomy of the tibial sesamoid bursa can also be very effective for long-term pain relief.
- The sesamoid itself can be shaved or excised, or the underlying deformity can be corrected, such as a dorsiflexion osteotomy of the first ray.

Arthritis

- First MTP arthrodesis, hallux valgus correction, etc. Care should be taken to ensure the sesamoid complex is reduced and stable.

8.1.5 Surgical Approaches

Direct Medial Incision

- This is the most common approach for tibial sesamoid excision (▶ Fig. 8.5).
- It is 3 cm in length from the base of the proximal phalanx to the proximal metatarsal head.
- Identify and protect the medial plantar cutaneous nerve.
- Identify and incise the capsule directly below abductor hallucis tendon.
- Resect the sesamoid subperiosteally.
- Identify the FHL and protect it.
- Close down the space left after excision with suture closure.

Dorsolateral

- It is useful for lateral fibular sesamoidectomy in the setting of hallux valgus.

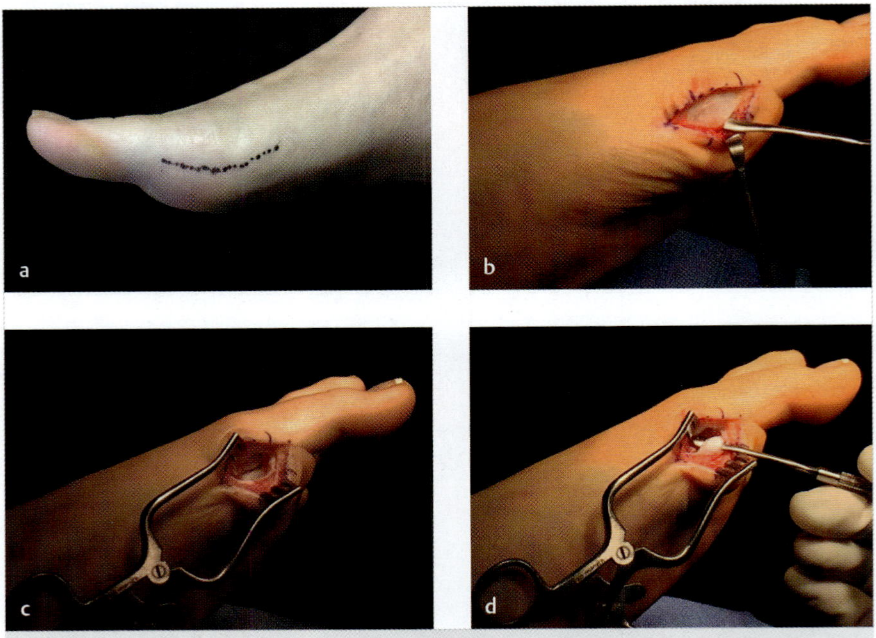

Fig. 8.5 (a) Medial-based incision, very slightly plantar from midline. **(b)** Medial plantar cutaneous nerve is identified and protected. **(c)** Sesamoid in situ, with articulation with the metatarsal head visible. **(d)** After the tibial sesamoid is excised, the flexor hallucis longus (FHL) tendon is carefully inspected.

- A 3-cm incision of the first intermetatarsal webspace.
- Identify the lateral capsule and adductor hallucis tendon.
- Release the adductor tendon and intersesamoid ligament from the sesamoid.
- Remember the lateral plantar digital nerve is plantar to the intermetatarsal ligament. Then the sesamoid can be removed.
- Reapproximate the adductor hallucis to the lateral capsule or to the base of the proximal phalanx.

Direct Plantar

- For removal of the lateral fibular sesamoid.
- Painful plantar scar is a concern.
- Incision should be intermetatarsal, just lateral to the metatarsal head.
- Identify and retract medially the lateral plantar digital nerve and the fat pad.
- Try to leave the adductor hallucis tendon intact.
- Use the scalpel blade to excise the sesamoid.

Arthroscopic Excision

- It is used mostly for nonunion and symptomatic bipartite sesamoid, usually removing the distal fragment only, although the whole sesamoid can be excised. Visualization of the lateral sesamoid is more difficult.[23]

8.1.6 Postoperative Care, Results, and Complications

- Care should be taken to allow soft tissues time to heal prior to weight bearing in a boot or postoperative shoe.

- With excision of both sesamoids, there is a high incidence of intrinsic minus cock-up deformity of the great toe due to disruption of the FHB insertion. As such, it is no longer recommended. If it is necessary, fusion of the interphalangeal joint is recommended at the same time.[24]
- About 10% of the time, the toe can drift into a hallux valgus deformity with tibial sesamoidectomy and hallux varus with fibular sesamoidectomy.[25] Maintaining joint capsule and adductor and abductor tendon integrity can help decrease this occurrence.
- About 50% of patients can have persistent pain.
- Other frequently reported complications include decreased plantar flexion strength (FHL moves closer to the center of rotation, thus weakening the moment arm) and decreased MTP range of motion.[26]

8.2 Accessory Bones of the Foot

- Common developmental variants with almost 40 described.
- Derived from unfused primary or secondary ossification centers.
- Higher incidence is reported in embryos than in adults.[27]
- Understanding them is key to avoiding misdiagnosis, although they can frequently be associated with different pathology.

8.2.1 Os Trigonum

Anatomy

- Located off the posterior body of the talus, lateral to the FHL groove, and can come in wide array of shapes and sizes.
- Can have varying densities of attachment to the talus, but has been described as a separate ossification center.[28]
- Easily mistaken as a fracture to the posterior body of the talus, but the majority are asymptomatic and found incidentally (▶ Fig. 8.6a).

Incidence

- Variably reported as present in 2 to 10% of radiographs of the normal feet.[29]

Clinical Significance and Treatment

- Plantar flexion, particularly forced plantar flexion, often seen in ballet

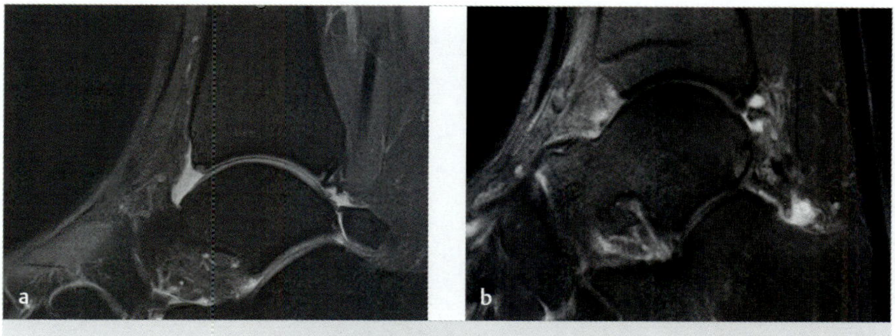

Fig. 8.6 (a) T2-weighted sagittal magnetic resonance imaging (MRI) of an incidental os trigonum. The patient was asymptomatic. No surrounding bone edema or bursitis is noted. **(b)** T2-weighted sagittal MRI of a symptomatic os trigonum. Note degenerative cystic and edema changes within the os trigonum, surrounding fluid collection and bursitis, and adjacent bony edema in the talus from impingement.

dancers, can cause retrocalcaneal pain and impingement (▶ Fig. 8.6b).

- Tenosynovitis of the FHL tendon can also occur secondary to friction and impingement.
- Pain is insidious in onset and usually activity related and located posteriorly.
- Differential diagnosis includes fracture of the posterior facet of the talus, retrocalcaneal bursitis, and the rare bipartite talus.[30]
- The os trigonum can be confused as an ununited fracture of the lateral tuberosity of the posterior body of the talus, called a Shepherd fracture.[31]

Treatment

- NSAIDs, rest, casting, and activity modification—particularly avoiding forced plantar flexion.
- Lateral approach excision (classic):
  - A 5-cm incision posterior to the fibula over the retrocalcaneal space.
  - Identify and protect the sural nerve.
  - Peroneal tendons retracted to expose space.
  - Trigonum denuded of all attachments.
  - FHL needs to be inspected and addressed if necessary.[32,33]
- Medial approach: Theoretically better for addressing FHL pathology.[34]
  - A 5-cm incision anterior to the Achilles tendon.
  - Neurovascular bundle is identified and retracted.
- Arthroscopic:
  - Viewed initially through the posteromedial portal with a high-speed burr in the posterolateral portal.
  - Very rarely reported posterior tibial nerve calcaneal branch neurapraxia.
  - Showing similar patient outcomes as open approaches.[35]

Complications

- Persistent pain, nerve injury, failure to address FHL pathology, and wound healing problems.

8.2.2 Accessory Navicular

Anatomy

- Also termed os tibiale externum, among other less used nomenclature.
- Results from a secondary ossification center from the tuberosity of the navicular and is not to be confused with a bipartite navicular, which has been rarely reported.
- Three types: type I well-defined oval shape, not attached to the main navicular bone (▶ Fig. 8.7); type II has a fibrocartilaginous connection less than 2 mm from the main navicular with irregular borders. These can be subclassified as IIA or IIB based on the angle of orientation to the talar process and size with A being smaller in size and less acute of an angle as compared to B.[36] Type III has a bony connection to the main navicular.

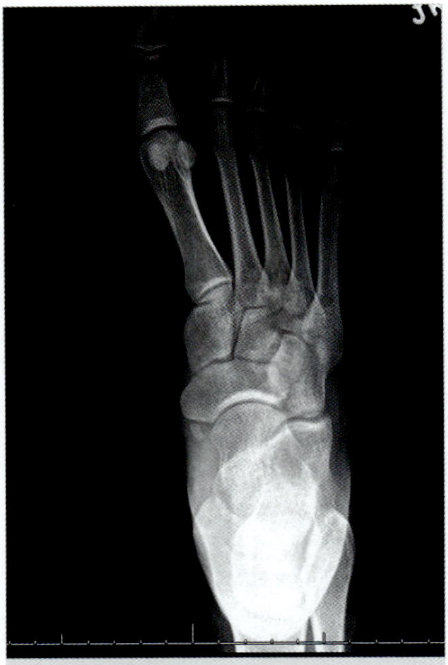

Fig. 8.7 A type I accessory navicular, also commonly referred to as a sesamoid of the posterior tibial tendon.

Incidence

Incidence range anywhere from 3 to 14%, with reported autosomal dominant inheritance.[37]

These are more commonly seen in children and adolescents, of which many go onto fuse to the navicular by adulthood.[38]

Clinical Significance and Treatment

- Type 1 is asymptomatic and also thought of as a sesamoid to the posterior tibial tendon.
- Type 2 is often symptomatic and mistaken for a fracture. They can be at risk of an avulsion injury at the synchondrosis, particularly in patients with associated pes planus as the navicular is placed under more stress.
  - Some think that altered forces in the posterior tibial tendon in patients with an accessory navicular may contribute to the development of pes planus by altering the force vector of the tendon into a more adductor role than a supinator role, thus flattening the longitudinal arch.[39]
- The bony prominence can also make shoe wear symptomatic.
- Patients uniformly have tenderness over the prominence on the medial aspect of the midfoot.
- Activity modification, shoe wear modifications, and casting/bracing can be helpful in the short term, but a large majority of symptomatic accessory naviculars are successfully treated with excision.
- Commonly used technique is the Kidner procedure,[40] where the accessory ossicle is removed from within the substance of the posterior tibial tendon and, depending on concomitant foot pathology, the tendon is either repaired directly to the remaining navicular or advanced through a drill hole plantar to dorsal and repaired back to itself.

8.2.3 Os Peroneum

Anatomy

- Referred to as the sesamoid of the peroneus longus.
- Found along the lateral wall of the calcaneus, at the level of the calcaneocuboid joint articulation, or just inferior to the cuboid.
- Multiple soft-tissue attachments, including the plantar fascia, the fifth metatarsal, peroneus brevis, and the cuboid.[41]

Incidence

- Five to 26% but can be more or less frequent depending on ossification.[41]

Clinical Significance and Treatment

- Because it is a sesamoid bone, it is subject to similar pathology as the hallucal sesamoids as stated above.
- Can cause pathology within the peroneal tendon itself, leading to tendinopathy, tears, and rupture.[42]
- Knowledge of a potential sesamoid presence in this location is important in order to differentiate it from a fracture of the cuboid.
- Nonsurgical treatment includes activity modification, casting, etc.
- Surgical treatment involves excision and possible tendon repair, tenodesis, etc.

8.2.4 Os Subtibiale

Anatomy

- A rounded ossicle, diameter greater than 4 mm, margins well defined, with close relationship to the posterior colliculus of the medial malleolus, most notable on lateral radiograph at the ankle.[43]
- If margins poorly defined, it is more likely an avulsion fragment of the deltoid ligament from trauma.

Incidence

- Accessory bones around the medial malleolus are noted in nearly 5% of ankle radiographs, but true os subtibiale as described above is much rarer with an incidence of 0.2 to 1.2%.[43]

Clinical Significance and Treatment

- Important to differentiate a routine accessory bone to that resulting from trauma and acute injury as well as from a secondary ossification center in children and adolescents.
- Rarely is surgical intervention required for any of the notable ossicles in this region.

8.2.5 Os Subfibulare

Anatomy

- Debate exists whether this is an accessory ossicle, a united apophysis of the distal fibula, or a sesamoid of the peroneus longus tendon.
- Radiologic studies report the true os subfibulare is posterior to the tip of the distal fibula, has smooth edges, and can be anywhere from 5 to 10 mm in size.
- The apophysis is anterior to the lateral malleolus on a lateral radiograph of the ankle.[27]

Incidence

- Rare: 0.2%.[27]

Clinical Significance and Treatment

- It needs to be differentiated from acute traumatic injury. Most are asymptomatic, and those rare symptomatic cases nearly always resolve with conservative treatment.

8.2.6 Os Calcaneus Secundarius

Anatomy

- Found on the dorsal beak of the calcaneus associated with the anterior process, near the junction of the head of the talus, the navicular, and the cuboid.[44]
- Typically, 3 to 4 mm in size and visualized on a lateral oblique hindfoot radiograph.

Incidence

- Two percent to 4%.

Clinical Significance and Treatment

- Needs to be differentiated from a fracture or nonunion of the anterior process of the calcaneus, as well as a talonavicular coalition.
- Can cause decreased hindfoot motion and impingement type pain.
- It can be excised in refractory cases.
- Bone scan can aid in differentiating a traumatic injury from an anatomic variant.

8.2.7 Os Vesalianum

Anatomy

- Located just proximal to the tip of a well-developed fifth metatarsal tuberosity.
- A fracture is transverse across the tuberosity.
- An ossification center of the apophysis is linearly and longitudinally oriented to the metatarsal shaft.[45]

Incidence

- Ranges from 0.1 to 1%.

Clinical Significance and Treatment

- These can be very difficult to differentiate from chronic traumatic injury and an ununited apophysis.
- Pain can be from a fracture, apophysitis, or a symptomatic os vesalianum.
- Regardless, treatment for all is the same: activity modification and immobilization, and most improve.
- Rarely, excision is required and is usually successful in symptomatic relief.[46]

8.2.8 Additional Rare Accessory Bones

► Fig. 8.6

Additional rare accessory bones are the following:

- Os cuboideum secundarium.
- Os sustentaculum.
- Os subcalcis and os aponeurosis plantaris.
- Os talonaviculare dorsale.
- Os supratalare.
- Os intercuneiforme.
- Os intermetatarseum.

8.3 Key Testing Facts

- **Sesamoids:** Pain at the plantar aspect of the foot, particularly during toe-off, could indicate sesamoid pathology. Detailed motor, sensory, and vascular exams are crucial, with tenderness under the first MTP joint being a key finding.
- **Common Sesamoid Pathologies:** Fractures, avascular necrosis, congenital absence, and bipartite sesamoids are common pathologies. Bipartite sesamoids, caused by incomplete ossification, often require differentiation from fractures.
- **Accessory Bones of the Foot:** Accessory bones are common developmental variants, with almost 40 described. The most frequent include the os trigonum, os navicular, and os peroneum. These bones often present as incidental findings but can be symptomatic under certain conditions.
- **Os Trigonum Syndrome:** The os trigonum is located posterior to the talus and may cause impingement during forced plantarflexion, especially in ballet dancers. Symptoms include posterior ankle pain, often aggravated by activity.
- **Accessory Navicular:** The accessory navicular, particularly type II, is often symptomatic, with tenderness over the medial midfoot. This bone can contribute to pes planus due to altered biomechanics of the posterior tibial tendon.
- **Surgical Approaches for Sesamoid and Accessory Bone Pathologies:** Surgery includes sesamoidectomy via medial, lateral, or plantar approaches. For accessory bones like the os trigonum, excision is indicated if symptomatic. Postoperative care includes protecting the soft tissues and careful monitoring to avoid complications like deformities or loss of function.

References

[1] Inge GAL, Ferguson AB. Surgery of the sesamoid bones of the great toe. Arch Surg. 1933; 27:466–488

[2] Dharap AS, Al-Hashimi H, Kassab S, Abu-Hijleh MF. Incidence and ossification of sesamoid bones in the hands and feet: a radiographic study in an Arab population. Clin Anat. 2007; 20(4):416–423

[3] Aseyo D, Nathan H. Hallux sesamoid bones. Anatomical observations with special reference to osteoarthritis and hallux valgus. Int Orthop. 1984; 8(1):67–73

[4] Potter HG, Pavlcv H, Abrahams TG. The hallux sesamoids revisited. Skeletal Radiol. 1992; 21(7): 437–444

[5] Nwawka OK, Hayashi D, Diaz LE, et al. Sesamoids and accessory ossicles of the foot: anatomical variability and related pathology. Insights Imaging. 2013; 4(5):581–593

[6] Yammine K. The sesamoids of the feet in humans: a systematic review and meta-analysis. Anat Sci Int. 2015; 90(3):144–160

[7] Coughlin MJ. Sesamoids and accessory bones of the foot. In: Coughlin MJ, Saltzman CL, Anderson RB, eds. Mann's Surgery of the Foot and Ankle. Philadelphia, PA: Saunders; 2014:492–568

[8] Orr TG. Fracture of great toe sesamoid bones. Ann Surg. 1918; 67(5):609–612

[9] Pretterklieber ML, Wanivenhaus A. The arterial supply of the sesamoid bones of the hallux: the

course and source of the nutrient arteries as an anatomical basis for surgical approaches to the great toe. Foot Ankle. 1992; 13(1):27–31

[10] Rath B, Notermans HP, Frank D, et al. Arterial anatomy of the hallucal sesamoids. Clin Anat. 2009; 22(6):755–760

[11] Richardson EG. Injuries to the hallucal sesamoids in the athlete. Foot Ankle. 1987; 7(4):229–244

[12] Kuwano T, Nagamine R, Sakaki K, Urabe K, Iwamoto Y. New radiographic analysis of sesamoid rotation in hallux valgus: comparison with conventional evaluation methods. Foot Ankle Int. 2002; 23(9): 811–817

[13] Walling AK, Ogden JA. Case report 666. Bipartite medial sesamoid below the head of the first metatarsal, a developmental variant. Skeletal Radiol. 1991; 20(3):233–235

[14] Frankel JP, Harrington J. Symptomatic bipartite sesamoids. J Foot Surg. 1990; 29(4):318–323

[15] McBryde AM, Jr, Anderson RB. Sesamoid foot problems in the athlete. Clin Sports Med. 1988; 7(1): 51–60

[16] Alshryda S, Lou T, Faulconer ER, Adedapo AO. Adolescent hallux valgus deformity with bilateral absence of the hallucal sesamoids: a case report. J Foot Ankle Surg. 2012; 51(1):80–82

[17] Mann RA, Mann JA. Keratotic disorders of the plantar skin. Instr Course Lect. 2004; 53:287–302

[18] Schon LC, Baxter DE. Neuropathies of the foot and ankle in athletes. Clin Sports Med. 1990; 9(2): 489–509

[19] Garber EK, Silver S. Pedal manifestations of DISH. Foot Ankle. 1982; 3(1):12–16

[20] Garrido IM, Bosch MN, González MS, Carsí VV. Osteochondritis of the hallux sesamoid bones. Foot Ankle Surg. 2008; 14(4):175–179

[21] Dobas DC, Silvers MD. The frequency of partite sesamoids of the first metatarsophalangeal joint. J Am Podiatry Assoc. 1977; 67(12):880–882

[22] Apley AG. Open sesamoid. A re-appraisal of the medial sesamoid of the hallux. Proc R Soc Med. 1966; 59(2):120–121

[23] Ahn JH, Choy WS, Lee KW. Arthroscopy of the first metatarsophalangeal joint in 59 consecutive cases. J Foot Ankle Surg. 2012; 51(2):161–167

[24] Alshouli MT, Lin A, Kadakia AR. Simultaneous first metatarsophalangeal joint arthrodesis and sesamoidectomy with a single dorsomedial incision. Foot Ankle Spec. 2014; 7(5):403–408

[25] Saxena A, Krisdakumtorn T. Return to activity after sesamoidectomy in athletically active individuals. Foot Ankle Int. 2003; 24(5):415–419

[26] Aper RL, Saltzman CL, Brown TD. The effect of hallux sesamoid excision on the flexor hallucis longus moment arm. Clin Orthop Relat Res. 1996 (325):209–217

[27] Trolle D. Accessory Bones of the Human Foot. Copenhagen: Munksgaard; 1948;194–195

[28] McDougall A. The os trigonum. J Bone Joint Surg Br. 1955; 37-B(2):257–265

[29] Coskun N, Yuksel M, Cevener M, et al. Incidence of accessory ossicles and sesamoid bones in the feet: a radiographic study of the Turkish subjects. Surg Radiol Anat. 2009; 31(1):19–24

[30] Weinstein SL, Bonfiglio M. Unusual accessory (bipartite) talus simulating fracture. A case report. J Bone Joint Surg Am. 1975; 57(8):1161–1163

[31] Karasick D, Schweitzer ME. The os trigonum syndrome: imaging features. AJR Am J Roentgenol. 1996; 166(1):125–129

[32] Abramowitz Y, Wollstein R, Barzilay Y, et al. Outcome of resection of a symptomatic os trigonum. J Bone Joint Surg Am. 2003; 85(6):1051–1057

[33] Nault ML, Kocher MS, Micheli LJ. Os trigonum syndrome. J Am Acad Orthop Surg. 2014; 22(9): 545–553

[34] Labs K, Leutloff D, Perka C. Posterior ankle impingement syndrome in dancers: a short-term follow-up after operative treatment. Foot Ankle Surg. 2002; 8(1):33–39

[35] Weiss WM, Sanders EJ, Crates JM, Barber FA. Arthroscopic excision of a symptomatic os trigonum. Arthroscopy. 2015; 31(11):2082–2088

[36] Sella EJ, Lawson JP. Biomechanics of the accessory navicular synchondrosis. Foot Ankle. 1987; 8(3): 156–163

[37] Geist ES. The accessory scaphoid bone. J Bone Joint Surg.. 1925; 7:570–574

[38] Knapik DM, Guraya SS, Conry KT, Cooperman DR, Liu RW. Longitudinal radiographic behavior of accessory navicular in pediatric patients. J Child Orthop. 2016; 10(6):685–689

[39] Kidner FC. The prehallux (accessory scaphoid) in its relation to flat foot. J Bone Joint Surg. 1929; 11: 831–837

[40] Cha SM, Shin HD, Kim KC, Lee JK. Simple excision vs the Kidner procedure for type 2 accessory navicular associated with flatfoot in pediatric population. Foot Ankle Int. 2013; 34(2):167–172

[41] Bianchi S, Bortolotto C, Draghi F. Os peroneum imaging: normal appearance and pathological findings. Insights Imaging. 2017; 8(1):59–68

[42] Thompson FM, Patterson AH. Rupture of the peroneus longus tendon. Report of three cases. J Bone Joint Surg Am. 1989; 71(2):293–295

[43] Coral A. The radiology of skeletal elements in the subtibial region: incidence and significance. Skeletal Radiol. 1987; 16(4):298–303

[44] Mann RW. Calcaneus secundarius. Variation of a common accessory ossicle. J Am Podiatr Med Assoc. 1989; 79(8):363–366

[45] Sarrafian SK. Osteology. In: Sarrafian SK, ed. Anatomy of the Foot and Ankle. Philadelphia, PA: JB Lippincott; 1983:35–106

[46] Ralph BG, Barrett J, Kenyhercz C, DiDomenico LA. Iselin's disease: a case presentation of nonunion and review of the differential diagnosis. J Foot Ankle Surg. 1999; 38(6):409–416

9 Flatfoot Deformity

Johnny L. Lin and Christopher E. Gross

Abstract

Flatfoot deformity, also known as pes planus, is a condition characterized by loss of the arch of the foot, as well as other associated deformities such as hindfoot valgus, that is, pes planovalgus. The most common cause of flatfoot deformity is posterior tibial tendon dysfunction, due to the important role the tendon plays in maintaining the arch of the foot. Most patients seen in a clinical setting with symptomatic flatfoot deformity are adults who have developed the deformity over time, hence the term adult-acquired flatfoot deformity.

Keywords: posterior tibial tendon dysfunction, pes planus

9.1 Etiology and Pathophysiology

- The posterior tibial tendon plays a key role in maintaining the arch of the foot; therefore, posterior tibial tendon dysfunction (PTTD) is the most common cause of flatfoot deformity (▶ Fig. 9.1).

9.1.1 Anatomy

- The tibialis posterior muscle originates from the posterior aspect of the tibia, interosseous membrane, and fibula, and passes posterior to the medial malleolus.
- The posterior tibial tendon not only has a significant insertion on the navicular tuberosity but also has broad insertions on the medial and plantar midfoot, which is organized into three limbs:
  - The anterior limb inserts on the navicular tuberosity and the medial cuneiform.
  - The middle limb inserts onto the middle and lateral cuneiforms, cuboid, and base of the second through the fifth metatarsals.
  - The posterior limb inserts on the sustentaculum tali.
- There is a zone of hypovascularity in the posterior tibial tendon approximately 2 to 6 cm proximal to its insertion on the navicular, which may play a role in degeneration of the tendon.[1]
- The primary function of the tibialis posterior is inversion of the hindfoot, and it acts as a secondary plantarflexor due to its course posterior to the medial malleolus.
- The primary antagonist of the tibialis posterior is the peroneus brevis.
- During the gait cycle, as the limb transitions from midstance to terminal stance, the posterior tibial tendon inverts the hindfoot, which locks the transverse

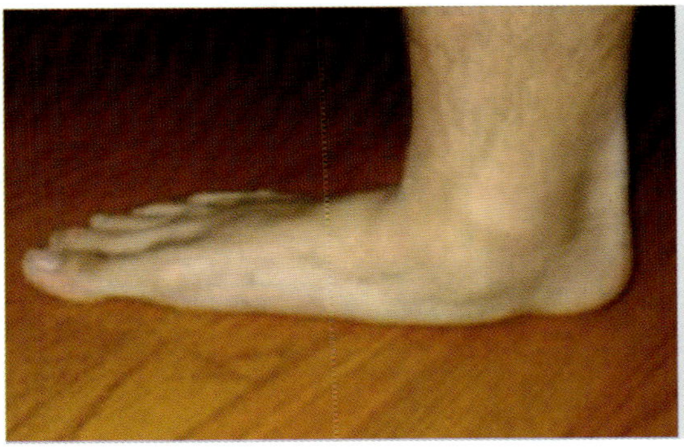

Fig. 9.1 Flatfoot deformity, with loss of medial arch, hindfoot valgus, and forefoot abduction.

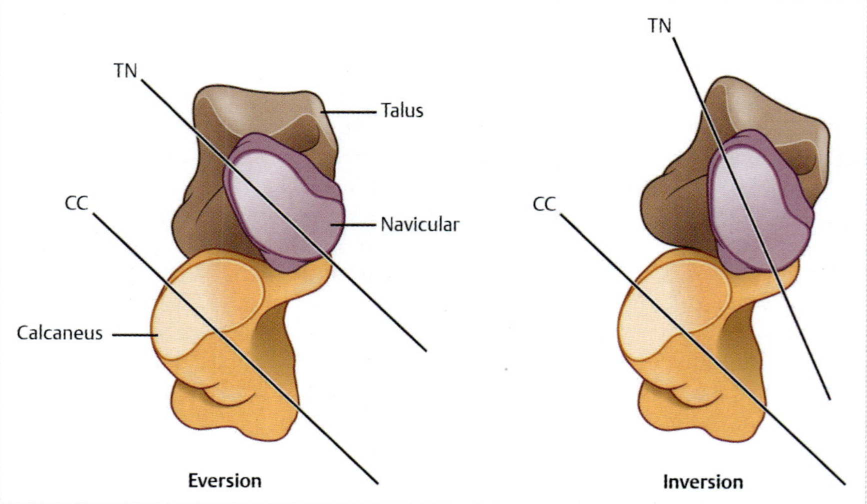

Fig. 9.2 During the gait cycle, the tibialis posterior inverts the hindfoot, locking the transverse tarsal joints and creating a rigid arch for push-off. CC, calcaneocuboid; TN, talonavicular.

tarsal joints and provides a rigid lever for push-off by the plantarflexors (▶ Fig. 9.2).

9.1.2 Etiology

- Flatfoot deformity is most common among females in the sixth decade of life and is associated with obesity and inflammatory disorders, due to increased loading and decreased strength of soft tissues, respectively.
- In PTTD, the posterior tibial tendon is weakened or degenerated, which leads to the loss of dynamic arch support and eventual collapse of the medial arch as the static soft tissue supporting structures attenuate over time. Ultimately, peritalar instability causes the progressive collapsing foot deformity.
- Inability to invert the hindfoot leads to hindfoot valgus, which can progress to tibiotalar valgus if the deltoid ligament complex is compromised.
- There is often forefoot abduction through the talonavicular joint as the surrounding soft tissues are weakened.
- The calcaneonavicular ligament, or spring ligament, is the primary static support of the talonavicular joint, and degeneration or injury to the spring ligament also contributes to loss of arch and progression of deformity.
- As the flatfoot deformity progresses, patients may develop degenerative changes or pathology in surrounding structures, such as subtalar arthritis, midfoot arthritis, or subfibular impingement as hindfoot valgus worsens.

9.1.3 Pediatric Pes Planus

- When flatfoot is found in pediatric patients, it is usually bilateral, asymptomatic, familial, and usually a flexible deformity. In this population, it can be associated with tarsal coalition, ligamentous laxity, or rotational limb deformities.
- Pediatric flatfoot is treated conservatively the majority of the time, with a period of immobilization if necessary, followed by use of arch supports or supportive shoes.
- If pediatric patients fail conservative treatment, they may undergo a lateral calcaneal lengthening osteotomy

combined with medial soft-tissue tightening, or a 3C procedure, which includes a medializing **calcaneal** osteotomy, opening wedge **cuboid** osteotomy, and plantarflexion medial **cuneiform** osteotomy.

9.2 Symptoms

- In early disease, patients may present with medial hindfoot and arch pain, with tenderness along the posterior tibial tendon and its insertion, with very little deformity.
- Some patients present with a history of chronic flatfoot deformity, which has become progressively symptomatic over time.
- In later stages, many complain of lateral foot and ankle pain due to subfibular impingement and medial-sided pain may actually improve.
- In addition to pain, patients may report weakness with activities requiring push-off strength such as running, jumping, or climbing stairs.
- Patients may also have complaints related to other conditions commonly coexisting with flatfoot, such as midfoot or subtalar arthritis.

9.3 Physical Examination

- Inspection of the bilateral feet and ankles from the front and the back while the patient is weight bearing in order to evaluate the overall alignment and compare the symptomatic side to the contralateral side.
- When looking at the feet from behind, hindfoot valgus can be assessed and forefoot abduction can often be identified when more of the toes can be seen on the affected side, which is also known as the "too many toes" sign (▶ Fig. 9.3).
- The patient may have tenderness to palpation along the course of the posterior tibial tendon and insertion on the navicular.
- The hindfoot valgus should be tested for rigidity by testing passive inversion and eversion of the subtalar joint to achieve a normal hindfoot valgus.
- If the hindfoot valgus is passively correctable, the forefoot should similarly be tested for rigidity by passively pronating and adducting the forefoot with the hindfoot corrected to achieve a plantigrade foot.
- Hypermobility of the first ray should be tested and accounted for when attempting to correct the forefoot supination.
- The gastrocnemius–soleus complex should be assessed for a relative equinus contracture with the hindfoot and forefoot held in a corrected position by passively dorsiflexing the ankle with the knee flexed and extended (Silfverskiöld's test).

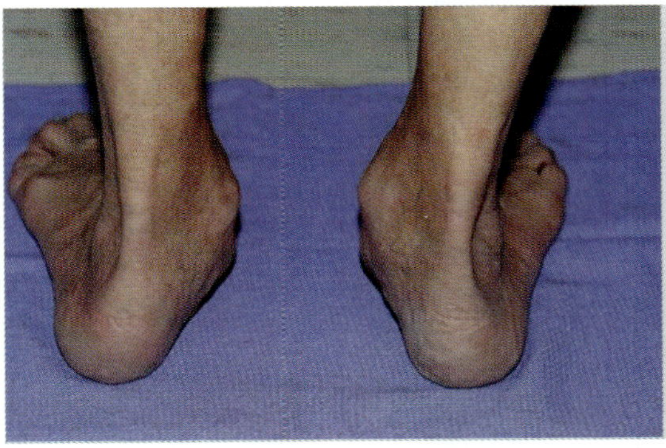

Fig. 9.3 The "too many toes sign," where multiple toes can be seen when looking at the feet from behind, indicating forefoot abduction.

- Resisted inversion is tested with the ankle in plantarflexion, in order to isolate the tibialis posterior and check for pain and weakness.
- The patient is asked to perform a double-leg heel rise with the knee extended to observe whether the hindfoot valgus corrects during heel rise (▶ Fig. 9.4):
  - The patient is also asked to perform a single-limb heel rise. If the patient is unable to perform a single-limb heel rise, then the patient has PTTD.
- The midfoot, sinus tarsi, and ankle joint are palpated in order to evaluate for pain due to concomitant midfoot, subtalar, or tibiotalar arthritis.

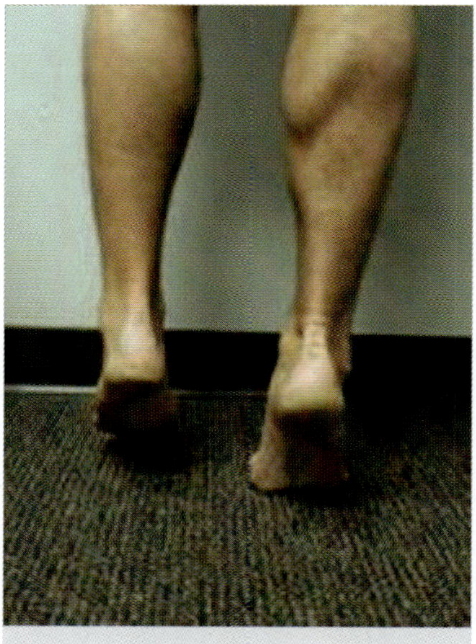

Fig. 9.4 Single-leg heel rise test.

9.4 Imaging

- Radiographic evaluation of a patient with flatfoot deformity should include weight-bearing views of the foot and ankle, including the anteroposterior (AP), lateral, and oblique views.
- Other potentially useful views include a hindfoot alignment view of the heel to assess heel valgus.
- On the lateral view of the foot, flatfoot is identified by a decrease in Meary's angle, formed by the axes of the talus and the first metatarsal, which is normally close to zero in a normally aligned foot (▶ Fig. 9.5a).
- The lateral view may also show a decrease in calcaneal pitch, formed by the inferior border of the calcaneus and a line parallel to the floor (▶ Fig. 9.5b).

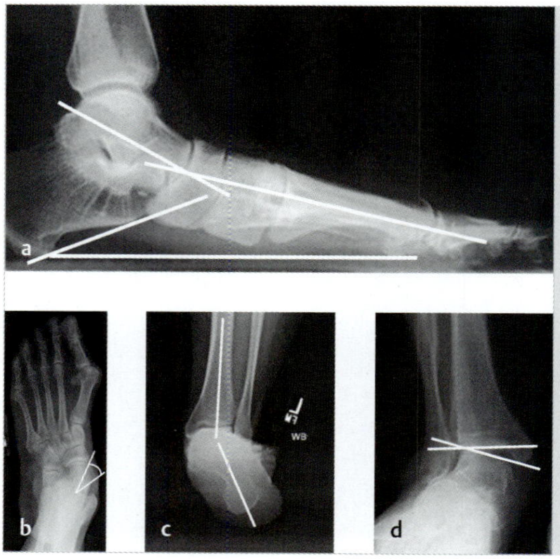

Fig. 9.5 **(a)** Meary's angle and calcaneal pitch; bottom left **(b)** Hindfoot alignment view showing calcaneovalgus; middle bottom **(c)** ankle valgus; bottom right **(d)** AP view of the foot demonstrating talonavicular uncoverage.

- Forefoot abduction can be seen on an AP view of the foot, measured by the percentage of the talar head, which is uncovered at the talonavicular joint, with greater than 40% uncovered indicating excessive forefoot abduction (▶ Fig. 9.5c).
- A hindfoot alignment view demonstrates the severity of calcaneovalgus relative to the rest of the lower limb (▶ Fig. 9.5d).
- A mortise of the ankle can be used to evaluate for valgus at the ankle joint, demonstrating increased talar tilt and suggesting deltoid incompetency, as well as concomitant tibiotalar arthritis.
- Magnetic resonance imaging (MRI) is not routinely required for evaluation of patients with flatfoot deformity, but it can be used to rule out other causes of hindfoot and ankle pain:
  - It can show evidence of degenerative changes in the posterior tibial tendon, such as partial or complete tear, tenosynovitis or fluid surrounding the tendon, and enlarged tendon potentially with heterogeneous signal within the tendon.
  - It can also illustrate degenerative or reactive changes in surrounding structures, such as findings consistent with subtalar or midfoot arthritis, or incompetence of the spring ligament.
    - Weightbearing CT scans are becoming more popular in understanding foot biomechanics in peritalar instability

9.5 Classification

- Appropriate classification of flatfoot deformity is important as stage of the disease helps guide the treatment options.
- Classification is based on a number of clinical and radiographic findings, summarized in ▶ Table 9.1.

Table 9.1 Classification of flatfoot deformity

Stage	Deformity	Physical Examination	Radiographs
Stage 1	• No deformity	• Medial hindfoot and arch pain • Tenderness along the posterior tibial tendon	• Normal radiographs
Stage 2	• Flexible hindfoot valgus	• Unable to perform a single-leg heel rise • Flexible hindfoot • Potential gastrocnemius tightness	• Loss of arch • Decreased calcaneal pitch • Calcaneal valgus
Stage 2A	• Stage 2 deformity without significant forefoot abduction		• Less than 40% uncovering of the talar head on the AP view
Stage 2B	• With forefoot abduction	• "Too many toes" sign	• More than 40% uncovering of talar head on the AP view
Stage 2C	• With forefoot supination	• First ray elevates when hind-foot valgus is corrected	•
Stage 3	• Rigid hindfoot valgus	• Loss of passive inversion and eversion • Tenderness at the sinus tarsi	• Subtalar arthritis
Stage 4	• Tibiotalar valgus or tibiotalar arthritis	• Deltoid insufficiency • Pain at the tibiotalar joint • Possible subfibular impingement	• Increased talar tilt • Tibiotalar degenerative changes

- As patients progress through the various stages, they may continue to have some findings of earlier stages, but the key distinguishing features are as shown in ▶ Table 9.1.

9.6 Treatment

- Treatment of PTTD is guided by stage, and while conservative and surgical treatment options are available for each stage, treatment tends to be more often conservative for early stages with increasing surgical intervention for later stages.

9.7 Conservative Management

- Stage 1:
  - A period of immobilization (4 weeks in a weight-bearing controlled ankle motion [CAM] boot or weight-bearing cast) may be necessary to reduce pain and inflammation, followed by use of orthotics with arch support and a medial heel wedge.
  - Physical therapy can provide therapeutic modalities in order to help control pain and inflammation.
- Stage 2:
  - In patients with a flexible deformity, physical therapy may be beneficial to improve strength about the ankle and reduce calf tightness, as well as provide therapeutic modalities.
  - Custom orthotics with medial arch support and medial posting can be used for definitive treatment.
  - A University of California Biomechanical Laboratory (UCBL) orthotic can also be utilized for more significant hindfoot deformities although this is oftentimes not tolerated by patients.
  - Patients with stage 2 disease that is resistant to below-the-ankle devices may also benefit from use of an ankle–foot orthosis (AFO) brace (i.e., Arizona brace, solid AFO, or articulated AFO) or a Richie brace.
- Stage 3:
  - In stage 3 disease, the deformity is rigid or not fully correctable and can be treated with an accommodating articulating Richie, AFO, or custom Arizona brace.
- Stage 4:
  - Bracing for stage 4 also consists of a rigid AFO or Arizona brace, with adequate support for ankle instability.

9.8 Surgical Intervention

- Stage 1:
  - Operative treatment of stage 1 disease is less common, but consists of tenosynovectomy of the posterior tibial tendon (open or camera assisted).
- Stage 2:
  - Reconstruction of the posterior tibial tendon by transfer of flexor hallucis longus (FHL) tendon or flexor digitorum longus (FDL) tendon into the navicular.[2]
  - Stage 2A: Correct hindfoot valgus with a medial slide calcaneal osteotomy (▶ Fig. 9.6).
  - Stage 2B: Correct forefoot abduction with lateral column lengthening, using an opening wedge osteotomy of the calcaneus (Evans osteotomy), potentially combined with a medial slide calcaneal osteotomy.
  - Stage 2C: Correct forefoot supination through plantarflexion of the first ray with a dorsal opening wedge osteotomy of the medial cuneiform (Cotton osteotomy) if the medial column is stable, or with a first tarsometatarsal (TMT) arthrodesis (Lapidus) if the medial column is unstable.
  - Assess for gastrocnemius contracture, and perform a gastrocnemius recession if necessary.
  - Spring ligament reconstruction can be performed in order to augment the strength of the overall reconstruction.

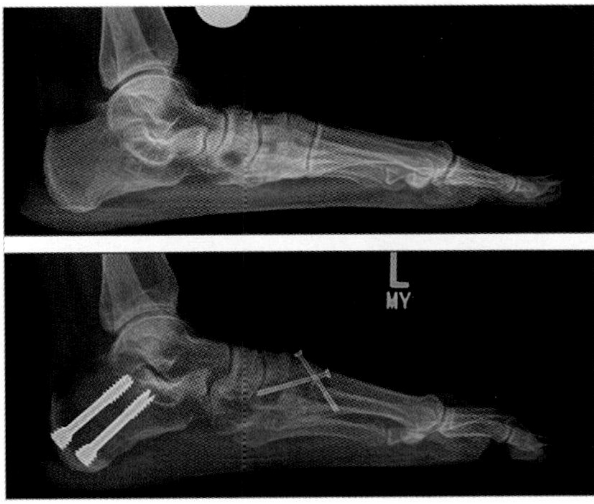

Fig. 9.6 Stage 2 pre-op and post-op X-rays.

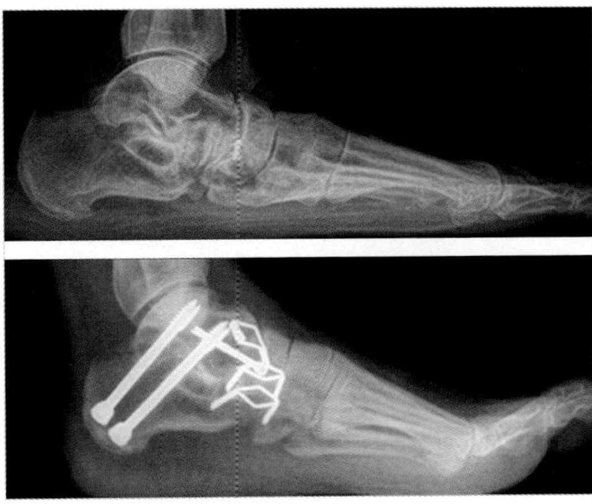

Fig. 9.7 Stage 3 pre-op and post-op X-rays.

- In patients with severe deformity (or a rigid deformity) or obesity, performing a triple arthrodesis primarily may be preferred.
- Stage 3:
  - Rigid deformity correction requires a triple arthrodesis (subtalar, talonavicular, and calcaneocuboid) for correction (▸ Fig. 9.7).[3]
  - Some surgeons prefer a combined subtalar and talonavicular fusion, which can be performed through a single medial incision, as correction of a significant deformity can put lateral soft tissues under tension.[4]
  - Medial column stabilization (a Cotton osteotomy or Lapidus) can also be performed to correct forefoot supination if necessary.
  - Correct equinus contracture with Achilles' tendon lengthening or a gastrocnemius recession if necessary.
- Stage 4:
  - If valgus at the tibiotalar joint is passively correctable and there are minimal degenerative changes to the tibiotalar joint, a deltoid ligament reconstruction can be performed in addition to reconstruction of the hindfoot.

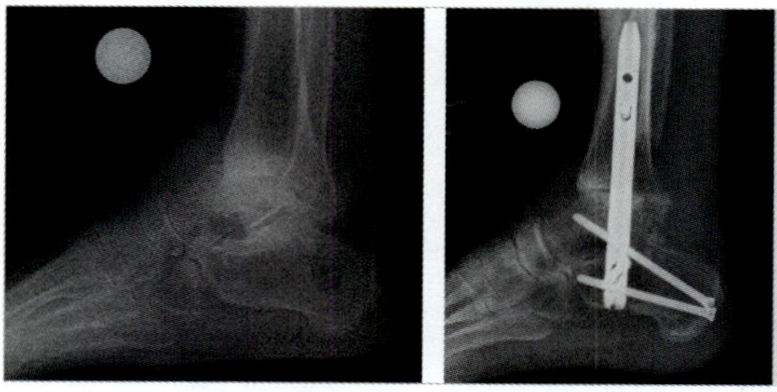

Fig. 9.8 Stage 4 pre-op and post-op X-rays.

 - If the deformity at the tibiotalar joint is not passively correctable or there is significant arthritis in the tibiotalar joint, a tibiotalocalcaneal (TTC) fusion produces more reliable correction of the deformity (▶ Fig. 9.8).
 - A total ankle replacement with a subtalar and talonavicular fusion can also provide good relief.

9.9 Rehabilitation

- Reconstruction of a flatfoot deformity requires a period of postoperative immobilization and non-weight-bearing in order for the tendon transfer, osteotomies, or fusions to heal, and the duration of each is determined by the procedures performed as well as patient-specific factors.
- In general, the patient is placed into a well-padded splint for the first 10 to 14 days after surgery, and then transitioned to a short leg cast.
- Transition from non-weight-bearing in a cast to gradual increase in weight bearing in a boot occurs between 6 and 10 weeks after surgery depending on the procedures performed, generally shorter for osteotomies and longer for fusions, and the progress of the patient.
- Resuming regular shoe wear usually occurs approximately 12 weeks postoperatively.
- Physical therapy focuses on range of motion initially, progressing to strengthening of limb and gait training as needed.

9.10 Key Testing Facts

- Flatfoot deformity (pes planovalgus) involves loss of the medial arch and hindfoot valgus, potentially with forefoot abduction and supination.
- The tibialis posterior is the primary dynamic stabilizer of the arch through hindfoot inversion, and the most common cause of flatfoot is PTTD.
- A hypovascular zone 2 to 6 cm proximal to the insertion of the PT tendon on the navicular is involved in its degeneration.
- Forefoot abduction can be seen as the “too many toes” sign and patients may be unable to perform a single-leg heel rise.
- Radiographs show decreased Meary’s angle, decreased calcaneal pitch, and decreased coverage of the talar head at the talonavicular joint.
- Treatment depends on the stage of the deformity, and flexibility or rigidity of the hindfoot deformity is a key distinction between stages 2 and 3.
- Nonoperative treatment includes physical therapy and orthotics such as inserts with arch support and medial wedge, UCBL orthotics, articulating or rigid AFO, or Arizona brace.
- Operative treatment is guided by stage and often involves a variety of procedures to correct the deformity.

References

[1] Frey C, Shereff M, Greenidge N. Vascularity of the posterior tibial tendon. J Bone Joint Surg Am. 1990; 72(6):884–888

[2] Chadwick C, Whitehouse SL, Saxby TS. Long-term follow-up of flexor digitorum longus transfer and calcaneal osteotomy for stage II posterior tibial tendon dysfunction. Bone Joint J. 2015; 97-B(3): 346–352

[3] Röhm J, Zwicky L, Horn Lang T, Salentiny Y, Hintermann B, Knupp M. Mid- to long-term outcome of 96 corrective hindfoot fusions in 84 patients with rigid flatfoot deformity. Bone Joint J. 2015; 97-B(5):668–674

[4] Sammarco VJ, Magur EG, Sammarco GJ, Bagwe MR. Arthrodesis of the subtalar and talonavicular joints for correction of symptomatic hindfoot malalignment. Foot Ankle Int. 2006; 27(9):661–666

10 Pes Cavus

Thomas I. Sherman and Gregory P. Guyton

Abstract

The etiology of pes cavus varies widely and most cases are idiopathic, but the condition can also be a sign of underlying neuromuscular disorder such as Charcot–Marie–Tooth disease and spinal cord abnormalities. It is important to recognize the underlying cavus deformity to direct neurologic referral when indicated and to manage treatment appropriately. Regardless of the etiology, pes cavus results from muscular imbalance that causes a foot position that effectively locks the transverse tarsal joints. The cavus foot is rigid and results in abnormal dissipation of stress with gait and weight-bearing activity. This can predispose individuals to both chronic and acute and overuse injuries, which are often the presenting complaints. Thorough physical and radiologic evaluation is mandated to fully characterize the deformity. Nonoperative management is often appropriate initially, but many patients ultimately require surgical intervention. The goal of all procedures is to obtain a painless, functional plantigrade foot, which is done with tendon transfers and/or osteotomies in supple deformities and corrective arthrodeses in rigid deformities. Early surgical intervention is often prudent to avoid progression from a supple to a rigid deformity. The choice of surgical procedures is dictated by the nature and severity of the deformity.

Keywords: pes cavus, high arch, hindfoot varus, cavovarus, Charcot–Marie–Tooth, foot deformity, ankle instability, lateral column overload, tendon transfer, osteotomies

10.1 Introduction

Pes cavus is an elevated arch maintained with weight bearing.

It is defined as forefoot equinus relative to the hindfoot and is comprised of contributing factors of variable degrees:

- Increased calcaneal pitch.
- Hindfoot varus.
- Excessive plantar flexion of the medial forefoot.
- Adduction of the entire forefoot.

Combined, these deformities disrupt the normal weight-bearing tripod comprising the calcaneus, first metatarsal, and fifth metatarsal. The result is a rigid conformation of the foot, which can precipitate acute injuries and overuse pathology.

10.2 Etiology and Pathophysiology

All cavus deformities result from a muscular imbalance and may involve the extrinsic and/or intrinsic muscle groups. Etiologies of cavus deformities are categorized as neuromuscular, congenital, traumatic, and idiopathic (▶ Table 10.1). The pathophysiology and pathomechanics are similar despite different etiologies.

- Rigidity of the transverse tarsal joint is the defining feature of cavus biomechanics and leads to a stiffer foot than is encountered with neutral or flat arches.
- The axes of talus and calcaneus are parallel because of internal rotation of the calcaneus.
- The cuboid moves with the calcaneus and is positioned inferior to the navicular rather than lateral to it. These deformities prevent pronation of the foot and lock the talar head on top of the calcaneus. This locks the transverse tarsal joints with cavus posture.[1]

Table 10.1 Summary of pes cavus etiologies

Neuromuscular	
Muscle disease	**Muscular dystrophy**
Peripheral nerve and lumbosacral root pathology	Charcot–Marie–Tooth disease (hereditary motor sensory neuropathy [HMSN]) Spinal dysraphism Polyneuritis Intraspinal tumor Spinocerebellar ataxia
Anterior horn cell disease of the spinal cord	Diastematomyelia Syringomyelia Spinal cord tumor Spinal musculature atrophy Spinal cord injury
Long tract and central disease	Friedreich ataxia Roussy–Lévy syndrome Primary cerebellar disease Cerebral palsy Multiple sclerosis Stroke; traumatic brain injury
Congenital	Residual of clubfoot Arthrogryposis Tarsal coalition
Traumatic	Compartment syndrome sequelae Lower extremity crush injury/burns Fracture malunion
Idiopathic	

Source: Adapted from Ibrahim K. Pes cavus. In: Evarts CM, ed. Surgery of the Musculoskeletal System. New York, NY: Churchill Livingstone; 1990:4015–4034.

- Limited rotation of the foot about the talus results in abnormal gait and prevents stress dissipation with weight-/load-bearing activities.
- The foot fails to pronate during early stance, which leads to stress concentration on the lateral foot and first metatarsal head.[2]
- Cavus motor imbalance before skeletal maturity can lead to changes in osseous morphology and rigid deformities.
- Development of rigid deformities in the skeletally mature individual may lead to accelerated degenerative changes and soft-tissue contractures.

10.2.1 Neuromuscular Causes

Charcot–Marie–Tooth/Hereditary Motor Sensory Neuropathy (HMSN)

Charcot–Marie–Tooth (CMT)/hereditary motor and sensory neuropathy (HMSN) is a group of disorders characterized by distal muscle weakness, sensory loss, depressed tendon reflexes, and pes cavus.

- CMT accounts for the majority of neuromuscular cases of pes cavus and is the most common hereditary polyneuropathy. The prevalence of CMT is 9.7/100,000 to 82.3/100,000.[3,4]
- CMT is classified into multiple evolving subtypes according to genetic transmission, electrophysiological characteristics, and/or nerve biopsy findings (▶ Table 10.2).
- CMT classically results in forefoot cavus due to a common pattern of motor imbalance.
- The typical imbalance of the lower extremity muscles is summarized in ▶ Table 10.3.

Poliomyelitis (Polio)

Polio was historically a primary etiology for cavus deformities, but it is seldom encountered today because of global vaccination programs.

- Polio is caused by poliovirus, a ribonucleic acid (RNA) virus that affects the central nervous system with a proclivity for the anterior horn cells of the spinal column. It results in lower extremity dysfunction and manifestations.
- Hindfoot cavus predominant deformities result from paralysis of the

Table 10.2 Summary of Charcot–Marie–Tooth (CMT) types and subtypes.[5,6,7,8]

Type	Inheritance	Proportion of CMT subtypes	Pattern	Most common genes	Features
CMT-1 CMT-1A subtype (80%)	AD	40–50%	Primarily demyelinating	**PMP22** (CMT-1A) MPZ (CMT-1B)	Muscle weakness and atrophy Sensory loss Slow NCV Usually slowly progressive Onset at 5–25 y; normal lifespan
CMT-2	AD, AR	10–15%	**Axonal**	MFN2 MPZ	Similar to CMT-1 but less severe Distal muscle weakness and atrophy Mild sensory loss **Normal NCV**
CMT-IM	AD	Rare	Axonal and demyelinating	MPZ	Overlapping features of both CMT-1 and CMT-2
CMT-X	**X-linked recessive**	10–14%	Axonal with demyelinating features	GJB1	More **severe** than CMT-1 Progressive motor and sensory neuropathy Males more severely affected than female carries **Hearing loss**
CMT-4	AR	**Rare**	Axonal or demyelinating	11 genes	Distal muscle weakness and atrophy; sensory loss

Abbreviations: AD, autosomal dominant; AR, autosomal recessive; NCV, nerve conduction velocity.
Note: Defining subtype features in bold.

Table 10.3 Summary of the typical muscle imbalances in patients with CMT

Deformity	Weak agonist muscle(s)	Intact antagonist muscle(s)	Imbalance effect
Equinus	Tibialis anterior	Gastrocnemius–soleus complex (triceps–surae)	Plantar flexion
Adduction and hindfoot varus	Peroneus brevis	Tibialis posterior	Adducts the foot, inverts the subtalar joint
Plantar flexion of the first ray	Tibialis anterior	Peroneus longus	Plantarflexes the first ray, creates a secondary forefoot cavus
Toe deformities	Foot intrinsics	Long toe flexors	Clawing occurs as the extrinsic forces are unmodified by the intrinsics; also depresses the metatarsal heads and accentuates cavus
Hallux claw toe	Foot intrinsics	EHL and FHL	Severe hallucal clawing occurs when a spared EHL is used to assist a weak tibialis anterior dorsiflexion of the foot

Abbreviations: CMT, Charcot–Marie–Tooth; EHL, extensor hallucis longus; FHL, flexor hallucis longus.

gastrocnemius–soleus complex (GSC). Overpull by the tibialis anterior (TA), depression of the metatarsals by the long toe flexors, and foreshortening of the distance between the attachment and origin of the intrinsic muscles result in a cavus foot with marked calcaneal pitch.
- Cases where forefoot cavus is predominant result from paralysis of the TA. Its unopposed antagonist, the peroneus longus (PL), plantarflexes the first ray. Dorsiflexion resulting from the compensatory extensor hallucis longus (EHL) and extensor digitorum longus (EDL) results in clawing of the toes, which further depresses the metatarsal heads.

Friedreich's Ataxia

- Friedreich's ataxia is an autosomal recessive progressive ataxia involving the FXN gene.
- Average clinical onset is between ages 10 and 15 years.
- Most commonly inherited ataxia in Europe, Middle East, South Asia, and North Africa.
- Frequency of 2:100,000 to 4:100,000 and a carrier frequency of 1:60 to 1:100.
- Ataxia is often the first manifestation.
- It is also characterized by dysarthria, scoliosis, bladder dysfunction, depressed lower limb reflexes, and sensory loss.
- Cardiology referral is necessary because approximately two-thirds of individuals have cardiomyopathy, and 30% have diabetes mellitus.[9]

Cerebral Palsy

- Cerebral palsy may precipitate cavovarus deformities due to spasticity of the posterior tibialis tendon (PTT).[10]

Spinal Pathology

Spinal pathology, potentially reversible, may present with a static or progressive cavus deformity.

- Diastematomyelia or myelodysplasia is associated with unilateral or bilateral deformities from gastrocnemius weakness.
- Syringomyelia is associated with unilateral deformity.
- Spinal cord tumor may initially and solely manifest with a cavus foot.
- Spinal cord injury and multiple sclerosis may lead to cavus deformities due to relative overpull of the tibialis posterior.[11]

10.2.2 Congenital Causes

Clubfoot Deformity

Clubfoot deformity is a combination of cavus, adductus, varus, and equinus.

- Modern treatment is appropriately initiated during infancy with serial Ponseti casting. Although this method is vastly successful, residual deformity may occur. This may result from failure to sufficiently elevate the first ray prior to abduction using the talar head as a fulcrum.[12]
- Previous surgical correction of the clubfoot, popularized in the 1970s and 1980s, may result in overcorrection or undercorrection, and sequelae may become symptomatic in the adulthood or adolescence.[13] These procedures are often associated with profound stiffness, often obligating a hindfoot fusion.[14]

Tarsal Coalitions

Tarsal coalition is most often associated with stiff pes planovalgus deformities in children, but this condition has been reported in children with cavovarus deformities.[15]

10.2.3 Traumatic Causes

Compartment Syndrome

- Compartment syndrome may result in an equinovarus deformity due to ischemic fibrosis of the deep posterior compartment contents.[16]

- The PTT develops increased medial and plantar pull on the navicular and positions the talus in relative dorsiflexion.
- Additionally, ischemic injury to the distal tibial nerve may result in intrinsic muscle weakness and claw toes.
- Compartment syndrome of the foot, most typically in the setting of crush injury or calcaneus fractures, is also associated with claw-toe deformity sequelae.[16,17]

Talar Neck Fracture

- Talar neck fracture with typical medial and dorsal comminution may result in a varus and dorsiflexed malunion.
- The calcaneus follows the talus into varus.
- Untreated calcaneus fractures may also progress to varus malunion.

10.2.4 Idiopathic Causes

- Most cases of pes cavus are idiopathic.
- The deformity is generally relatively mild and is popularly termed the "subtle cavus foot."[18]
- These conformations are bilateral and likely represent a normal variant on the population distribution of arch height.
- Some patients may have clinical weakness with atrophy, but the vast majority have normal neurophysiological profiles.[19]
- Primary complaints are most often related to or exacerbated by cavus posture, such as recurrent ankle sprains, peroneal tendinopathy, or metatarsalgia.

10.3 Symptoms

- Not all patients with cavus feet are symptomatic, and symptomatic patients may have a variety of primary complaints.

10.3.1 History

- After pes cavus is identified, a thorough history including a detailed family history is necessary to facilitate appropriate neurologic referral when indicated.
- Deformities that are progressive or asymmetric and those accompanied by profound weakness, abnormal reflexes, or sensory changes warrant neurologic referral.
  - If deformity is not severe, patients are typically not aware of any abnormality of their foot conformity.
- Common complaints are vague lateral forefoot pain, difficulty with footwear, or ankle instability.
  - These associated complaints are related to the unique biomechanical properties of the cavus foot, which affects function of the lower limb and predisposes individuals to acute and overuse injuries.[20,21,22]
- Hindfoot varus predisposes individuals to ankle instability and is associated with recurrence after lateral ligament repair if the underlying cavus deformity is not corrected.[22,23,24,25,26]
- Ankle pain, arthrosis, and joint surface injury results from rigidity of the subtalar and transverse tarsal joints, which concentrates contact stresses to the anteromedial ankle joint.
- Additionally, predisposition to recurrent instability events is associated with chondral injury.[24,27,28,29,30]
- Patients may develop forefoot overload and metatarsalgia due to excessive plantar flexion of the medial forefoot and associated GSC tightness.[31,32,33] Clawing of the digits, as seen in CMT, may exacerbate metatarsal pain due to distal migration of the plantar fat pad.
- Stress fractures occur frequently, particularly of the fourth and fifth metatarsals, due to overload of the lateral forefoot and decreased stress dissipation due to the underlying rigidity of the foot.[1,2,20,34,35,36]
- Complaints of sesamoiditis and sesamoid fracture are common due to the plantarflexed position of the first

metatarsal and resultant overload of the underlying sesamoids.

- Pathology of the fifth metatarsal base is common, including fracture, nonunion, and failure of operative management of the fifth metatarsal base fractures due to lateral column overload.[37,38]
- Peroneal tendinopathy from strain and friction at the calcaneal process and cuboid notch as a result of hindfoot varus posture is common. Additionally, recurrent instability episodes exacerbate this pathology.[32,39,40]
- An association between Lisfranc injuries and pes cavus has been described.[41]
- Cavus conformities have been implicated with medial tibial stress syndrome, tibial and femoral stress fractures, and iliotibial band syndrome.[42,43,44]

10.3.2 Physical Examination

- Physical examination is essential for surgical decision-making (▸ Fig. 10.1).
- Cavus is best identified and quantified by heel varus, which is most clearly evaluated by viewing the patient from the front. Visualization of the medial heel pad is diagnostic of heel varus and termed the "peek-a-boo" heel sign[18] (▸ Fig. 10.2).
- Lateral column overload may manifest through callus formation and lateral metatarsal tenderness or dorsal swelling from underlying stress fractures.
- Asymmetry, long-tract signs (clonus, hyperreflexia, or upgoing Babinski's reflex), hyperreflexia, and intrinsic wasting in the hands warrant neurological referral.

Rigid Deformities

Rigid deformities are identified by assessing active and, more importantly, passive motion of the entire foot and ankle. Limited motion may be due to a coalition, arthrosis, or contractures. Limited ankle motion may also be due to a tight GSC or anterior ankle impingement.

Flexible Deformities

Flexible deformities are passively correctable. They are further differentiated based upon whether the primary cause of the deformity is plantar flexion of the first ray or varus heel (▸ Fig. 10.3). It is performed by evaluating the persistence of heel varus with the patient standing on the heel and lateral column but not the medial column (Coleman block test). Typically, a heel that corrects requires only intervention to the forefoot (▸ Fig. 10.1).

- Assessing muscle strength is paramount to surgical decision-making for potential tendon transfers. Muscles with strength of less than 4 out of 5 are not candidates for transfer.
- Patients with a weak TA, as seen in CMT, have compensatory EHL and EDL activity during the swing phase of the gait cycle. This may cause a dynamic cock-up deformity initially, but this deformity may become fixed with time.

10.4 Diagnostics and Classification

10.4.1 Radiographs

Weight-bearing radiographs should be performed with the patient in normal stance and should include views of the foot and ankle. In addition to assessing the typical parameters of pes cavus, all radiographs should be carefully reviewed for commonly associated pathology, such as lateral metatarsal stress fractures and anteromedial ankle arthritis.

Lateral Foot/Ankle Radiographs

- Calcaneal pitch/inclination angle is elevated with hindfoot varus. An angle of greater than 28 degrees represents the upper 10% of the normal population distribution (▸ Fig. 10.4).[45]
- Meary's angle (talar–first metatarsal angle) assesses forefoot plantar flexion and is elevated (concave plantar) in

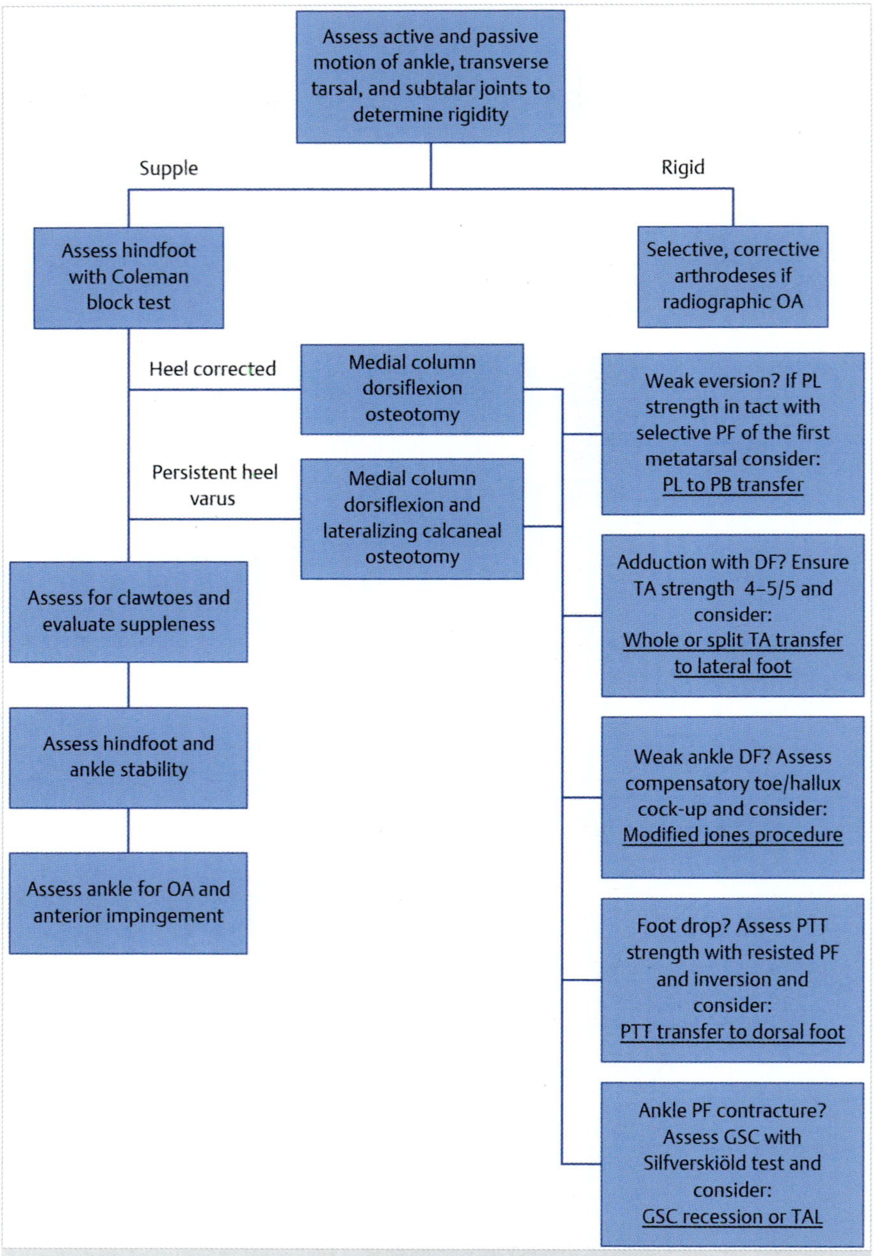

Fig. 10.1 Pes cavus physical examination algorithm to assist in surgical decision-making. OA, osteoarthritis; TAL, tendo-Achilles lengthening.

forefoot cavus. Normal values are 0 ± 4 degrees, but this value is more typically 15 degrees or more in the cavus feet.

More elevated values correspond to anteromedial ankle arthrosis and more rigid deformities.[29,46]

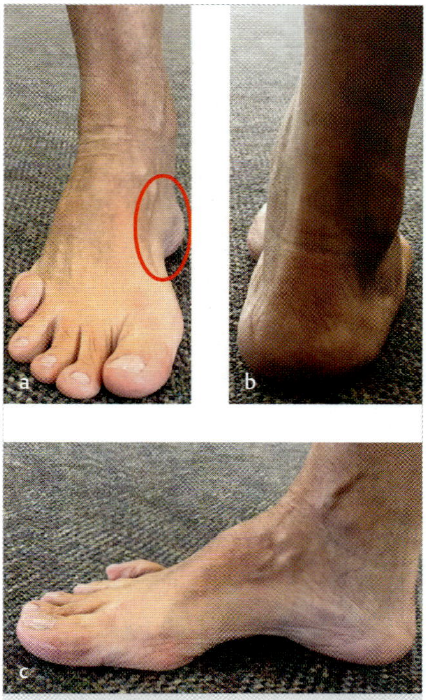

Fig. 10.2 Clinical photographs of a patient with idiopathic pes cavus. **(a)** The “peek-a-boo” heel sign (*red oval*) is visualized facing the patient. **(b)** Inspection from behind reveals a varus orientation to the heel. **(c)** A high medial arch maintained with weight bearing is apparent in profile.

- The Hibbs, or first metatarsal–calcaneal, angle is lower than normal (150 degrees)[47] in cavus deformities.
- The medial cuneiform and navicular are elevated relative to the fifth metatarsal base.
- Posterior positioning of the fibula and a relative flat-top appearance of the talar dome are artifacts that result from the relative external rotation of tibia in a lateral radiograph of the foot (a lateral view of the foot is an oblique ankle view in a cavus deformity).
- The metatarsals appear stacked due to the greater declination of the medial metatarsals compared to the lateral metatarsals.

Anteroposterior Foot Radiograph

Kite’s angle (talocalcaneal angle) approaches parallelism in the cavus foot (▶ Fig. 10.5).

Overcoverage of the talonavicular joints is often observed.

Anteroposterior and Mortise Ankle Radiographs

Careful attention should be given to evaluate for signs of ankle arthritis, particularly to the

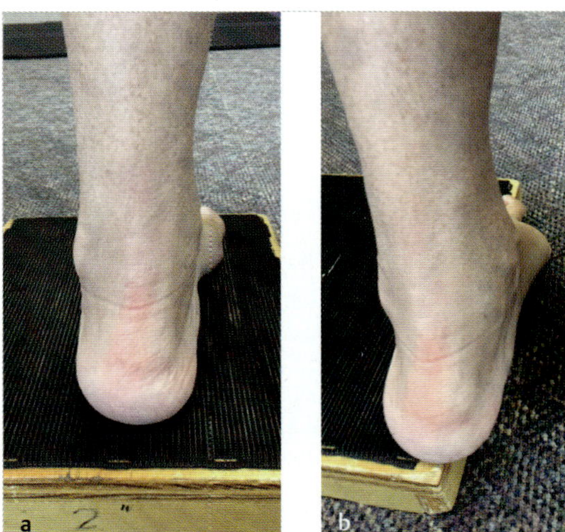

Fig. 10.3 Clinical photographs of a patient with idiopathic pes cavus. **(a,b)** Coleman block testing reveals partial correction of the hindfoot varus, indicating this deformity is primarily driven by a plantarflexed first ray.

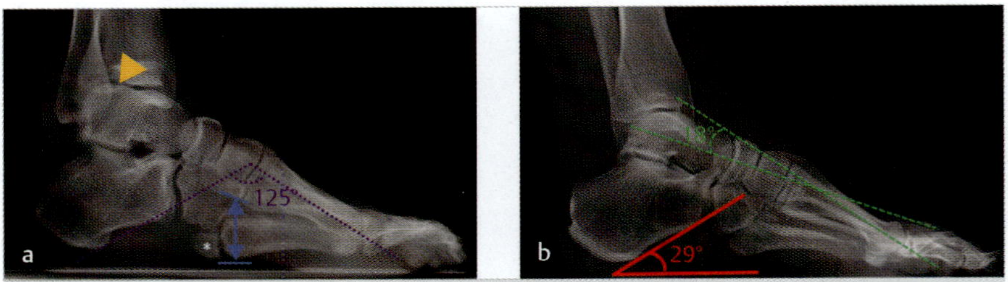

Fig. 10.4 **(a)** Lateral weight-bearing foot and ankle radiographs of a patient with Charcot–Marie–Tooth disease type 1A (CMT-1A) and **(b)** idiopathic cavus deformities. The fibula appears posterior and the talus flat due to rotational artifact (**a**; *yellow arrowhead*). Hibbs angle (**a**; *purple dashed line*) is less than depressed. A nonunion of a fifth metatarsal base fracture (**a**; *) is identified due to persistent lateral column overload. The medial cuneiform is elevated in relation to the base of the fifth metatarsal (**a**; *blue arrow*). Meary's angle is concave plantar and elevated (**b**; *green dashed lines*). Calcaneal inclination is elevated (**b**; *red line*). The metatarsal appears stacked (**a,b**).

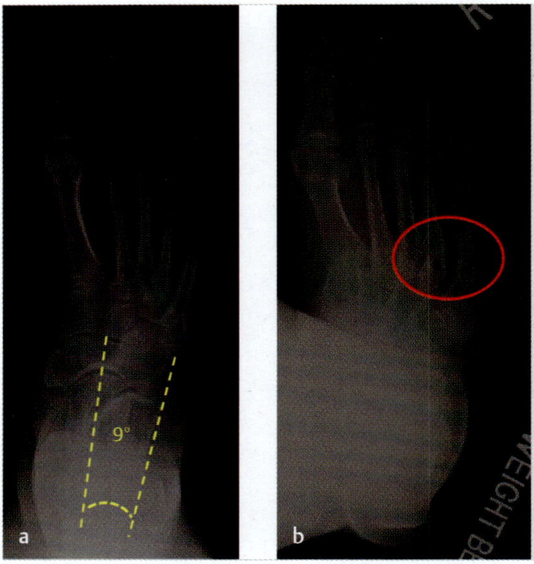

Fig. 10.5 Weight-bearing anteroposterior radiographs of two patients with idiopathic pes cavus. Relative parallelism of the **(a)** talocalcaneal angle (*yellow lines*) and **(b)** lateral metatarsal stress fractures (*red circle*) are characteristic of pes cavus.

anteromedial region. Varus talar tilt may indicate chronic lateral ankle instability.

10.4.2 Computed Tomography

Computed tomography (CT) should be obtained in rigid deformities and those that do not correct with the Coleman block testing to assess for tarsal coalitions and occult arthrosis.[15]

10.4.3 Magnetic Resonance Imaging

Magnetic resonance imaging (MRI) is not routinely needed. It is primarily useful for evaluation of the lateral ankle ligaments, osteochondral injuries, and peroneal tendons, although reliability for this purpose is degraded due to the course of the tendons relative to the magnetic vector.[38,48]

10.5 Conservative Management

- Nonsurgical management should be attempted initially in most patients.
- However, progressive deformities often benefit from early surgical management, while soft-tissue procedures are still feasible to prevent progression to a rigid deformity.
- In general, treatment should be tailored to the specific complaints and patients should be counseled regarding the effect of their pes cavus on associated pathology.
- For example, an acute ankle sprain and associated pes cavus may be treated with a short period of rest followed by physical therapy for peroneal strengthening, proprioceptive training, bracing as needed, and possibly a corrective orthotic.
  - Success with this approach may be tempered by the underlying deformity. Stretching focused on dorsiflexion and eversion is beneficial in all cases to maintain a supple foot.

10.5.1 Orthotics

- Foot orthotics for pes cavus may include a recess to accommodate first ray plantar flexion, a low arch to allow eversion, a heel wedge for the tight gastrocnemius soleus, and a lateral forefoot wedge to offload the lateral column.
- Orthotics do not alter the natural history or progression of the deformity.
- Orthotics improve function, alleviate pain, and decrease elevated plantar pressure in patients with cavus feet.[49,50,51]
- Orthotics may be an effective treatment adjunct in addition to modalities aimed at managing the primary complaint.[38,43]
- Corrective orthotics are not well tolerated in rigid deformities.

10.5.2 Orthoses

- Ankle–foot orthoses (AFO) are options in the setting of severe dorsiflexion weakness.
- Modifications with a hinge and dynamic dorsiflexion assist can facilitate normal gait.

10.6 Surgical Intervention

- The goal of surgery is correction of the cavus deformity with maintenance of a supple plantigrade foot.
- Treatment includes the following:
  - Transfer of deformity inducing tendons to more functional locations.
  - Release of contracted structures.
  - Corrective osteotomies for realignment in a supple foot.
  - Arthrodeses for a rigid or arthritic foot.
- Procedures are seldom indicated or performed in isolation, and the surgical algorithm should be appropriately directed to each deformity. In general, motion- and joint-sparing procedures are preferable to fusion procedures to avoid further motion restriction in the already stiff pes cavus foot[52] (► Fig. 10.6).

10.6.1 Forefoot Corrective Procedures

Modified Jones Procedure

- The EHL provides compensatory dorsiflexion in the setting of a weak TA, which leads to cock-up deformity of the hallux.
- Transfer of the EHL to the proximal aspect of the first metatarsal alleviates the clawing deformity at the hallux and facilitates ankle dorsiflexion.[53]
- A modification of this procedure with concomitant arthrodesis of the first interphalangeal joint is typically performed to prevent a floppy toe.[54,55,56]

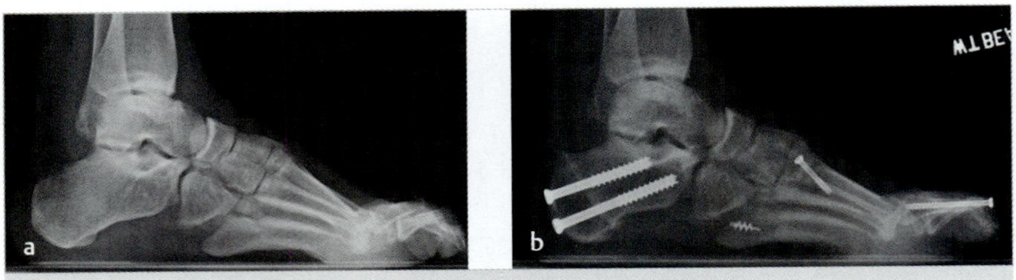

Fig. 10.6 **(a)** Preoperative and **(b)** postoperative weight-bearing lateral radiographs of the foot and ankle of a patient with Charcot–Marie–Tooth disease type 1A (CMT-1A). Surgical reconstruction included a lateral closing wedge calcaneal osteotomy, a dorsiflexion osteotomy of the proximal first metatarsal, a modified Jones transfer, and peroneus longus to peroneus brevis transfer.

- This procedure is most effective for symptoms related to claw toe than for metatarsalgia.[57,58]

Claw-Toe Correction

- Flexible claw toe often spontaneously resolves after correction of the midfoot deformity.
- For deformities that are supple but do not fully correct, a viable option is Girdlestone–Taylor transfer in which the lesser FDL tendon is transferred to the extensor hood.[59,60]
- Proximal interphalangeal joint fusions or metatarsal shortening osteotomies may be considered for those with more rigid deformities.

10.6.2 Soft-Tissue Procedures and Tendon Transfers

Plantar Fascia Release/Steindler Stripping

- The plantar fascia becomes contracted in the chronic cavus foot and may prevent elevation of the metatarsals and contribute to varus positioning of the calcaneus.
- Release of the plantar fascia and abductor hallucis fascia for associated adduction deformities alleviates this.
- More extensive release of structures, including the flexor digitorum brevis, quadratus plantae, and abductor digiti quinti may be performed if required for more complete correction.

Tibialis Anterior Transfer

- TA transfer to the lateral cuneiform converts the inversion moment associated with dorsiflexion to slight eversion moment.
- Strength of at least 4 out of 5 is required for this transfer because one grade of strength is usually lost with transfer.[61]
- A split tendon transfer was traditionally performed to avoid overcorrection. However, transfer of the entire tendon is more reliable, easier to perform, and does not lead to overcorrection.[52,62,63]

Posterior Tibialis Tendon Transfer

- Transfer of the PTT is indicated in patients with profound dorsiflexion weakness, precluding transfer of the TA.[64]
- The tendon is routed to the dorsum of the foot through the interosseous membrane, thereby diminishing the cavus-inducing forces and providing dorsiflexion.
- Alternatively, a spastic posterior tibialis may contribute to deformity in

conditions such as cerebral palsy. A fractional lengthening of the myotendinous junction can be used to address this overpull.

Peroneus Longus to Brevis Transfer

- PL to peroneus brevis (PB) transfer is based upon the concept that the PL plantarflexes the first ray and exacerbates forefoot equinus, and the PB is weak in many neuromuscular pes cavus cases.
- Thus, transfer of the PL to PB removes the deforming force on the first ray and supplements eversion.[52]
- This transfer is of particular importance in cases of CMT.[65]

10.6.3 Bony Procedures

- Osteotomies are needed when there is a bone deformity inhibiting the ability to obtain a plantigrade foot with soft-tissue procedures only.
- They are also used in conjunction with additional procedures to protect or offload concomitant reconstructive procedures.

Medial Column Dorsiflexion Osteotomy

- A plantarflexed first ray creates a valgus position of the foot and relative inversion of the middle and lateral columns.
- This results in more stress on the lateral hindfoot.
- This deformity can be corrected with a dorsal closing wedge osteotomy of the first metatarsal base or medial cuneiform as long as the hindfoot is supple.
- Very favorable outcomes have been reported with this procedure.[52,54,66]
- Arthrodesis with incorporated dorsiflexion may be performed if arthritic changes are present in the tarsometatarsal joint.
- A plantar opening wedge osteotomy may also be attempted in the setting of a relatively short first metatarsal, but dorsal closing wedge osteotomies are inherently stable due to compression with weight bearing.
- Sufficient correction is obtained when the first and fifth metatarsal heads are on the same plane as the calcaneus with neutral ankle dorsiflexion.

Calcaneal Osteotomies

- A lateralizing osteotomy of the calcaneus is indicated in the setting of hindfoot varus and the absence of substantial subtalar arthritis.
- This redistributes weight bearing through the ankle, restores the normal tripod of the foot, and provides a mechanical advantage to the strained lateral foot and ankle structures.
- The Dwyer osteotomy removes a lateral-based wedge to achieve these goals, but similar effects can be obtained with a lateral slide.
- Both a wedge and displacement may be performed if greater correction is desired.
- Care should be taken during these procedures to avoid iatrogenic injury to the strained tibial nerve after realignment.[67]

Midtarsal Osteotomies

- Midtarsal corrective osteotomies are theoretically advantageous in that they are often performed at the apex of the primary deformity.
- However, they are challenging and invariably disrupt midfoot joints.
- Multiple techniques have been described, including Akron dome osteotomies and the Japas V-osteotomy, which requires removal of a dorsal wedge of bone from the midfoot.[68]

- These osteotomies are appropriately considered salvage procedures in severe or recalcitrant cases.[69,70]

Triple Arthrodesis

- Triple arthrodesis is reserved for patients with severe degenerative changes of the hindfoot or extreme rigidity.
- An increased rate of nonunion has been reported in the setting of cavus foot.[65,71,72]
- Late-onset arthritis of the adjacent joints, including the ankle, is a common finding in patients who have undergone a triple arthrodesis for pes cavus, particularly in the setting of CMT.[71,72]
- It should be noted that operative correction of the heel into valgus often induces further plantar flexion of the first ray, and a dorsiflexion osteotomy of the medial column may need to be performed to offset this effect.

Rehabilitation

- Rehabilitation is dictated by the procedures performed.
- In general, patients are initially immobilized postoperatively in a splint and are restricted to non-weight-bearing for 6 weeks after surgery if an osteotomy was performed to allow for sufficient bony healing.
- A removable controlled ankle motion (CAM) walking boot is beneficial when concomitant tendon transfers are performed.
- Gentle non-weight-bearing motion can be started early out of the boot to help prevent formation of adhesions.

10.7 Key Testing Facts

- The pes cavus conformation results in a rigid foot, which inhibits stress dispersion with load bearing and predisposes individuals to acute and overuse injuries.
- Most cases of pes cavus are idiopathic, but pes cavus may also be a sign of underlying neurologic pathology such as CMT and spinal disease.
- A careful history and thorough physical examination is required to direct appropriate neurologic referral and select appropriate treatment.
- Nonoperative management typically consists of a corrective foot orthotic or ankle brace.
- Surgical algorithms are based upon physical examination and radiologic findings.
- In general, motion-preserving procedures such as tendon transfers augmented with corrective osteotomies are preferred over arthrodesis procedures.

References

[1] Aminian A, Sangeorzan BJ. The anatomy of cavus foot deformity. Foot Ankle Clin. 2008; 13(2): 191–198, v

[2] Mann RA. Biomechanical approach to the treatment of foot problems. Foot Ankle. 1982; 2(4): 205–212

[3] Barreto LC, Oliveira FS, Nunes PS, et al. Epidemiologic study of Charcot-Marie-Tooth disease: a systematic review. Neuroepidemiology. 2016; 46(3):157–165

[4] Combarros O, Calleja J, Polo JM, Berciano J. Prevalence of hereditary motor and sensory neuropathy in Cantabria. Acta Neurol Scand. 1987; 75(1):9–12

[5] Bird TD. Charcot-Marie-Tooth hereditary neuropathy overview. 2016. Accessed March 5, 2018 at: https://www.ncbi.nlm.nih.gov/books/NBK1358/

[6] Bird TD. Charcot-Marie-Tooth neuropathy type 1. 2015. Accessed March 5, 2018 at: https://www.ncbi.nlm.nih.gov/books/NBK1205/

[7] Bird TD. Charcot-Marie-Tooth neuropathy type 2. 2016. Accessed March 5, 2018 at: https://www.ncbi.nlm.nih.gov/books/NBK1285/

[8] Bird TD. Charcot-Marie-Tooth neuropathy X type 1. 2016. Accessed March 5, 2018 at: https://www.ncbi.nlm.nih.gov/books/NBK1374/

[9] Bidichandani SI, Delatycki MB. Friedreich ataxia. 1993. Accessed March 1, 2018 at: https://www.ncbi.nlm.nih.gov/books/NBK1281/

[10] Medina PA, Karpman RR, Yeung AT. Split posterior tibial tendon transfer for spastic equinovarus foot deformity. Foot Ankle. 1989; 10(2):65–67

[11] Rivera-Dominguez M, DiBenedetto M, Frisbie JH, Rossier AB. Pes cavus and claw toes deformity in patients with spinal cord injury and multiple sclerosis. Paraplegia. 1979; 16(4):375–382

[12] Morcuende JA, Dolan LA, Dietz FR, Ponseti IV. Radical reduction in the rate of extensive corrective surgery for clubfoot using the Ponseti method. Pediatrics. 2004; 113(2):376–380

[13] Henn RF, III, Crawford DC, Eberson CP, Ehrlich MG. Subtalar release in clubfeet: a retrospective study of 10-year outcomes. Foot Ankle Int. 2008; 29(4): 390–395

[14] Huber H, Dutoit M. Dynamic foot-pressure measurement in the assessment of operatively treated clubfeet. J Bone Joint Surg Am. 2004; 86 (6):1203–1210

[15] Stuecker RD, Bennett JT. Tarsal coalition presenting as a pes cavo-varus deformity: report of three cases and review of the literature. Foot Ankle. 1993; 14(9):540–544

[16] Lintz F, Colombier JA, Letenneur J, Gouin F. Management of long-term sequelae of compartment syndrome involving the foot and ankle. Foot Ankle Int. 2009; 30(9):847–853

[17] Santi MD, Botte MJ. Volkmann's ischemic contracture of the foot and ankle: evaluation and treatment of established deformity. Foot Ankle Int. 1995; 16(6): 368–377

[18] Manoli A, II, Graham B. The subtle cavus foot, "the underpronator." Foot Ankle Int. 2005; 26(3): 256–263

[19] Di Fabio R, Lispi L, Santorelli FM, et al. Idiopathic pes cavus in adults is not associated with neurophysiological impairment in the lower limbs. Neurol Sci. 2015; 36(12):2287–2290

[20] Buldt AK, Levinger P, Murley GS, Menz HB, Nester CJ, Landorf KB. Foot posture is associated with kinematics of the foot during gait: a comparison of normal, planus and cavus feet. Gait Posture. 2015; 42(1):42–48

[21] Riskowski JL, Dufour AB, Hagedorn TJ, Hillstrom HJ, Casey VA, Hannan MT. Associations of foot posture and function to lower extremity pain: results from a population-based foot study. Arthritis Care Res (Hoboken). 2013; 65(11):1804–1812

[22] Van Bergeyk AB, Younger A, Carson B. CT analysis of hindfoot alignment in chronic lateral ankle instability. Foot Ankle Int. 2002; 23(1):37–42

[23] Csizy M, Hintermann B. Dwyer osteotomy with or without lateral stabilization in calcaneus varus with lateral ligament insufficiency of the upper ankle joint. Sportverletz Sportschaden. 1996; 10 (4):100–102

[24] Fortin PT, Guettler J, Manoli A, II. Idiopathic cavovarus and lateral ankle instability: recognition and treatment implications relating to ankle arthritis. Foot Ankle Int. 2002; 23(11):1031–1037

[25] Strauss JE, Forsberg JA, Lippert FG, III. Chronic lateral ankle instability and associated conditions: a rationale for treatment. Foot Ankle Int. 2007; 28 (10):1041–1044

[26] Vienne P, Schöniger R, Helmy N, Espinosa N. Hindfoot instability in cavovarus deformity: static and dynamic balancing. Foot Ankle Int. 2007; 28 (1):96–102

[27] Irwin TA, Anderson RB, Davis WH, Cohen BE. Effect of ankle arthritis on clinical outcome of lateral ankle ligament reconstruction in cavovarus feet. Foot Ankle Int. 2010; 31(11):941–948

[28] Jung HG, Jeon SH, Kim TH, Park JT. Total ankle arthroplasty with combined calcaneal and metatarsal osteotomies for treatment of ankle osteoarthritis with accompanying cavovarus deformities: early results. Foot Ankle Int. 2013; 34(1):140–147

[29] Krause F, Windolf M, Schwieger K, Weber M. Ankle joint pressure in pes cavovarus. J Bone Joint Surg Br. 2007; 89(12):1660–1665

[30] Schmid T, Zurbriggen S, Zderic I, Gueorguiev B, Weber M, Krause FG. Ankle joint pressure changes in a pes cavovarus model: supramalleolar valgus osteotomy versus lateralizing calcaneal osteotomy. Foot Ankle Int. 2013; 34(9):1190–1197

[31] DiGiovanni CW, Kuo R, Tejwani N, et al. Isolated gastrocnemius tightness. J Bone Joint Surg Am. 2002; 84(6):962–970

[32] Maskill MP, Maskill JD, Pomeroy GC. Surgical management and treatment algorithm for the subtle cavovarus foot. Foot Ankle Int. 2010; 31(12): 1057–1063

[33] Morales-Muñoz P, De Los Santos Real R, Barrio Sanz P, Pérez JL, Varas Navas J, Escalera Alonso J. Proximal gastrocnemius release in the treatment of mechanical metatarsalgia. Foot Ankle Int. 2016; 37 (7):782–789

[34] Bluth B, Eagan M, Otsuka NY. Stress fractures of the lateral rays in the cavovarus foot: indication for surgical intervention. Orthopedics. 2011; 34(10): e696–e699

[35] Cavanagh PR, Morag E, Boulton AJ, Young MJ, Deffner KT, Pammer SE. The relationship of static foot structure to dynamic foot function. J Biomech. 1997; 30(3):243–250

[36] McCluskey WP, Lovell WW, Cummings RJ. The cavovarus foot deformity. Etiology and management. Clin Orthop Relat Res. 1989(247):27–37

[37] Lee KT, Park YU, Jegal H, Kim KC, Young KW, Kim JS. Factors associated with recurrent fifth metatarsal stress fracture. Foot Ankle Int. 2013; 34 (12):1645–1653

[38] Raikin SM, Slenker N, Ratigan B. The association of a varus hindfoot and fracture of the fifth metatarsal metaphyseal-diaphyseal junction: the Jones fracture. Am J Sports Med. 2008; 36(7):1367–1372

[39] Brandes CB, Smith RW. Characterization of patients with primary peroneus longus tendinopathy: a review of twenty-two cases. Foot Ankle Int. 2000; 21(6):462–468

[40] Sobel M, Geppert MJ, Warren RF. Chronic ankle instability as a cause of peroneal tendon injury. Clin Orthop Relat Res. 1993(296):187–191

[41] Podolnick JD, Donovan DS, DeBellis N, Pino A. Is pes cavus alignment associated with Lisfranc injuries of the foot? Clin Orthop Relat Res. 2017; 475(5): 1463–1469

[42] Fields KB, Sykes JC, Walker KM, Jackson JC. Prevention of running injuries. Curr Sports Med Rep. 2010; 9(3):176–182

[43] Simkin A, Leichter I, Giladi M, Stein M, Milgrom C. Combined effect of foot arch structure and an orthotic device on stress fractures. Foot Ankle. 1989; 10(1):25–29

[44] Williams DS, III, McClay IS, Hamill J. Arch structure and injury patterns in runners. Clin Biomech (Bristol, Avon). 2001; 16(4):341–347

[45] Steel MW, III, Johnson KA, DeWitz MA, Ilstrup DM. Radiographic measurements of the normal adult foot. Foot Ankle. 1980; 1(3):151–158

[46] Gould N. Graphing the adult foot and ankle. Foot Ankle. 1982; 2(4):213–219

[47] Robinow M, Johnston M, Anderson M. Feet of normal children: a study of lateral X-rays of the weight-bearing foot. J Pediatr. 1943; 23:141–149

[48] O'Neill PJ, Van Aman SE, Guyton GP. Is MRI adequate to detect lesions in patients with ankle instability? Clin Orthop Relat Res. 2010; 468(4): 1115–1119

[49] Burns J, Crosbie J, Ouvrier R, Hunt A. Effective orthotic therapy for the painful cavus foot: a randomized controlled trial. J Am Podiatr Med Assoc. 2006; 96(3):205–211

[50] Hawke F, Burns J, Radford JA, du Toit V. Custom-made foot orthoses for the treatment of foot pain. Cochrane Database Syst Rev. 2008(3):CD006801

[51] LoPiccolo M, Chilvers M, Graham B, Manoli A, II. Effectiveness of the cavus foot orthosis. J Surg Orthop Adv. 2010; 19(3):166–169

[52] Ward CM, Dolan LA, Bennett DL, Morcuende JA, Cooper RR. Long-term results of reconstruction for treatment of a flexible cavovarus foot in Charcot-Marie-Tooth disease. J Bone Joint Surg Am. 2008; 90(12):2631–2642

[53] Paulos L, Coleman SS, Samuelson KM. Pes cavovarus. Review of a surgical approach using selective soft-tissue procedures. J Bone Joint Surg Am. 1980; 62(6):942–953

[54] Faldini C, Traina F, Nanni M, et al. Surgical treatment of cavus foot in Charcot-Marie-tooth disease: a review of twenty-four cases: AAOS exhibit selection. J Bone Joint Surg Am. 2015; 97(6):e30

[55] Giannini S, Girolami M, Ceccarelli F, Maffei G. Modified Jones operation in the treatment of pes cavovarus. Ital J Orthop Traumatol. 1985; 11(2): 165–170

[56] M'Bamali EI. Results of modified Robert Jones operation for clawed hallux. Br J Surg. 1975; 62(8): 647–650

[57] Breusch SJ, Wenz W, Döderlein L. Function after correction of a clawed great toe by a modified Robert Jones transfer. J Bone Joint Surg Br. 2000; 82 (2):250–254

[58] Tynan MC, Klenerman L. The modified Robert Jones tendon transfer in cases of pes cavus and clawed hallux. Foot Ankle Int. 1994; 15(2):68–71

[59] Barbari SG, Brevig K. Correction of clawtoes by the Girdlestone-Taylor flexor-extensor transfer procedure. Foot Ankle. 1984; 5(2):67–73

[60] Cyphers SM, Feiwell E. Review of the Girdlestone-Taylor procedure for clawtoes in myelodysplasia. Foot Ankle. 1988; 8(5):229–233

[61] Samilson RL, Dillin W. Cavus, cavovarus, and calcaneocavus. An update. Clin Orthop Relat Res. 1983(177):125–132

[62] Henderson CP, Parks BG, Guyton GP. Lateral and medial plantar pressures after split versus whole anterior tibialis tendon transfer. Foot Ankle Int. 2008; 29(10):1038–1041

[63] Knutsen AR, Avoian T, Sangiorgio SN, Borkowski SL, Ebramzadeh E, Zionts LE. How do different anterior tibial tendon transfer techniques influence forefoot and hindfoot motion? Clin Orthop Relat Res. 2015; 473(5):1737–1743

[64] Dreher T, Wolf SI, Heitzmann D, Fremd C, Klotz MC, Wenz W. Tibialis posterior tendon transfer corrects the foot drop component of cavovarus foot deformity in Charcot-Marie-Tooth disease. J Bone Joint Surg Am. 2014; 96(6):456–462

[65] Mann DC, Hsu JD. Triple arthrodesis in the treatment of fixed cavovarus deformity in adolescent patients with Charcot-Marie-Tooth disease. Foot Ankle. 1992; 13(1):1–6

[66] Leeuwesteijn AE, de Visser E, Louwerens JW. Flexible cavovarus feet in Charcot-Marie-Tooth disease treated with first ray proximal dorsiflexion osteotomy combined with soft tissue surgery: a short-term to mid-term outcome study. Foot Ankle Surg. 2010; 16(3):142–147

[67] VanValkenburg S, Hsu RY, Palmer DS, Blankenhorn B, Den Hartog BD, DiGiovanni CW. Neurologic deficit associated with lateralizing calcaneal osteotomy for cavovarus foot correction. Foot Ankle Int. 2016; 37 (10):1106–1112

[68] Japas LM. Surgical treatment of pes cavus by tarsal V-osteotomy. Preliminary report. J Bone Joint Surg Am. 1968; 50(5):927–944

[69] Bennett GL, Weiner DS, Leighley B. Surgical treatment of symptomatic accessory tarsal navicular. J Pediatr Orthop. 1990; 10(4):445–449

[70] Wicart P, Seringe R. Plantar opening-wedge osteotomy of cuneiform bones combined with selective plantar release and Dwyer osteotomy for pes cavovarus in children. J Pediatr Orthop. 2006; 26(1):100–108

[71] Wetmore RS, Drennan JC. Long-term results of triple arthrodesis in Charcot-Marie-Tooth disease. J Bone Joint Surg Am. 1989; 71(3):417–422

[72] Wukich DK, Bowen JR. A long-term study of triple arthrodesis for correction of pes cavovarus in Charcot-Marie-Tooth disease. J Pediatr Orthop. 1989; 9(4):433–437

11 Heel Pain

Austin R. Davidson and Clayton C. Bettin

Abstract

Heel pain is a very common presenting complaint to both the foot and ankle specialist and the general health care provider. A significant number of people will deal with heel pain during their life. Most causes of heel pain are self-limiting (although may be slow to resolve) and amenable to a variety of conservative treatment modalities.

Keywords: heel pain, plantar fasciitis, neuropathy, tarsal tunnel

11.1 Introduction

- Heel pain is a very common presenting complaint accounting for nearly 2 million patient visits per year.[1,2,3,4,5]
- Between 4 and 7% of adults will endorse heel pain at some point during their adult life.[6,7]
- History often gives diagnosis prior to physical examination.
- Careful physical examination will often pinpoint etiology based on point of maximal tenderness (▸ Fig. 11.1).
- Imaging is usually not necessary at initial visit (unless warning signs are present).

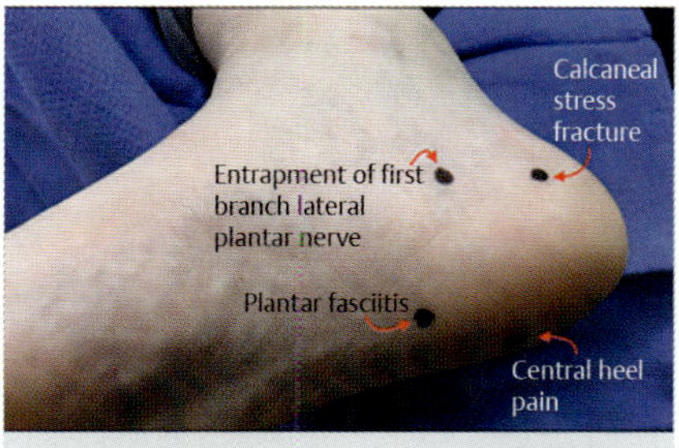

Fig. 11.1 Photograph demonstrating point of maximal tenderness in the heel and corresponding diagnosis.

11.2 Plantar Fasciitis

- **Etiology:**
  - From a histologic perspective, plantar fasciitis is a fibrofatty degeneration and microtearing of the plantar fascia origin with collagen necrosis.[8]
- **Anatomy:**
  - *Plantar fascia:* inelastic fibrous bands from anteromedial calcaneus to proximal phalanges.
  - Responsible for the windlass mechanism of the foot: dorsiflexion of the metatarsophalangeal (MTP) joints with heel rise from gastrocnemius contraction during gait leads to arch elevation and supination of the foot, which stabilizes the medial column during gait propulsion.
- **Symptoms:**
  - Classic description is startup inferior heel pain (typically first thing in the morning or after prolonged sitting).
  - Patients will often ambulate on toes with the first few steps.
  - They will commonly have a gastrocnemius contracture.[9]
- **Diagnosis:**
  - The patient's history and symptoms will typically give the diagnosis, but it can be confirmed with physical examination.
  - Point of maximal tenderness is located at the proximal medial origin of the plantar fascia.
  - The examination sensitivity is increased with dorsiflexion of the toes and ankle while palpating the origin of the plantar fascia.
  - Given the significant association of tightness in dorsiflexion, the ankle should be assessed for gastrocnemius tightness with the **Silfverskiöld** test: dorsiflexion tested with both the knee flexed and extended.

- *Imaging:*
  - As with most causes of heel pain, plain radiographs will often be normal.
  - Radiographs may reveal heel spur, which patients will often associate with the pain. Many patients may concurrently have both heel pain and a heel spur, but the general population will have an asymptomatic heel spur at a very similar rate.[10]
  - Bone formation is the end result of chronic inflammation, which is why "bone spurs" may be found in the substance of the plantar fascia in long-standing plantar fasciitis.
  - There have been reports suggesting intrasubstance spurs as being a marker of plantar fasciitis severity; however, more investigation is needed to clearly link a classification of heel spurs as a causative factor (rather than result) of plantar fasciitis.[11]
  - Magnetic resonance imaging (MRI) may show thickening of plantar fascia with or without edema, but is not typically necessary for diagnosis.
  - Laboratory studies provide limited additional information except for those patients in which other etiologies are suspected, such as hypovitaminosis D and stress fracture.

- **Conservative management:**
  - In all cases of plantar fasciitis, nonsurgical treatment should be the initial pathway as over 90% of patients will improve with nonoperative management.[12]
  - American Orthopaedic Foot and Ankle Society (AOFAS) recommends a minimum of 6 to 12 months of nonoperative treatment prior to operative intervention due to high success of various treatment modalities and natural history of plantar fasciitis.[13]
  - *Shoe wear and activity modifications are important:*
    - Avoiding barefoot activities: properly cushioned and supportive shoes should be worn.
    - Rocker bottom sole to reduce first MTP dorsiflexion, which in turn reduces peak tensile strength of plantar fascia.
    - Prefabricated inserts have shown equivalent improvement compared with custom insoles.[14]
  - *Plantar fascia-specific stretching (PFSS)*:
    - Maintain passive ankle and toe dorsiflexion position with concurrent palpation/massage of taut bands of plantar fascia.
    - Shown to have improved results at 8 weeks when compared with Achilles stretching program, although results are similar at the 2-year mark (▶ Fig. 11.2).[15,16]
  - *Night splint*:
    - Functions by keeping the ankle in dorsiflexed position during sleep to prevent the plantar fascia from contracting.
    - Night splints show good results, especially with decreasing the first-step pain within the first month, but studies show a significant percentage of patients do not tolerate the splints (i.e., discomfort, interrupting

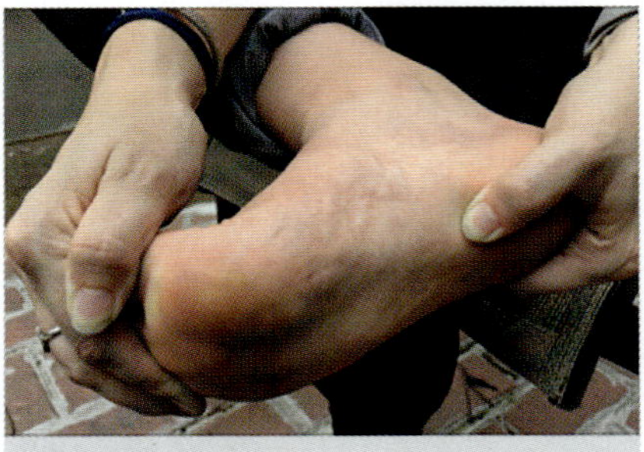

Fig. 11.2 Photograph demonstrating plantar fascia–specific stretching: dorsiflexion of the ankle and first ray, slight eversion, and massage of the plantar fascia origin.

sleeping habits) and will discontinue use even with positive results.[17,18]
- *Corticosteroid injections*:
  - Generally not recommended due to lack of evidence for long-term benefit and association with complications (plantar fascia ruptures, plantar fat pad atrophy).[19]
  - Might see some improvement at 1 month but no better results at 3 or 6 months.[20,21]
- *Other treatment options*:
  - Nonsteroidal anti-inflammatory drugs (NSAIDs): commonly used in the treatment of plantar fasciitis, but reliable evidence of usefulness is limited.
  - Extracorporeal shock wave therapy: encouraging initial results with success rates between 50 and 65% although further study is needed. Additionally, at this time most insurance companies do not cover the treatment and may result in out-of-pocket expense for the patient.[22]
  - Positive results have been seen with botulinum toxin injections into both the plantar fascia and gastrocnemius–soleus complex at 1, 6, and 12 months.[23,24]
  - Platelet-rich plasma (PRP) injections have shown promise in long-term relief of chronic plantar fasciitis[25]; however, head-to-head studies between PRP and corticosteroid injections show mixed results—either no difference between the two[26] or better improvement short term with corticosteroid and improved long-term outcomes with PRP.[27]

- **Surgery**:
  - An option if the patient has failed 9 to 12 months of nonoperative management.
  - *Open versus endoscopic release of plantar fascia:*
    - Goal is releasing the medial one-third to two-thirds of fascia.
    - Endoscopic release patients returned to work quicker when compared to open release patients (6 vs. 10 weeks) with a slightly higher complication rate; similar long-term results.[28,29]
  - *Gastrocnemius recession*:
    - Popular option as many patients with plantar fasciitis often have concomitant gastrocnemius contracture.
    - Majority of surgeons choose to include gastrocnemius recession as part of the operative intervention, either as isolated procedure or in combination with plantar fascia release.[30]
    - Positive results with quicker recovery and higher patient satisfaction have been reported with isolated proximal medial gastrocnemius recession when compared with partial plantar fascia release.[31]
  - *Complications:* damage to lateral plantar nerve, complete fascia rupture (which leads to loss of medial longitudinal arch), stress reaction of dorsolateral midfoot, and continued pain.

11.3 Fat Pad Atrophy/Contusion

- **Etiology**:
  - Typically begins in the fifth decade of life if there is no history of trauma or inciting event (e.g., blunt trauma).
  - Decreased levels of water, collagen, and elastic tissue within the fat pad lead to atrophy of fat pad.
  - Can be associated with corticosteroid injections, inflammatory disease, or trauma that damages the fibroelastic septa.
- **Anatomy**:
  - Fat pad consists of honeycomb fibroelastic septa anchored to

calcaneus and skin with transverse fibers serving as reinforcement (▶ Fig. 11.3).
  - The calcaneus sees 110% of body weight during heel strike while walking, up to 250% while running.[32]
- **Symptoms**:
  - More central and proximal heel pain when compared with plantar fasciitis.
  - Erythema and inflammation may occur in this condition.
  - Exacerbated while walking barefoot, relieved by absence of heel pressure.
- **Diagnosis**:
  - Clinical diagnosis; radiographs are typically not necessary.
  - May see increased mobility of fat pad from calcaneal tuberosity.
  - Pain is often not reproducible during examination.
- **Conservative management**:
  - Nonoperative management is the mainstay of treatment.
  - Symptomatic relief with heel cups or full-length insoles that offload the heel.
- **Surgery**:
  - No proven techniques have been found.
  - Some reports of success with subdermal silicone injection to recreate the anatomy, however there are no high-quality studies evaluating safety or efficacy.[33]

11.4 Calcaneal Stress Fracture

- **Etiology**:
  - Caused by repetitive loading of calcaneus and an inability for the bone formation to match resorption.[34]
  - Calcaneus remains primarily cancellous bone despite chronic loading during gait cycle.
  - Highest incidence of calcaneal stress fracture is seen in female military recruits and athletes.[35]
  - The pull of the Achilles in resisted plantar flexion leads to the characteristic fracture line.
- **Symptoms**:
  - Often will present with insidious onset around 7 to 10 days after increase in physical activity.
  - Noted to have high incidence in military recruits, especially those who had been relatively sedentary prior to beginning training.
  - Pain is worsened with activity and weight bearing.
  - If acute, swelling in the region of the precalcaneal bursa may be present; however, there is often little to no swelling due to a delayed presentation.
  - The "female athlete triad" of disordered eating, amenorrhea, and osteoporosis may be present.

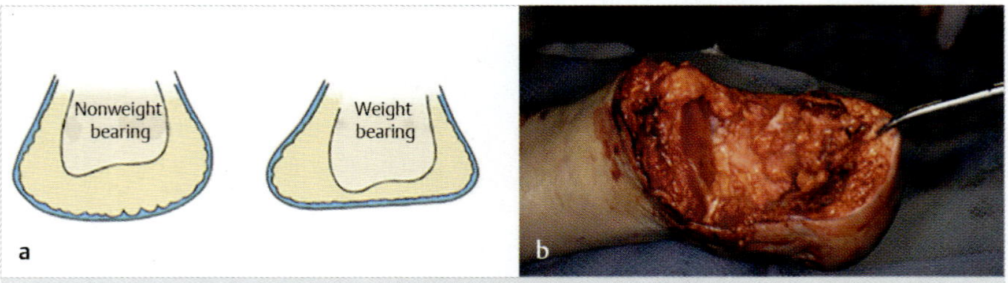

Fig. 11.3 (a) Illustration displaying coronal view of the heel pad, both non-weight-bearing and weight bearing. **(b)** Intraoperative photograph from Syme amputation, hemostat pointing to heel pad with calcaneus and talus removed. (Reproduced with permission of Azar FM, Beaty JH, Canale ST, eds. Campbell's Operative Orthopaedics. 13th ed. Philadelphia, PA: Elsevier; 2017:669.)

- **Diagnosis**:
  - Pathognomonic sign is a positive calcaneal squeeze test: pain on compression of the medial and lateral calcaneal tuberosities.
  - ***Imaging:***
    - Findings on plain radiographs may be present 10 to 14 days after onset, but will often be interpreted as negative initially.
    - Characteristic (although uncommon) finding is fracture line in the posterosuperior aspect of the calcaneus that is perpendicular to the trabecular stress lines of the calcaneus.
    - Highest likelihood of abnormal radiographs is at 6 weeks.
    - Technetium bone scans can detect stress fracture as early as 2 to 8 days after onset.
    - MRI may reveal edema in the posterior aspect of the calcaneus[36] (▶ Fig. 11.4).
    - Both bone scans and MRI have a relatively high false-positive rate.
- **Conservative management**:
  - Mainstay of treatment is activity modification with avoidance of high-impact or painful activities and for 4 to 8 weeks.
  - If significant pain during ambulation, a weight-bearing cast or boot may be useful.
  - As symptoms improve, transition to regular shoes and nonimpact activity.
  - Not necessary to follow radiographically as clinical resolution serves as the marker of healing.
  - If the patient has a previous history of stress fracture or any other warning signs of metabolic disorder, consider a metabolic workup including vitamin D. High prevalence of hypovitaminosis D in the general population even without predisposing risk factors.[37]
- **Surgery**:
  - No role for surgical intervention in most cases.
  - Only indication would be displacement of fracture, which is exceedingly rare.

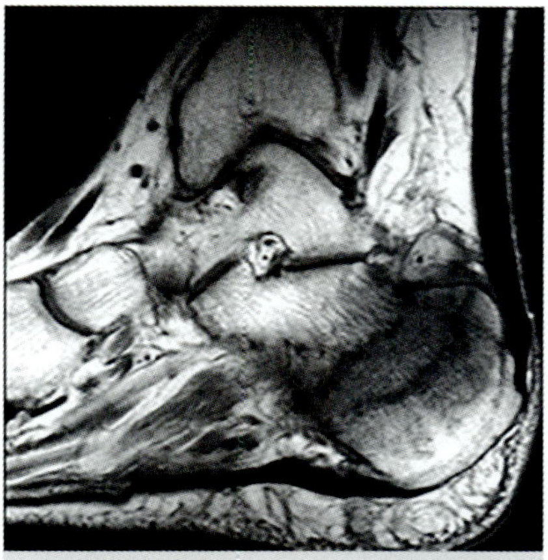

Fig. 11.4 Magnetic resonance imaging (MRI) showing characteristic edema tracking along fracture line.

11.5 Entrapment of the First Branch of the Lateral Plantar Nerve (Baxter's Nerve) (also refer to chapter 17)

- **Etiology**:
  - Most common etiology is compression of the first branch of the lateral plantar nerve between the deep fascia of the abductor hallucis and the inferomedial margin of the quadratus plantae.[38,39]
  - Has also been described as occurring between the flexor digitorum brevis and calcaneus, adjacent to the medial calcaneal tuberosity.
  - More common in athletes on their toes for substantial amount of time (i.e., sprinters, ballet dancers).
- **Anatomy**:
  - First branch of the lateral plantar nerve is a distal branch of the tibial nerve providing motor and sensory functions.

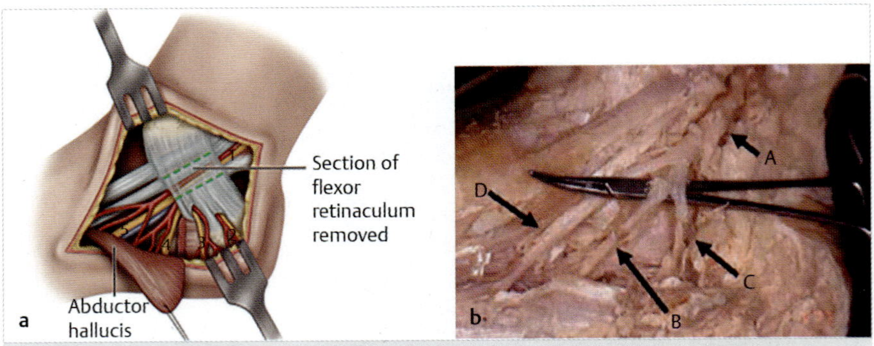

Fig. 11.5 **(a)** Illustration of tibial nerve branching: tibial nerve (1), medial calcaneal branches (2 and 3), first branch of lateral plantar nerve (4), and lateral plantar nerve (5). (Reproduced with permission of Azar FM, Beaty JH, Canale ST, eds. Campbell's Operative Orthopaedics. 13th ed. Philadelphia, PA: Elsevier; 2017:4216.) **(b)** Cadaveric specimen displaying tibial nerve branching: tibial nerve (A), lateral plantar nerve (B), first branch of lateral plantar nerve (C), and medial plantar nerve (D). (Reproduced with permission from Leiberman.[2])

 - Branches deep to the fascia of the abductor hallucis and the flexor hallucis brevis, just distal to the medial process of the calcaneal tuberosity (▶ Fig. 11.5).
 - Innervates the calcaneal periosteum, flexor digitorum brevis, and abductor digiti quinti.
- **Symptoms**:
 - Presents as chronic medial plantar heel pain.
 - Patients will complain of medial-based heel pain that may radiate proximally or distally along the course of the tibial nerve with possible burning or tingling quality.
 - Similar location of pain to that of plantar fasciitis; however, the first branch lateral plantar nerve entrapment neuropathy will tend to worsen with activity and exacerbated by eversion and abduction of the foot.
 - Some patients will describe paresthesias with running.
- **Diagnosis**:
 - Physical examination finding may include a pain with the "dorsiflexion–eversion test" (dorsiflexion and eversion of the ankle in combination with full extension of the MTP joints), although this test is more specific to tarsal tunnel syndrome.
 - Tender to palpation deep to the abductor hallucis, which might cause radiation of pain proximally or distally.
 - Might see positive Tinel's sign in the nerve distribution.
 - Although long-standing cases may produce atrophy of the abductor digiti quinti, this finding is difficult to detect.
 - *Imaging:*
   - Radiographs add little to diagnosis; however, they may reveal bony abnormalities that are contributing to the compression.
   - MRI may show space-occupying lesion or muscle denervation (either acute or chronic); however, MRI is not necessary for diagnosis.
- **Conservative management**:
 - Similar treatment algorithm as to plantar fasciitis: rest, NSAIDs, activity modification, stretching, and ice for at least 6 months.
 - Cross-training to decrease high-impact exercises that could exacerbate symptoms.

 - Insoles that provide medial longitudinal arch support may prove beneficial, especially with patients who exhibit excessive pronation.
 - Local irritation from the insert is possible.
- **Surgery**:
 - Indicated after failure of prolonged conservative management unless space-occupying lesion found on MRI.
 - Perform open decompression of nerve releasing the abductor hallucis fascia and follow nerve both proximally and distally releasing any other areas of entrapment.
 - May also perform partial plantar fascia release at the same time as there will often be some compression from the plantar fascia and some patients will have concomitant plantar fasciitis.[40]
 - Reports of 90% patient satisfaction with combined nerve decompression and partial plantar fascia release.[40,41]

11.6 Tarsal Tunnel Syndrome (also refer to chapter 17)

- **Etiology**:
 - Chronic compression of the tibial nerve as it passes through the tarsal tunnel on the medial portion of the ankle.
 - Associated with pes planus due to the increased stress and tension placed on the nerve due to the hindfoot valgus and forefoot abduction.[42]
 - Other potential causes of compression include fracture, space-occupying lesions, tenosynovitis, accessory abductor hallucis muscle, and iatrogenic tethering after lateral displacement calcaneal osteotomy.
- **Anatomy**:
 - Fibro-osseous space located posterior and distal to the medial malleolus.
 - Bordered by the flexor retinaculum as the roof; medial wall of the calcaneus serves as the floor.
 - *Contents of tarsal tunnel:* posterior tibial neurovascular bundle, posterior tibial tendon, flexor digitorum longus tendon, and flexor hallucis longus tendon.
- **Symptoms**:
 - Often vague medial ankle and heel pain that radiates distally into the foot.
 - Discomfort exacerbated by activity, alleviated with rest.
 - Pain, paresthesias, and dysesthesias may be present.
 - Weakness and atrophy noted first in hallux abduction; rarely clinically evident until the very end stages of the disease process.
- **Diagnosis**:
 - Similar physical examination as entrapment of the first branch of the lateral plantar nerve although findings will be more proximal.
 - The patient will typically have positive Tinel's sign along the tarsal tunnel.
 - Provocative tests include the dorsiflexion–eversion test placing the tibial nerve on tension and triple compression test (plantar flexion and inversion with pressure on the posterior tibial nerve shows sensitivity of 85% and specificity of 100%).[43]
 - *Imaging:*
   - Radiographs will occasionally highlight bony/structural abnormality contributing to compression.
   - Ultrasonography may reliably identify compression in a cost-effective manner; however, results are heavily operator dependent.[44]
   - MRI will show detailed anatomy of tarsal tunnel as well as detecting possible space-occupying lesion.
   - Nerve conduction velocity (NCV) and electromyographic (EMG) studies may be used to assist in the diagnosis, although there is a high false-negative rate.[45]

- **Conservative management**:
  - Initial treatment should include a combination of rest, NSAIDs, activity modification, stretching, and ice.
  - Given the association of pes planus and tarsal tunnel syndrome, orthoses that provide good medial support may alleviate symptoms.
  - Some authors recommend corticosteroid injections; these injections introduce potential complications of intravascular infiltration and tendon rupture.
- **Surgery**:
  - Failure of prolonged conservative treatment or space-occupying lesion serves as indication for surgical intervention (▶ Fig. 11.6).
  - Complete release of flexor retinaculum overlying the tarsal tunnel is critical to success; incomplete release may lead to recurrence or continued pain.
  - Release of plantar fascia overlying the distal branches of the tibial nerve has been advocated as the method for ensuring complete decompression.
  - Early decompression may lead to improved results; however, conservative management should be attempted in all patients.
  - Potential complications include continued symptoms secondary to an incomplete release or scar formation and iatrogenic neurovascular injury.

11.7 Complex Regional Pain Syndrome

- This is a complex constellation of neurologic-type symptoms occasionally presenting as heel pain.[46]
- It is often a result of minor trauma or possibly precipitated by a surgical procedure; occasionally, no discernible inciting event is identified.
- Symptoms include allodynia, hyperesthesia, dysesthesias, edema, erythema, hyperhidrosis, dryness/scaling, toenail changes, hair-growth changes, skin atrophy, skin rash, and skin temperature changes.
- Treatment involves a combination of physical therapy (with desensitization), topical analgesics, oral tricyclic

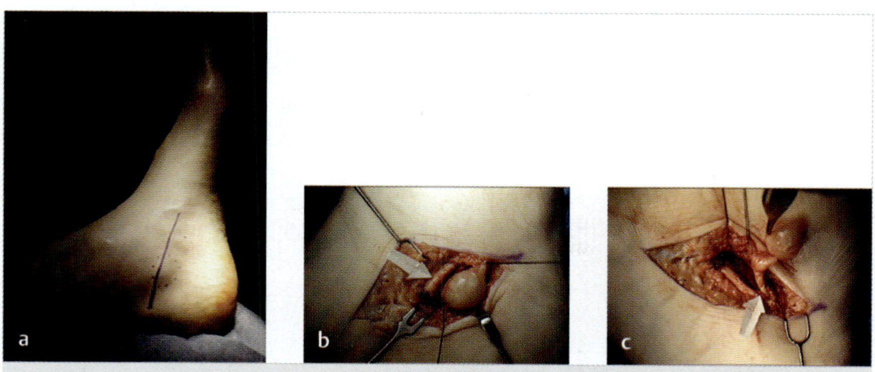

Fig. 11.6 Images depicting removal of tarsal tunnel ganglion. **(a)** Planned surgical incision. **(b)** Ganglion clearly present in tarsal tunnel; the *arrow* points to the lateral plantar nerve. **(c)** Removal of mass allows for effective decompression. (Reproduced with permission of Azar FM, Beaty JH, Canale ST, eds. Campbell's Operative Orthopaedics. 13th ed. Philadelphia, PA: Elsevier; 2017:4217.)

antidepressants or neuromodulators (gabapentin, pregabalin), and/or regional anesthesia.

11.8 Tumor

- Most common tumor of the calcaneus is osteoid osteoma.[47]
  - Most commonly found in males, aged 5 to 25 years.
  - Classic symptom of nocturnal pain relieved by NSAIDs; may complain of activity-related pain as well.
  - Plain radiographs may be normal (may reveal cortical thickening); computed tomography (CT) considered diagnostic and provides the clearest detail of the lesion.[48]
  - It may regress spontaneously; however, symptoms will dictate the need for intervention.
  - Key to successful treatment is removal of nidus, either with radiofrequency ablation or curettage; en bloc resection is rarely necessary.
- Simple (unicameral) bone cysts (UBC) may be found in the anterolateral calcaneus.
  - Radiolucent bone cyst with benign appearing features (▶ Fig. 11.7).

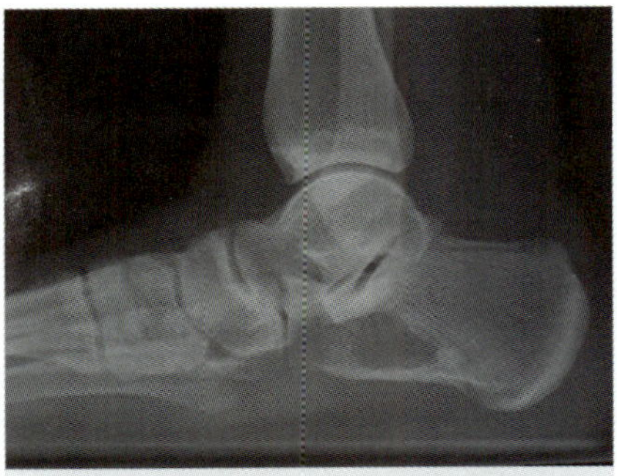

Fig. 11.7 Radiograph displaying calcaneal bone cyst.

  - Most commonly asymptomatic and found incidentally, but may occasionally cause heel pain.
  - Will often persist into adulthood, unlike most other UBCs.
  - Typically followed radiographically; intervention only needed if it becomes symptomatic or pathologic fracture.
  - Treatment involves corticosteroid injections, injection of allograft, or curettage and grafting.[49]

11.9 Key Testing Facts

- Most causes of heel pain are self-limited (although slow to resolve) or amenable to nonsurgical management
- Plantar fascia–specific stretching has shown superior results to other methods of stretching the foot and ankle for relief of plantar fascia pain
- Corticosteroid injections as treatment of plantar fasciitis bring with them complications and no long-term benefits
- Promising conservative treatment modalities for plantar fasciitis include PRP injections, botulinum A injections, and extracorporeal shock wave therapy
- Calcaneal squeeze test is pathognomonic for calcaneus stress fractures
- The tibial nerve may be entrapped within the tarsal tunnel or more distally after the first branch of the lateral plantar nerve
- Entrapment of the first branch of the lateral plantar nerve most commonly occurs between the deep fascia of the abductor hallucis and the inferomedial margin of the quadratus plantae
- The most common cause of recurrence of entrapment neuropathies after surgical release is inadequate release during the original procedure
- Atypical presentations of heel pain require more thorough workup, including advanced imaging and blood work, to rule out insufficiency fractures or tumors

References

[1] DiGiovanni BF, Dawson LK, Baumhauer JF. Plantar heel pain. In: Coughlin MJ, Saltzman CL, Anderson RB, eds. Mann's Surgery of the Foot and Ankle. Philadelphia, PA: Elsevier Saunders; 2014:685–701

[2] JR Lieberman: AAOS Comprehensive Orthopaedic Review 3. Wolters Kluwer Health: American Academy of Orthopaedic Surgeons; 2019

[3] Lareau CR, Sawyer GA, Wang JH, DiGiovanni CW. Plantar and medial heel pain: diagnosis and management. J Am Acad Orthop Surg. 2014; 22(6): 372–380

[4] Pfeffer G, Bacchetti P, Deland J, et al. Comparison of custom and prefabricated orthoses in the initial treatment of proximal plantar fasciitis. Foot Ankle Int. 1999; 20(4):214–221

[5] Riddle DL, Schappert SM. Volume of ambulatory care visits and patterns of care for patients diagnosed with plantar fasciitis: a national study of medical doctors. Foot Ankle Int. 2004; 25(5): 303–310

[6] Dunn JE, Link CL, Felson DT, Crincoli MG, Keysor JJ, McKinlay JB. Prevalence of foot and ankle conditions in a multiethnic community sample of older adults. Am J Epidemiol. 2004; 159(5):491–498

[7] Hill CL, Gill TK, Menz HB, Taylor AW. Prevalence and correlates of foot pain in a population-based study: the North West Adelaide health study. J Foot Ankle Res. 2008; 1(1):2

[8] Lemont H, Ammirati KM, Usen N. Plantar fasciitis: a degenerative process (fasciosis) without inflammation. J Am Podiatr Med Assoc. 2003; 93 (3):234–237

[9] Patel A, DiGiovanni B. Association between plantar fasciitis and isolated contracture of the gastrocnemius. Foot Ankle Int. 2011; 32(1):5–8

[10] Williams PL, Smibert JG, Cox R, Mitchell R, Klenerman L. Imaging study of the painful heel syndrome. Foot Ankle. 1987; 7(6):345–349

[11] Zhou B, Zhou Y, Tao X, Yuan C, Tang K. Classification of calcaneal spurs and their relationship with plantar fasciitis. J Foot Ankle Surg. 2015; 54(4):594–600

[12] Davis PF, Severud E, Baxter DE. Painful heel syndrome: results of nonoperative treatment. Foot Ankle Int. 1994; 15(10):531–535

[13] American Orthopaedic Foot and Ankle Society. AOFAS information page on plantar fasciitis. Accessed March 4 2017 at: http://www.aofas.org/footcaremd/treatments/Pages/Plantar-Fascia-Release.aspx

[14] Landorf KB, Keenan AM, Herbert RD. Effectiveness of foot orthoses to treat plantar fasciitis: a randomized trial. Arch Intern Med. 2006; 166(12): 1305–1310

[15] DiGiovanni BF, Nawoczenski DA, Lintal ME, et al. Tissue-specific plantar fascia-stretching exercise enhances outcomes in patients with chronic heel pain. A prospective, randomized study. J Bone Joint Surg Am. 2003; 85(7):1270–1277

[16] Digiovanni BF, Nawoczenski DA, Malay DP, et al. Plantar fascia-specific stretching exercise improves outcomes in patients with chronic plantar fasciitis. A prospective clinical trial with two-year follow-up. J Bone Joint Surg Am. 2006; 88(8):1775–1781

[17] Martin JE, Hosch JC, Goforth WP, Murff RT, Lynch DM, Odom RD. Mechanical treatment of plantar fasciitis. A prospective study. J Am Podiatr Med Assoc. 2001; 91(2):55–62

[18] Roos E, Engström M, Söderberg B. Foot orthoses for the treatment of plantar fasciitis. Foot Ankle Int. 2006; 27(8):606–611

[19] Acevedo JI, Beskin JL. Complications of plantar fascia rupture associated with corticosteroid injection. Foot Ankle Int. 1998; 19(2):91–97

[20] Crawford F, Atkins D, Young P, Edwards J. Steroid injection for heel pain: evidence of short-term effectiveness. A randomized controlled trial. Rheumatology (Oxford). 1999; 38(10):974–977

[21] Grice J, Marsland D, Smith G, Calder J. Efficacy of foot and ankle corticosteroid injections. Foot Ankle Int. 2017; 38(1):8–13

[22] Gollwitzer H, Saxena A, DiDomenico LA, et al. Clinically relevant effectiveness of focused extracorporeal shock wave therapy in the treatment of chronic plantar fasciitis: a randomized, controlled multicenter study. J Bone Joint Surg Am. 2015; 97(9): 701–708

[23] Ahmad J, Ahmad SH, Jones K. Treatment of plantar fasciitis with botulinum toxin. Foot Ankle Int. 2017; 38(1):1–7

[24] Elizondo-Rodriguez J, Araujo-Lopez Y, Moreno-Gonzalez JA, Cardenas-Estrada E, Mendoza-Lemus O, Acosta-Olivo C. A comparison of botulinum toxin a and intralesional steroids for the treatment of plantar fasciitis: a randomized, double-blinded study. Foot Ankle Int. 2013; 34(1):8–14

[25] Vahdatpour B, Kianimehr L, Moradi A, Haghighat S. Beneficial effects of platelet-rich plasma on improvement of pain severity and physical disability in patients with plantar fasciitis: a randomized trial. Adv Biomed Res. 2016; 5:179

[26] Jain SK, Suprashant K, Kumar S, Yadav A, Kearns SR. Comparison of plantar fasciitis injected with platelet-rich plasma vs corticosteroids. Foot Ankle Int. 2018; 39(7):780–786

[27] Shetty SH, Dhond A, Arora M, Deore S. Platelet-rich plasma has better long-term results than corticosteroids or placebo for chronic plantar fasciitis: randomized control trial. J Foot Ankle Surg. 2019; 58(1):42–46

[28] Kinley S, Frascone S, Calderone D, Wertheimer SJ, Squire MA, Wiseman FA. Endoscopic plantar fasciotomy versus traditional heel spur surgery: a prospective study. J Foot Ankle Surg. 1993; 32(6): 595–603

[29] Fallat LM, Cox JT, Chahal R, Morrison P, Kish J. A retrospective comparison of percutaneous plantar fasciotomy and open plantar fasciotomy with heel spur resection. J Foot Ankle Surg. 2013; 52(3):288–290

[30] DiGiovanni BF, Moore AM, Zlotnicki JP, Pinney SJ. Preferred management of recalcitrant plantar fasciitis among orthopaedic foot and ankle surgeons. Foot Ankle Int. 2012; 33(6):507–512

[31] Monteagudo M, Maceira E, Garcia-Virto V, Canosa R. Chronic plantar fasciitis: plantar fasciotomy versus gastrocnemius recession. Int Orthop. 2013; 37(9):1845–1850

[32] Jahss MH, Kummer F, Michelson JD. Investigations into the fat pads of the sole of the foot: heel pressure studies. Foot Ankle. 1992; 13(5):227–232

[33] Wallace WD, Balkin SW, Kaplan L, Nelson S. The histologic host response to liquid silicone injections for prevention of pressure-related ulcers of the foot: a 38-year study. J Am Podiatr Med Assoc. 2004; 94 (6):550–557

[34] Anderson RB, Cohen BE. Stress fractures of the foot and ankle. In: Coughlin MJ, Saltzman CL, Anderson RB, eds. Mann's Surgery of the Foot and Ankle. Philadelphia, PA: Elsevier Saunders; 2014:1688–1722

[35] Hopson CN, Perry DR. Stress fractures of the calcaneus in women marine recruits. Clin Orthop Relat Res. 1977(128):159–162

[36] Chang CD, Wu JS. MR imaging findings in heel pain. Magn Reson Imaging Clin N Am. 2017; 25(1):79–93

[37] Michelson JD, Charlson MD. Vitamin D status in an elective orthopedic surgical population. Foot Ankle Int. 2016; 37(2):186–191

[38] Baxter DE, Thigpen CM. Heel pain: operative results. Foot Ankle. 1984; 5(1):16–25

[39] Pomeroy G, Wilton J, Anthony S. Entrapment neuropathy about the foot and ankle: an update. J Am Acad Orthop Surg. 2015; 23(1):58–66

[40] DiGiovanni BF, Abuzzahab FS, Gould JS. plantar fascia release with proximal and distal tarsal tunnel release: a surgical approach to chronic, disabling plantar fasciitis with associated nerve pain. Tech Foot Ankle Surg. 2003; 2(4):254–261

[41] Sinnaeve F, Vandeputte G. Clinical outcome of surgical intervention for recalcitrant infero-medial heel pain. Acta Orthop Belg. 2008; 74(4):483–488

[42] Daniels TR, Lau JT, Hearn TC. The effects of foot position and load on tibial nerve tension. Foot Ankle Int. 1998; 19(2):73–78

[43] Abouelela AA, Zohiery AK. The triple compression stress test for diagnosis of tarsal tunnel syndrome. Foot. 2012; 22(3):146–149

[44] Lopez-Ben R. Imaging of nerve entrapment in the foot and ankle. Foot Ankle Clin. 2011; 16(2): 213–224

[45] Patel AT, Gaines K, Malamut R, Park TA, Toro DR, Holland N, American Association of Neuromuscular and Electrodiagnostic Medicine. Usefulness of electrodiagnostic techniques in the evaluation of suspected tarsal tunnel syndrome: an evidence-based review. Muscle Nerve. 2005; 32(2):236–240

[46] Harris J, Fallat L, Schwartz S. Characteristic trends of lower-extremity complex regional pain syndrome. J Foot Ankle Surg. 2004; 43(5):296–301

[47] Shereff MJ, Cullivan WT, Johnson KA. Osteoid-osteoma of the foot. J Bone Joint Surg Am. 1983; 65 (5):638–641

[48] Shukla S, Clarke AW, Saifuddin A. Imaging features of foot osteoid osteoma. Skeletal Radiol. 2010; 39 (7):683–689

[49] Park IH, Micic ID, Jeon IH. A study of 23 unicameral bone cysts of the calcaneus: open chip allogeneic bone graft versus percutaneous injection of bone powder with autogenous bone marrow. Foot Ankle Int. 2008; 29(2):164–170

12 Hallux Rigidus: Osteoarthritis of the First Metatarsophalangeal Joint

Thomas B. Bemenderfer and Kent Ellington

Abstract

Hallux rigidus is a noninflammatory degenerative arthropathy of the first metatarsophalangeal (MTP) joint resulting in mild to severe degenerative arthritis. Functionally, it may produce minimal symptoms to complete debilitation. Treatments range from supportive care to a cheilectomy or a 1st MTP fusion.

Keywords: hallux rigidus, first MTP joint arthritis

12.1 History

Hallux rigidus is a noninflammatory degenerative arthropathy of the first metatarsophalangeal (MTP) joint resulting in mild to severe degenerative arthritis. Functionally, it may produce minimal symptoms to complete debilitation. Hallux rigidus is the second most common deformity of the first MTP joint after hallux valgus in the general population. It is the most common MTP deformity in both amateur and professional athletes believed to be a sequelae of turf toe and repetitive MTP hyperextension.[1]

At least 45% of professional football players have sustained a turf toe injury,[2] and studies have demonstrated long-term sequelae with up to a 50% incidence of early hallux rigidus in athletes with prior turf toe injuries at greater than 5 years of follow-up.[3]

Orthopaedic versus podiatry nomenclature: Note that the orthopaedic literature uses the term "hallux rigidus" rather than "hallux limitus." The podiatric literature refers to hallux rigidus as the end stage of hallux limitus when motion is absent or severely restricted to the point of near ankylosis.

12.2 Pathophysiology

- Classic presentation of arthritis:
  - Joint space narrowing (cartilage degeneration/eburnation).
  - Subchondral cysts.
  - Altered joint mechanics.
  - Osteophyte formation most prominently on the dorsal aspect of the first metatarsal head.
- Pain is secondary to intrinsic mechanical intra-articular impingement, synovial inflammation, as well as shod-related extrinsic pressure on prominent osteophytes.
- The etiology is incompletely understood and broadly categorized into classic idiopathic versus posttraumatic arthritic process.
- In neutral alignment of the first metatarsophalangeal (MTP) joint, contact stresses are greatest concentrically and with toe-off during gait phase t→ greatest amount of force is distributed through the dorsal aspect of the MTP joint leading to increase subchondral bone density, formation of dorsal periarticular osteophytes, and cystic changes.
- *Cleave lesion:* Dorsal defect in the articular cartilage of the first metatarsal head can to lead to early chondritis dissecans and progress toward further cartilage eburnation and ultimately hallux rigidus.[4]
- *Dorsal cartilage wear patterns:* In an in vitro study, the contact distribution of the metatarsal articular surface shifted dorsally with increasing degrees of extension.[5]
- *Dorsal osteophytes:* Similar to osteoarthritis found elsewhere, dorsal osteophytes are the natural reactive

process by which the body attempts to increase surface area and diminish focal contact pressure. However, the abnormal loading further alters biomechanics that accelerates the degenerative process, leading to further eburnation of the articular cartilage, subchondral sclerosis and/or cyst formation, and osteophytes.
- *Turf toe injuries:* In the younger patient population, repetitive microtrauma associated with hyperextension secondary to toe-off positions during sprinting, acute changes in direction, and planting may increase the risk of patients sustaining turf toe injuries. Turf toe injuries allow for supraphysiologic range of motion (ROM) in the sagittal plane that accelerates the degenerative process and contributes to the high incidence in the athlete patient population.

12.3 Natural History

- The incidence hallux rigidus increases with age, affecting 10% of patients aged 20 to 24 years and 35 to 60% of the population over the age of 65 years.[6]
- For some, hallux rigidus is a fairly benign condition. Smith et al retrospectively reviewed 24 patients with long-term follow-up at 12 to 19 years following diagnosis of hallux rigidus. Despite evidence of radiographic progression, only 25% wished to consider surgery at the final review and in 23 (96%) patients the pain improved or remained constant.[7] However, in a randomized controlled trial comparing corticosteroid versus hyaluronate injections for hallux rigidus, 16 of 32 (50%) patients underwent surgery at 1 year.[8]
- The natural history is unpredictable, and it is unclear to predict who will ultimately require operative management.

12.4 Etiology

- Unknown genesis of degenerative changes:
  - The true cause of hallux rigidus remains unknown.
  - A traumatic episode or chronic repetitive microtrauma is considered the most likely cause of unilateral hallux rigidus.[9]
- Risk factors:
  - Studies do demonstrate an association between hallux rigidus and hallux valgus interphalangeus.
  - Family history (in bilateral cases of hallux rigidus).
  - Trauma (in unilateral cases of the condition).[9]
- Increased risk with athletes. Hallux rigidus is the most common deformity of the first ray in athletes:
  - Sequelae of turf toe and repetitive MTP hyperextension.[1]
  - Fifty percent incidence of early hallux rigidus in athletes with prior turf toe injuries at greater than 5 years of follow-up.[3]
- No evidence to support increased risk with running:
  - It is unknown whether running is a true cause of the disorder or an aggravating factor.

12.5 Symptoms

- Patients present with the following:
  - Localized pain of the first MTP joint.
  - Plantar calluses.
  - Stiffness with diminished ROM in the sagittal plane.
  - Enlargement of the joint.
- Eighty percent of symptoms are unilateral but increase to 80% bilateral involvement at the 9-year follow-up.[9]
- Stiffness is rarely the primary complaint unless the patient is a young athlete.
- Transfer metatarsalgia.
- Mass effect of dorsal osteophyte.

- Hallux dysesthesias: extrinsic compression by shoes or stretching of the dorsomedial cutaneous nerve.

12.5.1 Physical Examination

- Physical examination of the lower extremity should always be performed with the shoes off.
- Mid-arc of motion pain and crepitus indicates late-stage degenerative arthritis of the first MTP joint.
- Tenderness to palpation overlying the first MTP joint accompanied by restricted ROM in the sagittal plane should raise suspicion for hallux rigidus.
- Dorsal pain with maximum plantar flexion is common and is likely secondary to irritation of the extensor hallucis longus as it passes over the dorsal osteophyte.
- Antalgic gait with diminished first MTP dorsiflexion at toe-off stance.

12.6 Diagnosis and Classification

- No reliable or valid classification system (▶ Table 12.1).

12.7 Imaging

- Three views: anteroposterior (AP), lateral, oblique foot radiographs. Plain film radiographs in combination with physical examination are commonly sufficient to diagnose.
- Spectrum of radiographic changes:
  - Early changes: typically include marginal osteophyte formation of the dorsal metatarsal head and proximal phalanx with well-maintained joint space.
  - More severe degenerative changes including joint space narrowing, articular irregularities, loose bodies, osteochondral defects, subchondral cysts, and irregular hypertrophied sesamoids.
  - Forefoot deformities including hallux valgus (valgus angulation of the first MTP joint) and valgus interphalangeus (valgus angulation of the interphalangeal joint) may be identified (▶ Fig. 12.1).

12.8 Management

- Early conservative management:

Table 12.1 Classification system for hallux rigidus[9]

<table>
<tr><th></th><th>Dorsiflexion</th><th>Articular morphology</th><th>Osteophytes</th><th>Pain</th></tr>
<tr><td>Grade 0 (mild)</td><td>40–60 degrees</td><td>Normal radiographic results</td><td rowspan="2">None</td><td rowspan="3">None</td></tr>
<tr><td>Grade 1 (moderate)</td><td>30–40 degrees</td><td>Dorsal osteophytes</td></tr>
<tr><td>Grade 2 (severe)</td><td>10–30 degrees</td><td>Mild flattening of the MTP joint, mild to moderate joint narrowing, or sclerosis</td><td rowspan="3">Dorsal, lateral, and/or medial osteophytes</td></tr>
<tr><td>Grade 3</td><td><10 degrees</td><td>Hypertrophied cysts or erosions or with irregular sesamoids</td><td>Constant moderate to severe pain, and pain at the extremes of the ROM</td></tr>
<tr><td>Grade 4</td><td>Ankylosed</td><td>Loose bodies or osteochondritis dissecans</td><td>Pain throughout the entire ROM</td></tr>
</table>

NOTE: Normal passive ROM of the MTP joint is 45 degrees of flexion to 70 degrees of extension.

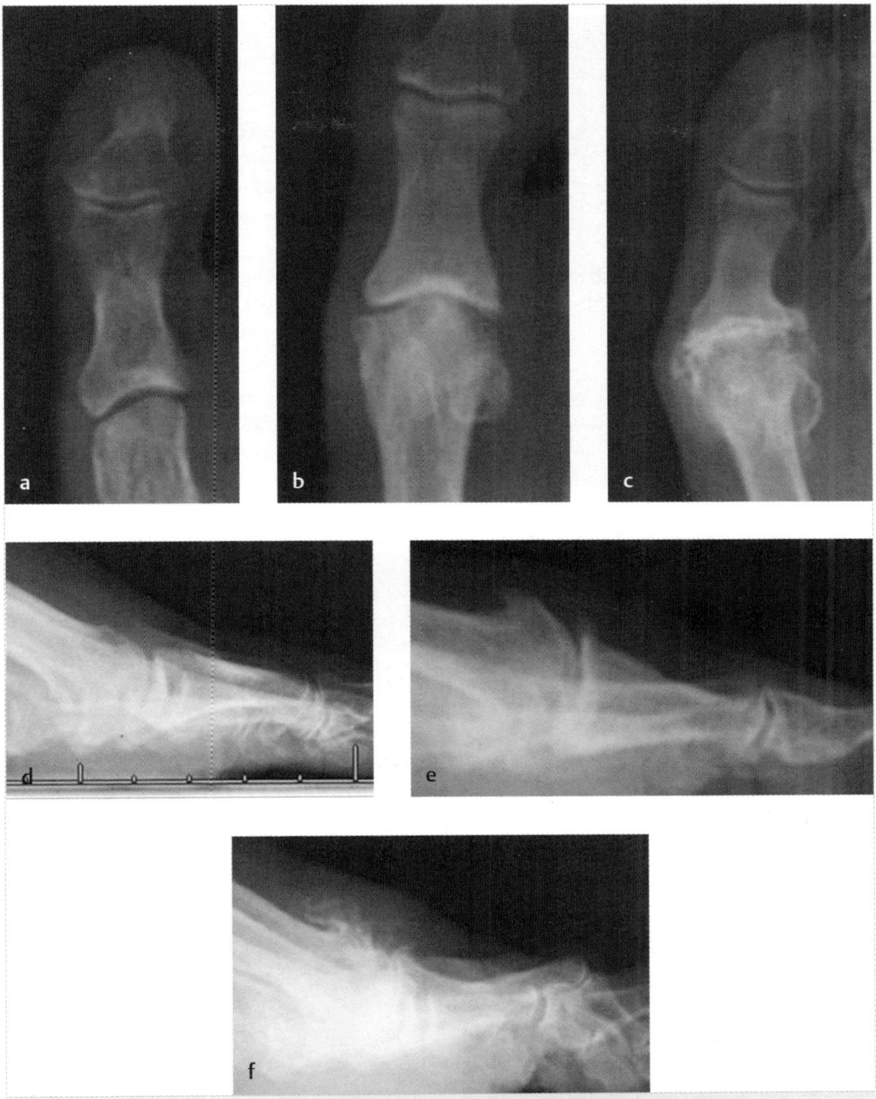

Fig. 12.1 Hattrup and Johnson classification weight-bearing anteroposterior (AP) and lateral radiographic examples. **(a,d)** Grade 1 (mild) with maintained joint space. **(b,e)** Grade 2 (moderate) with joint space narrowing, dorsal osteophyte, and subchondral sclerosis or cysts. **(c,f)** Grade 3 (severe) with significant joint space narrowing, extensive bony proliferation, and loose bodies.

   - Early detection and alleviation of symptoms.
- **Nonoperative**:
   - Nonsteroidal anti-inflammatory medicines.
   - Cryo- or thermotherapy.
   - Intra-articular corticosteroid (IACS) injections to reduce pain and stiffness.
      - Limited efficacy at a median of 6 months in low-grade hallux rigidus and progressively limited

symptomatic relief in patients with higher-grade osteoarthritis.[10]
  - Modifications of footwear to limit the first MTP joint motion include the following:
    - Avoid thin-soled shoes or high heels.
    - Rocker bottom shoes with wider curved sole.[11]
    - In-shoe orthotics (Morton's extension insert) promote medial stiffness that limits the motion at the MTP joint.[12]
  - Activity modifications:
    - Avoiding extremes of dorsiflexion of the great toe, such as those caused by kneeling, squatting, and running with the toes in an extended position.
  - May provide symptomatic relief but have not been demonstrated to reduce progression of hallux rigidus.
- **Operative**:
  - Several options for surgical management depending on the degree of involvement, the ROM limitations, the individual's activity level, and the surgeon's and patient's preference.
- Options include the following:
  - Cheilectomy.
  - Joint-sparing procedures (e.g., proximal phalanx osteotomy and metatarsal osteotomy).
  - Partial or total arthroplasty.
  - Arthroscopy.
  - Arthrodesis.
- **Dorsal cheilectomy (see ▶ Fig. 12.2):** Cheilectomy involves the excision of all irregular bony spurs (osteophytes) that limit motion. For minor hallux rigidus with mild to moderate arthritic changes, most authors recommend dorsal cheilectomy, particularly in young or active patients who demonstrate less than 50% articular cartilage involvement intraoperatively.[13]
  - *Joint-sparing techniques*:
    - **Proximal phalangeal osteotomy with dorsal cheilectomy:** This may increase dorsiflexion in patients with sufficient baseline plantar flexion; prerequisite to the procedure is the presence of adequate plantar flexion.
    - **Arthroscopic removal of dorsal osteophytes.**[14,15]
    - **Proximal phalanx/distal metatarsal hemiarthroplasty or total MTP arthroplasty (see** ▶ Fig. 12.3, ▶ Fig. 12.4, ▶ Fig. 12.5**):** Excisional arthroplasty (i.e., Keller's procedure involving excision of the base of the proximal phalanx), capsular interposition arthroplasty, silicone implant arthroplasty, and metallic hemi- or total arthroplasty are associated with a number of potential complications and are not generally recommended in orthopaedics[16,17,18,19] (see ▶ Fig. 12.3, ▶ Fig. 12.4, ▶ Fig. 12.5 for radiographic examples of failed arthroplasties).
    - **Arthrodesis** is the gold standard treatment for advanced hallux rigidus and serves as a reliable salvage procedure when other surgical methods fail.

12.9 Outcomes

- Variable success:
  - Current available evidence is poor given the clinical heterogeneity in combination with the low number of prospective trials.
  - Grade of recommendation for each procedure is low and the choice of the procedure remains largely based on prior training and individual preference of the treating surgeon.
- **Limited evidence:** With limited evidence to support any model for decision-making, joint-preserving operations are appealing, because if they fail to relief the symptoms, joint-sacrificing operations can still be performed.

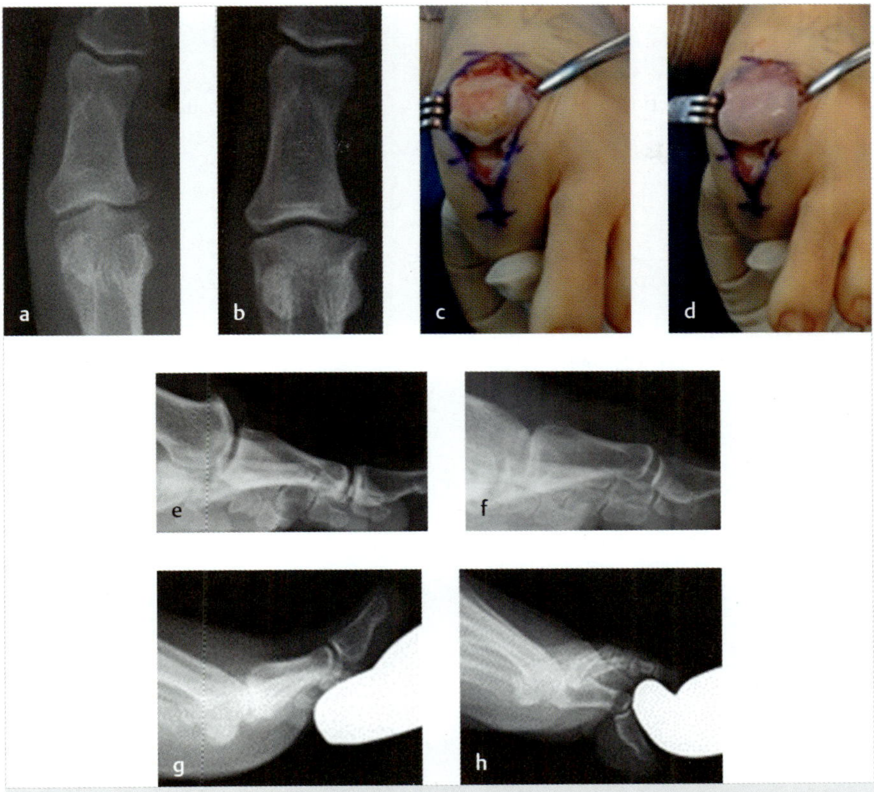

Fig. 12.2 Dorsal cheilectomy for grade 1 (mild) hallux rigidus. **(a–h)** Anteroposterior (AP) and lateral radiographs pre- and postoperatively with investigational orthobiologic examples and examples of postoperative range of motion.

12.10 Key Testing Facts

- Hallux rigidus is degenerative osteoarthritis of the first MTP joint with unknown pathologic etiology and demonstrates an increased incidence in older patient populations as well as athletes.
- Nonoperative options include standard osteoarthritic therapies (e.g., anti-inflammatories, activity modifications, and corticosteroid injection) as well as steel shank or other medial forefoot immobilization techniques.
- The most common and accepted techniques in orthopaedic literature include dorsal cheilectomy with or without Moberg's osteotomy for mild to moderate hallux rigidus to MTP arthrodesis for severe hallux rigidus once painful mid-range arc of motion occurs.
- Patient education with anticipatory guidance is important in order for patients to be appropriately informed for shared decision-making.

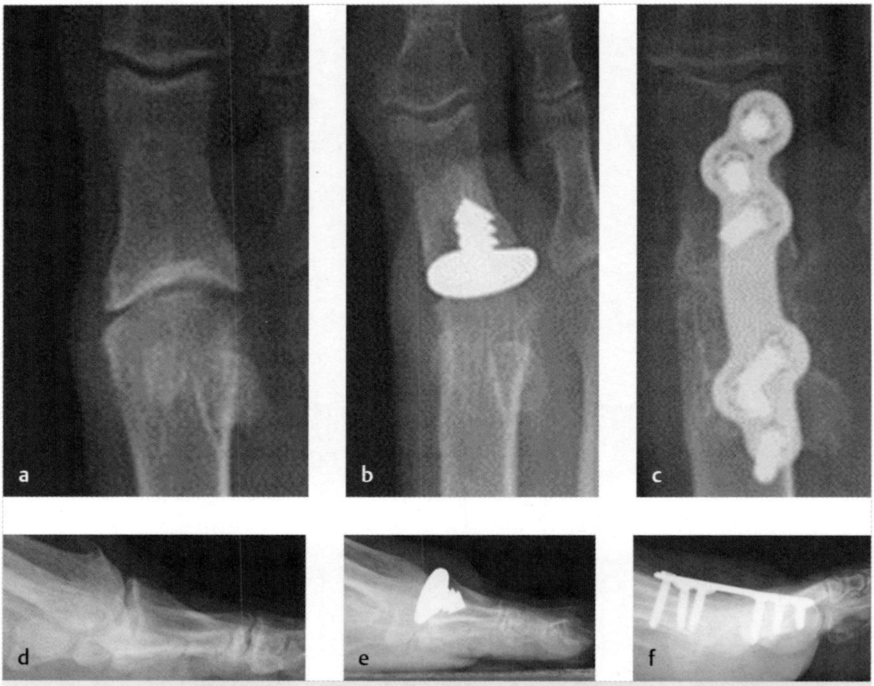

Fig. 12.3 (a–f) Failed proximal phalanx hemi-arthroplasty with conversion to arthrodesis with bone graft for hallux rigidus.

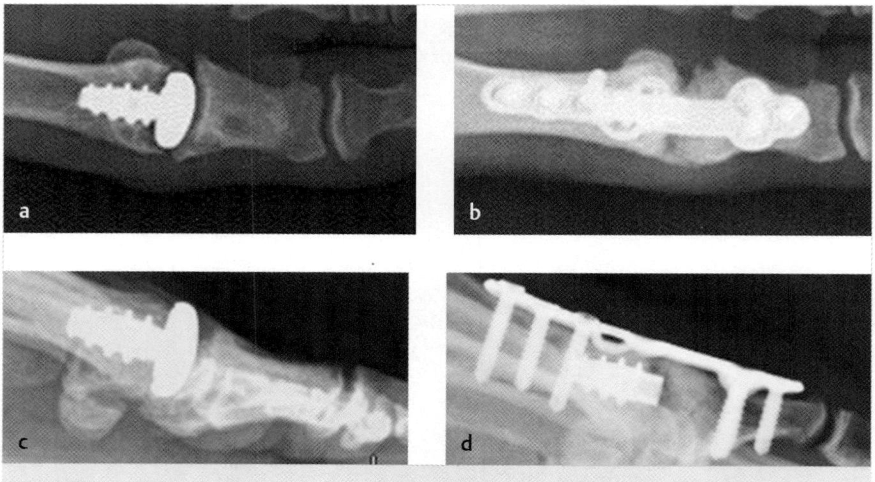

Fig. 12.4 (a–d) Failed distal metatarsal hemi-arthroplasty with conversion to arthrodesis with bone graft for hallux rigidus.

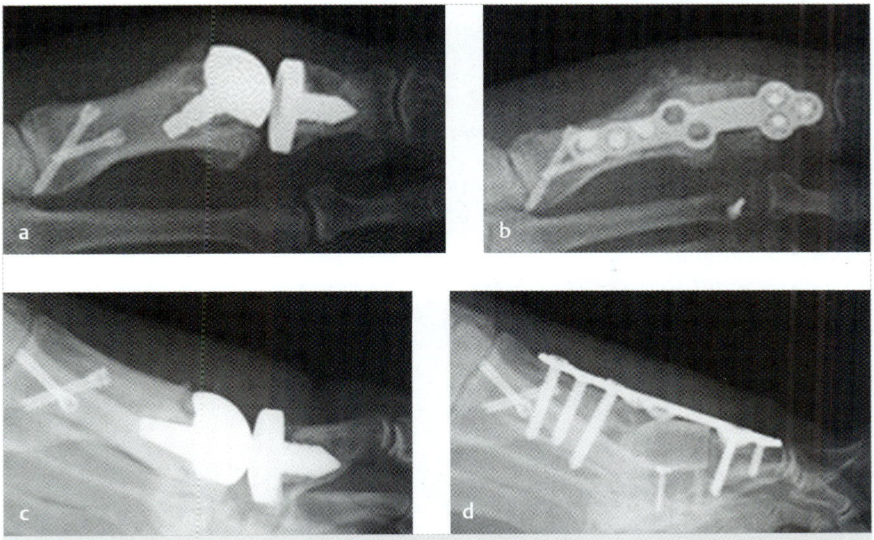

Fig. 12.5 (a–d) Failed first total metatarsophalangeal arthroplasty with conversion to arthrodesis with bone graft for hallux rigidus.

References

[1] Shankar NS. Silastic single-stem implants in the treatment of hallux rigidus. Foot Ankle Int. 1995; 16(8):487–491

[2] Rodeo SA, O'Brien S, Warren RF, Barnes R, Wickiewicz TL, Dillingham MF. Turf-toe: an analysis of metatarsophalangeal joint sprains in professional football players. Am J Sports Med. 1990; 18(3):280–285

[3] Clanton TO, Ford JJ. Turf toe injury. Clin Sports Med. 1994; 13(4):731–741

[4] McMaster MJ. The pathogenesis of hallux rigidus. J Bone Joint Surg Br. 1978; 60(1):82–87

[5] Ahn TK, Kitaoka HB, Luo ZP, An KN. Kinematics and contact characteristics of the first metatarsophalangeal joint. Foot Ankle Int. 1997; 18(3): 170–174

[6] van Saase JL, van Romunde LK, Cats A, Vandenbroucke JP, Valkenburg HA. Epidemiology of osteoarthritis: Zoetermeer survey. Comparison of radiological osteoarthritis in a Dutch population with that in 10 other populations. Ann Rheum Dis. 1989; 48(4):271–280

[7] Smith RW, Katchis SD, Ayson LC. Outcomes in hallux rigidus patients treated nonoperatively: a long-term follow-up study. Foot Ankle Int. 2000; 21(11):906–913

[8] Pons M, Alvarez F, Solana J, Viladot R, Varela L. Sodium hyaluronate in the treatment of hallux rigidus. A single-blind, randomized study. Foot Ankle Int. 2007; 28(1):38–42

[9] Coughlin MJ, Shurnas PS. Hallux rigidus: demographics, etiology, and radiographic assessment. Foot Ankle Int. 2003; 24(10):731–743

[10] Solan MC, Calder JD, Bendall SP. Manipulation and injection for hallux rigidus. Is it worthwhile? J Bone Joint Surg Br. 2001; 83(5):706–708

[11] Cusack J, Shtofmakher G, Kilfoil RL, Jr, Vu S. Improved step length symmetry and decreased low back pain with the use of a rocking-soled shoe in a patient with unilateral hallux rigidus. BMJ Case Rep. 2014; 2014

[12] Stinus H, Weber F. Inserts for foot deformities. Orthopade. 2005; 34(8):776–778, 780–781

[13] Lin J, Murphy GA. Treatment of hallux rigidus with cheilectomy using a dorsolateral approach. Foot Ankle Int. 2009; 30(2):115–119

[14] van Dijk CN, Veenstra KM, Nuesch BC. Arthroscopic surgery of the metatarsophalangeal first joint. Arthroscopy. 1998; 14(8):851–855

[15] Ahn JH, Choy WS, Lee KW. Arthroscopy of the first metatarsophalangeal joint in 59 consecutive cases. J Foot Ankle Surg. 2012; 51(2):161–167

[16] Can Akgun R, Sahin O, Demirors H, Cengiz Tuncay I. Analysis of modified oblique Keller procedure for

severe hallux rigidus. Foot Ankle Int. 2008; 29(12): 1203–1208

[17] Schenk S, Meizer R, Kramer R, Aigner N, Landsiedl F, Steinboeck G. Resection arthroplasty with and without capsular interposition for treatment of severe hallux rigidus. Int Orthop. 2009; 33(1):145–150

[18] Cook E, Cook J, Rosenblum B, Landsman A, Giurini J, Basile P. Meta-analysis of first metatarsophalangeal joint implant arthroplasty. J Foot Ankle Surg. 2009; 48(2):180–190

[19] Konkel KF, Menger AG, Retzlaff SA. Results of metallic hemi-great toe implant for grade III and early grade IV hallux rigidus. Foot Ankle Int. 2009; 30(7):653–660

13 Ankle Arthritis

Derrick Foge, Joseph Chavarria, and Kenneth J. Hunt

Abstract
Ankle arthritis is a debilitating disease, most commonly a result of traumatic injury, usually characterized by pain, decreased range of motion, and changes in gait pattern. There are multiple operative and nonoperative methods to treat this condition. Conservative management is typically indicated for patients with mild symptoms. Surgical management is indicated when a patient fails conservative management. For patients with pain related to loose bodies or inflamed synovium, arthroscopic debridement may be indicated. In patients with asymmetric ankle arthritis, a supramalleolar osteotomy may be indicated. Arthrodesis has traditionally been the gold standard for end-stage ankle arthritis in many patients, with a recommended fusion positioning of neutral dorsi-/plantar flexion, hindfoot valgus of 5 degrees, and equal rotation with contralateral ankle. Ankle arthroplasty is indicated in many patients with ankle arthritis, with the advantage of maintained ankle range of motion.

Keywords: arthritis, subtalar distraction arthrodesis, supramalleolar osteotomy, ankle arthrodesis, ankle arthroplasty

13.1 The Problem of Arthritis

- Arthritis is the most common joint disease, and affects greater 30 million people in the United States.[1,2]
  - It is the leading cause of chronic disability in older adults with a cost of greater than $185 billion annually.
  - More than 50% of adults older than 65 years are affected by osteoarthritis.

Table 13.1 Risk factors for ankle arthritis[1]

• Trauma
• Ligamentous injury
• Obesity
• Rheumatoid disease
• Hemochromatosis, hemophilia
• Infection
• Neuropathic disorders leading to Charcot joint (syringomyelia, tabes dorsalis, diabetes)
• Previous inflammatory arthritis or crystalline disease (e.g., gout)
• Avascular necrosis
• Previous surgical procedures

- Most commonly it results from injury, joint damage, abnormal mechanics, and inflammation, leading to the breakdown of articular cartilage (▶ Table 13.1).
  - *Primary osteoarthritis* is related to the aging process, typically in older individuals; occurs in previously intact joints without apparent inciting factor.
  - *Secondary arthritis* is a joint disease resulting from a predisposing condition that altered joint tissues.

13.2 Etiology and Pathophysiology

- Ankle arthritis is less common than osteoarthritis of the hip or knee.
- Common causes include the following[3,4,5,6]:
  - Posttraumatic arthritis is the most common cause accounting for approximately 70% of cases.[2]
    - Prior fracture that results in joint damage or heals in a nonanatomic position alters joint mechanics and changes the weight-bearing surfaces at the ankle joint.[4]

- *Other causes* are rheumatoid arthritis, primary degenerative disease, infection, peripheral neuropathy, Charcot neuropathic arthropathy, osteonecrosis of talus, infection, and gout.
- Inflammation and joint degeneration occur as cytokines and metalloproteinases are released into the joints, leading to excessive matrix degradation and cartilage degeneration.
  - *Early:* Swelling of cartilage because of increased synthesis of proteoglycans (effort by chondrocytes to repair cartilage damage).
  - *Late:* Level of proteoglycans drops and cartilage becomes soft, loses its elasticity, and begins to die.
    - As cartilage dies and sloughs off, this leads to decreased joint space.
  - *Subchondral sclerosis:* Subchondral bone reacts to increased stress with increased vascular supply, increased cellularity, and eventually becoming thick and dense.
  - *Subchondral cysts:* Abnormal stresses to bone may lead to cystic degeneration.
  - *Osteophyte formation:* At the margins of the cartilage surface, increased vascularity of the subchondral tissues in response to stress can lead to irregular outgrowths of new bone (▸ Fig. 13.1).

13.3 Symptoms and Physical Examination

- Decreased range of motion. Always compare to the contralateral side.
- Antalgic gait.
- Pain with weight-bearing activity, with push-off, and with motion.
- Pain often localized to the anterior aspect of the ankle.
- *Ankle joint effusion* may manifest with swelling, warmth, and erythema.
- Pain is worse with increased activity; typically worse in the morning or after rest.
- Pain and crepitus with ankle ROM.

13.4 Diagnostics and Classification

- Thorough history and physical examination, including any history of prior trauma to the affected ankle.
- *Recommended radiographs:* weight-bearing anteroposterior (AP), lateral, and oblique views ▸ Table 13.2.
- Consider standing limb length view to evaluate the proximal alignment abnormalities (e.g., genu varum).

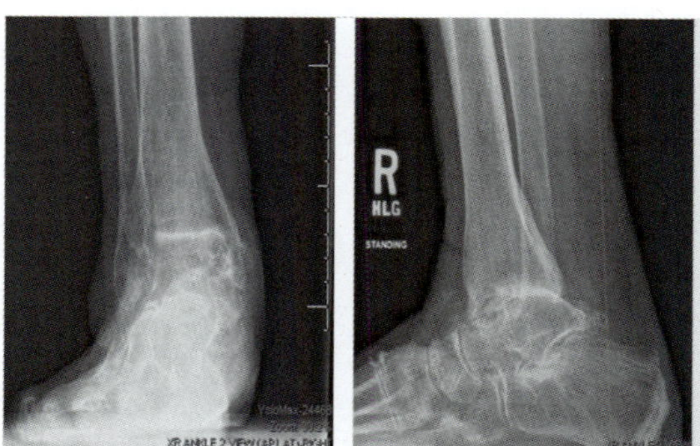

Fig. 13.1 Weight-bearing ankle radiographs demonstrating end-stage ankle arthritis.

Table 13.2 Takakura's classification

Stage I	Early sclerosis and osteophyte formation (no joint space narrowing)
Stage II	Narrowing of the medial joint space (no subchondral bone contact)
Stage IIIA	Obliteration of joint space at the medial malleolus, with subchondral bone contact)
Stage IIIB	Obliteration of joint space over the roof of the talar dome, with subchondral bone contact
Stage IV	Obliteration of joint space with complete bone contact

13.5 Conservative Management

- Indications: first-line treatment.
- Lifestyle modifications:
  - Minimizing activity that causes pain.
  - Minimizing high-impact activities or reducing their duration.
  - Weight loss to reduce stress on joint.
  - Low-impact exercise is recommended. Bicycle riding is particularly helpful.
- *Physical therapy* is aimed at improving ROM and strengthening muscles of the ankle and lower extremities.
  - It may aggravate pain from arthritis.
- Assistive devices:
  - Bracing (solid ankle cushion heel, lace-up ankle braces, ankle–foot orthoses [AFOs], Arizona brace, patella tendon-bearing braces, etc.).
  - Assistive devices (such as a cane).
  - Rocker sole shoe modification.
- Medications:
  - *Nonsteroidal anti-inflammatory drugs (NSAIDs):* inhibit activity of cyclooxygenase enzymes.
  - *Corticosteroid injections:* restrict accumulation of polymorphonuclear neutrophils in the joint.
- Biologics:
  - Platelet-rich plasma and stem cell injections are currently experimental but promising as a potential treatment.[7]
  - Hyaluronic acid injections have equivocal evidence of effectiveness for mild to moderate arthritis. Generally, use is not supported.
- There is no cure for arthritis, but therapies are directed at relieving pain and limiting disability.

13.6 Surgical Intervention

- *Indications:* failure of conservative management.
- *Arthroscopic debridement:* removal of loose cartilage, inflamed synovial tissue, inflamed tissue bands, and excision of osteophytes.
  - *Indications:* mild symptoms and pain during push-off.
  - May worsen symptoms as removal of osteophytes leads to more joint motion, which may precipitate cartilage wear.
  - Most effective when pain due to contact from osteophytes and/or synovial inflammation.
  - Not effective in advanced arthritis with joint space compromise.
  - Portals:
    - Most commonly used anterior portals are anteromedial and anterolateral.
    - Posterior portals typically lateral to Achilles tendon; trans-Achilles and posteromedial portals contraindicated in most cases.
- *Arthrodiastasis:* Reduces pain and increases motion without sacrificing the joint.[8,9,10]
  - *Indications:* Young patient with healthy bone and painful ankle joint.
  - Use of external fixator to distract ankle joint that is meant to give cartilage ability to repair itself and prevent further damage.

  - Limited large, long-term studies evaluating outcomes, and proper patient selection.[10]
- *Subtalar distraction arthrodesis:* Used in the treatment of symptomatic subtalar arthritis, which is most commonly a result of a previous calcaneus fracture.[11]
  - Realigns the hindfoot, which mechanically unloads diseased joint and restores proper anatomic relationships.
  - Multiple described techniques.
  - *Indications:* Moderate to severe symptoms from posttraumatic osteoarthritis, in a patient with the need for subtalar arthrodesis, but with a loss of hindfoot height (usually from calcaneus fracture), with loss of ROM (▸ Fig. 13.2a,b ▸ Fig. 13.3, and ▸ Fig. 13.4).
- *Supramalleolar osteotomy:* Correct deformity (congenital or acquired) of distal tibia to offload focal arthritis and increase contact on normal cartilage.[12,13,14]
  - *Indications:* Nearly full ROM with mild to moderate ankle arthritis, eccentric articular surface wear, and with a malalignment present (mild talar tilt or varus/valgus heel alignment, ankle arthritis subtypes Takakura stage II or IIIA).
    - There is no consensus on the acceptable degree of angular deformity of the distal tibia, but recent literature would suggest that patients with malalignment of at least 10 degrees and accompanying pain benefit.[14]
  - Offloads eccentric wear patterns (joint sparing).
  - Want to make osteotomy as close to apex of deformity (center of rotation and angulation [CORA]) as possible to return angles to as normal as possible and improve the biomechanics of ankle joint.
    - The CORA is the intersection of two lines that represent the mechanical axes of the proximal and distal segments or the apex of deformity. Osteotomy at this level achieves the most powerful correction possible (▸ Fig. 13.3).
- Arthrodesis[15,16,17,18,19]:
  - *Indications:* Historically the gold standard of end-stage ankle arthritis treatment in young patients, laborers, and some elderly, less active patients.
    - This notion is being challenged.
  - *Techniques*: arthroscopic, mini-arthrotomy, open with either internal or external fixation. Open technique when larger deformity to correct with fusion. Screws or plates.
  - The recommended ankle position during ankle arthrodesis is neutral dorsiflexion/plantar flexion, hindfoot valgus of 5 degrees, and equal rotation with contralateral ankle.
  - *Outcomes:* Good evidence of effective means to decrease pain and allow for return to activities of daily living.[18,19]
  - May include subtalar joint in fusion if it is also arthritic. Retrograde intramedullary nail or plate constructs often used in these hindfoot fusion scenarios.
  - *Complications:* Nonunion (1–17% historically, with recent literature demonstrating a rate of 9.2%), adjacent hindfoot (subtalar) joint degeneration, hardware irritation, and infection.
    - Overall 3 to 25% rate of complication depending on study.
    - Some have noted a lower nonunion rate when performed arthroscopically (▸ Fig. 13.4, ▸ Fig. 13.5).
    - ▸ Fig. 13.4a, b, ▸ Fig. 13.5
- Arthroplasty[20,21,22,23,24]:
  - *Indications:* elderly patient, nonobese posttraumatic or inflammatory arthritis.
  - *Contraindications:* active infection, peripheral vascular diseases, inadequate soft-tissue envelope, and Charcot arthropathy.
    - *Relative:* Young/active/laborers, previous infection, severe uncorrected malalignment, significant ankle instability,

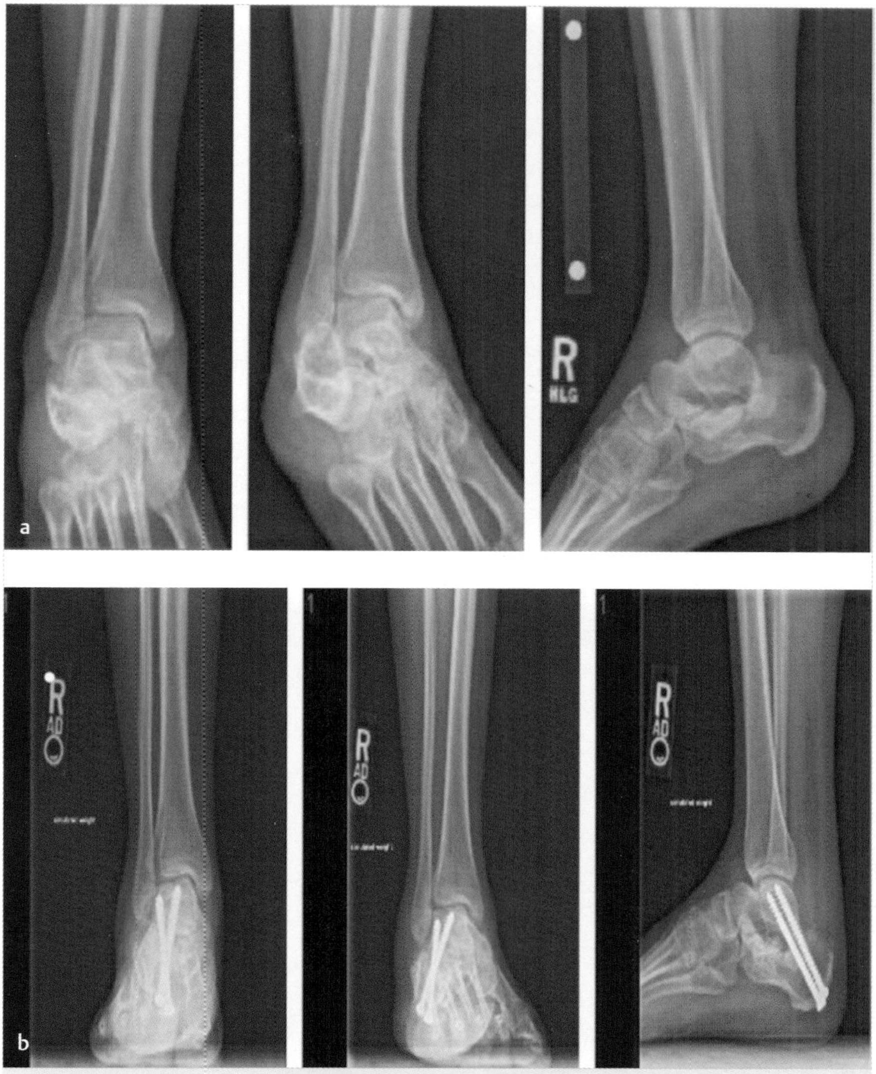

Fig. 13.2 A 36-year-old woman with posttraumatic arthrosis of the subtalar joint and debilitating pain following malunion of previous calcaneus fracture underwent distraction subtalar arthrodesis with iliac crest structural autograft. **(a)** Preoperative imaging. **(b)** Postoperative imaging.

significant osteoporosis, and osteonecrosis of talus.

- *Technique:* Anterior approach for most implant systems, interval between extensor digitorum longus (EDL) and tibialis anterior tendons. Many systems currently available.
- *Outcomes:* improved gait speed and stride length.
- *Complications:* infection, osteolysis, polyethylene wear, malleolar fracture, and superficial peroneal nerve injury (▶ Fig. 13.6).

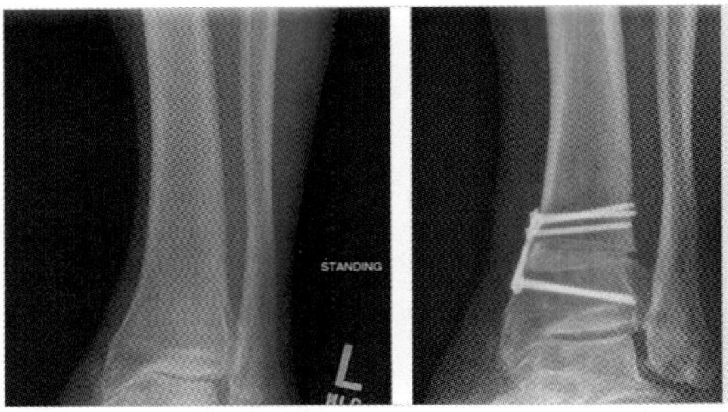

Fig. 13.3 A 63-year-old man with ankle arthritis and varus at the tibial plafond. Medial opening wedge osteotomy shifts the loads within the tibiotalar joint away from the advanced arthrosis and toward the healthier lateral articular cartilage.

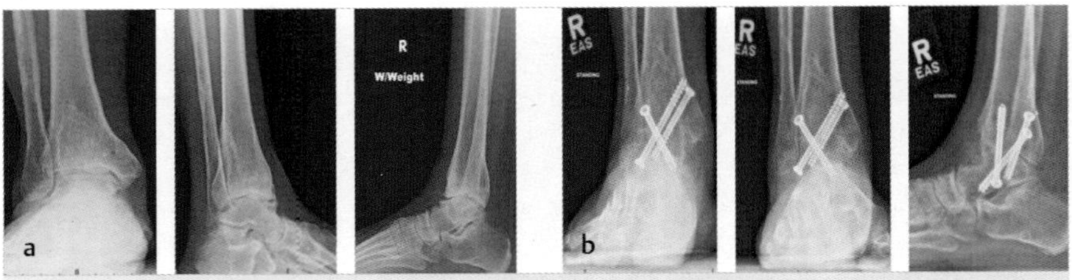

Fig. 13.4 A 37-year-old woman with posttraumatic right ankle arthritis after ankle fracture treated with open reduction and internal fixation (ORIF) who subsequently developed infection, requiring removal of hardware, debridement, and antibiotic therapy. The patient underwent right ankle arthroscopic arthrodesis with iliac crest bone graft for persistent symptoms. **(a)** Preoperative and **(b)** postoperative imaging.

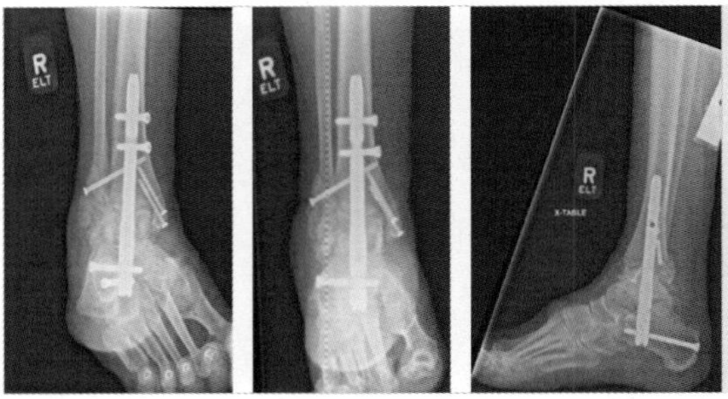

Fig. 13.5 Ankle radiographs from a patient with significant arthritis who underwent tibiotalocalcaneal arthrodesis.

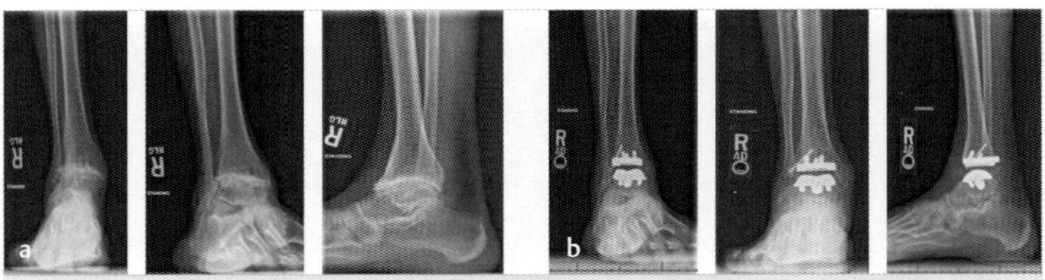

Fig. 13.6 A patient with significant arthritis who desired pain relief and had no contra-indications to ankle arthroplasty. The patient underwent ankle arthroplasty. **(a)** Preoperative imaging. **(b)** Postoperative imaging.

13.7 Rehabilitation

- Procedure/surgeon dependent.
- *Arthroplasty:* Early ROM, typically 2 to 6 weeks non-weight-bearing.
- *Ankle arthrodesis:* 6 weeks of non weight bearing. Computed tomography (CT) scan helpful to confirm healing (usually obtained at 3 months post-op).

13.8 Key Testing Facts

- Most arthritides of the ankle are the result of a previous traumatic injury (70%)
- Single rocker sole shoe modification can be an effective nonoperative treatment to improve gait and decrease pain in patients with mild ankle arthritis
- Ankle arthritis disease subtypes (Takakura stage II or IIIA) with varus of valgus deformity may be treated with supramalleolar osteotomy
- Arthrodesis is the gold standard of end-stage ankle arthritis treatment in elderly, less active patients
- The recommended ankle position during ankle arthrodesis is neutral dorsiflexion/plantar flexion, hindfoot valgus of 5 degrees, and equal rotation with contralateral ankle
- Overall complication rate of 3–25% with arthrodesis including nonunion, adjacent joint disease, infection, and hardware irritation
- Arthroplasty is a good option for elderly, nonobese patients and has been shown to increase gait speed and stride length
- Contraindications to arthroplasty include active infection, peripheral vascular diseases, inadequate soft-tissue envelope, and Charcot arthropathy

References

[1] Barg A, Pagenstert GI, Hügle T, et al. Ankle osteoarthritis: etiology, diagnostics, and classification. Foot Ankle Clin. 2013; 18(3):411–426

[2] Saltzman CL, Salamon ML, Blanchard GM, et al. Epidemiology of ankle arthritis: report of a consecutive series of 639 patients from a tertiary orthopaedic center. Iowa Orthop J. 2005; 25:44–46

[3] Daniels T, Thomas R. Etiology and biomechanics of ankle arthritis. Foot Ankle Clin. 2008; 13(3): 341–352, vii

[4] Demetriades L, Strauss E, Gallina J. Osteoarthritis of the ankle. Clin Orthop Relat Res. 1998(349): 28–42

[5] Hintermann B, Valderrabano V. Total ankle replacement. Foot Ankle Clin. 2003; 8(2):375–405

[6] Thomas RH, Daniels TR. Ankle arthritis. J Bone Joint Surg Am. 2003; 85(5):923–936

[7] Fukawa T, Yamaguchi S, Akatsu Y, Yamamoto Y, Akagi R, Sasho T. Safety and efficacy of intra-articular injection of platelet-rich plasma in patients with ankle osteoarthritis. Foot Ankle Int. 2017; 38(6):596–604

[8] Tellisi N, Fragomen AT, Kleinman D, O'Malley MJ, Rozbruch SR. Joint preservation of the osteoarthritic ankle using distraction arthroplasty. Foot Ankle Int. 2009; 30(4):318–325

[9] Kluesner AJ, Wukich DK. Ankle arthrodiastasis. Clin Podiatr Med Surg. 2009; 26(2):227–244

[10] Xu Y, Zhu Y, Xu XY. Ankle joint distraction arthroplasty for severe ankle arthritis. BMC Musculoskelet Disord. 2017; 18(1):96

[11] Fletcher AN, Liles JL, Steele JJ, Pereira GF, Adams SB. Systematic review of subtalar distraction arthrodesis for the treatment of subtalar arthritis. Foot Ankle Int. 2020; 41(4):437–448

[12] Barg A, Pagenstert GI, Horisberger M, et al. Supramalleolar osteotomies for degenerative joint disease of the ankle joint: indication, technique and results. Int Orthop. 2013; 37(9):1683–1695

[13] Becker AS, Myerson MS. The indications and technique of supramalleolar osteotomy. Foot Ankle Clin. 2009; 14(3):549–561

[14] Stamatis ED, Cooper PS, Myerson MS. Supramalleolar osteotomy for the treatment of distal tibial angular deformities and arthritis of the ankle joint. Foot Ankle Int. 2003; 24(10):754–764

[15] Scranton PE, Jr. An overview of ankle arthrodesis. Clin Orthop Relat Res. 1991(268):96–101

[16] Abidi NA, Gruen GS, Conti SF. Ankle arthrodesis: indications and techniques. J Am Acad Orthop Surg. 2000; 8(3):200–209

[17] Saltzman CL. Ankle arthritis. In: Coughlin MJ, Mann RA, Saltzman CL, eds. Surgery of the Foot and Ankle. Philadelphia, PA: Mosby-Elsevier; 2007:923–984

[18] Norvell DC, Ledoux WR, Shofer JB, et al. Effectiveness and safety of ankle arthrodesis versus arthroplasty: a prospective multicenter study. J Bone Joint Surg Am. 2019; 101(16):1485–1494

[19] Kerkhoff YRA, Keijsers NLW, Louwerens JWK. Sports participation, functional outcome, and complications after ankle arthrodesis: midterm follow-up. Foot Ankle Int. 2017; 38(10):1085–1091

[20] Saltzman CL, Kadoko RG, Suh JS. Treatment of isolated ankle osteoarthritis with arthrodesis or the total ankle replacement: a comparison of early outcomes. Clin Orthop Surg. 2010; 2(1):1–7

[21] DiDomenico LA, Anania MC. Total ankle replacements: an overview. Clin Podiatr Med Surg. 2011; 28(4):727–744

[22] Reeves CL, Shane AM, Vazales R. Current concepts regarding total ankle replacement as a viable treatment option for advanced ankle arthritis: what you need to know. Clin Podiatr Med Surg. 2017; 34(4):515–527

[23] Gougoulias NE, Khanna A, Maffulli N. History and evolution in total ankle arthroplasty. Br Med Bull. 2009; 89:111–151

[24] Bonasia DE, Dettoni F, Femino JE, Phisitkul P, Germano M, Amendola A. Total ankle replacement: why, when and how? Iowa Orthop J. 2010; 30: 119–130

14 Disorders of the Tendons

Gonzalo F. Bastias and Lew C. Schon

Abstract
Tendons of the foot and ankle are complex and balanced structures that play an important role in maintaining functional status both in daily activities and in situations of maximum demand such as high-endurance sports. Highly specialized to withstand large cyclical loads due to their great tensile strength, tendons on this region are especially susceptible to overuse injuries. Tendinopathies of the foot and ankle have a wide spectrum of clinical manifestations and represent a common cause of morbidity producing important functional impairment with high chronicity potential. On the other hand, their intrinsic subcutaneous nature makes them also specifically vulnerable to foot and ankle trauma and lacerations.

Keywords: tendinopathy, tenosynovitis, tendon rupture, tendonitis

14.1 Achilles Tendon

14.1.1 Anatomy

- The Achilles tendon is the body's strongest and longest tendon, measuring approximately 12 to 15 cm. The Achilles tendon is the confluence of the gastrocnemius and soleus muscles, beginning at the midportion of the calf and then internally rotating 90 degrees, coursing distally in the posterior aspect of the leg inserting in a broad area of the posterior tibial tuberosity of the calcaneus.[1]
- Below the musculotendinous junction, the tendon is surrounded by the paratenon throughout its course composed of flexible connective tissue that allows for 1.5 cm of tendon gliding with activity. The tendon lacks a true synovial sheath.
- Similar to other tendons, the Achilles tendon is composed of predominantly type I collagen.[2]
- The tendon's blood supply is segmental and is predominantly derived from anterior branches of the paratenon. Other sources include intratendinous vessels, the posterior tibial artery, and distal osseous and periosteal branches. A relatively avascular zone exists within 2 to 6 cm proximal to its calcaneal insertion, corresponding to the site of most Achilles tendon ruptures and noninsertional tendinitis.[3]
- The paratenon and tendon are innervated by nerves from muscles and local cutaneous nerves, especially the sural nerve, which crosses the tendon approximately 11 cm proximal to the calcaneal tuberosity and 3.5 cm distal to the musculotendinous junction. This makes it particularly vulnerable to iatrogenic injuries.[4]
- Two bursae are associated with the insertional area of the Achilles tendon: the retrocalcaneal bursa that lies between the distal Achilles tendon and the posterior superior calcaneal tuberosity, and the Achilles bursa, which is located between the skin and the tendon.[5]
- The tendon spans three different joints, being fundamental for knee flexion, tibiotalar flexion, and subtalar inversion, but making it notably more susceptible to injury than muscles that span a single joint.

14.1.2 Etiology and Risk Factors

- Usually multifactorial, with both intrinsic and extrinsic factors being recognized (▶ Table 14.1).[6,7,8]

14.1.3 Noninsertional Achilles Tendinopathy

- *Symptoms:* Characterized by pain and swelling elicited in the midportion of the tendon (between 2 and 6 cm proximal to the Achilles insertion) at the beginning of exercise and shortly after completion (▶ Fig. 14.1).[8,9]
- It is usually divided into three histopathologic and clinical entities[1]:
  - *Peritendinitis:* Peritendinitis is inflammation of only the paratenon with thickening and adhesions of peritendinous tissue to normal tendon. Tenderness remains in one location throughout the ankle range of motion.
  - *Peritendinitis with tendinosis:* It represents further inflammation with associated intratendinous degeneration. Pain and tenderness are marked and constant.
  - *Tendinosis or noninflammatory atrophic degeneration:* This is associated with normal aging and typically is accelerated with overuse. Calcifications and nodularity may be present as well as a point of tenderness that moves proximally and distally as the ankle is dorsiflexed or plantarflexed (▶ Fig. 14.2).
- Imaging:
  - Diagnosis is mainly based on history and clinical examination. Nevertheless, imaging techniques can be useful to assess the degree of severity and distinguish associated concomitant pathologies.[10]
  - Radiographs should be included in order to determine any bony abnormalities or intrasubstance tendon calcifications.
  - Magnetic resonance imaging (MRI) and ultrasound can be helpful to locate degeneration within the tendon or focal tendon ruptures (▶ Fig. 14.3).[8]
- Treatment:
  - Conservative:
    - Noninsertional tendinopathy usually responds to nonoperative measures as decreasing activity, cryotherapy, nonsteroidal anti-inflammatory drugs (NSAIDs), heel lifts, or shock-absorbing shoes/orthotics.[11]
    - Severe symptoms may benefit from a short period of compression,

Table 14.1 Intrinsic and extrinsic risk factors for Achilles tendon pathology

Intrinsic	Extrinsic
Increasing age (over 40 y)	Repetitive impact: loading activities
Male sex	Improper training techniques
Obesity	Inappropriate footwear
Postural problems (cavus, pes planus)	Corticosteroid or fluoroquinolone use
Inflammatory arthropathies	

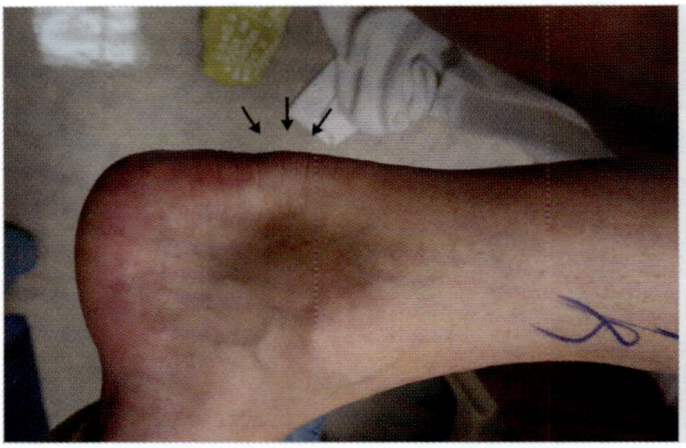

Fig. 14.1 Noninsertional Achilles tendinopathy (*black arrows*).

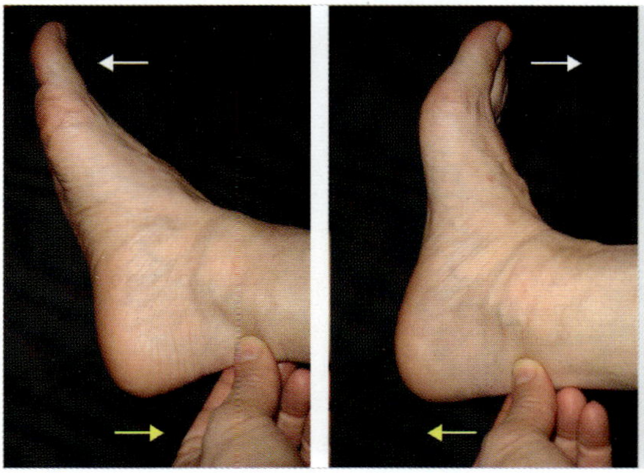

Fig. 14.2 Noninsertional Achilles tendinopathy. The point of tenderness moves proximally and distally (*yellow arrows*) as the ankle is dorsiflexed and plantarflexed (*white arrows*).

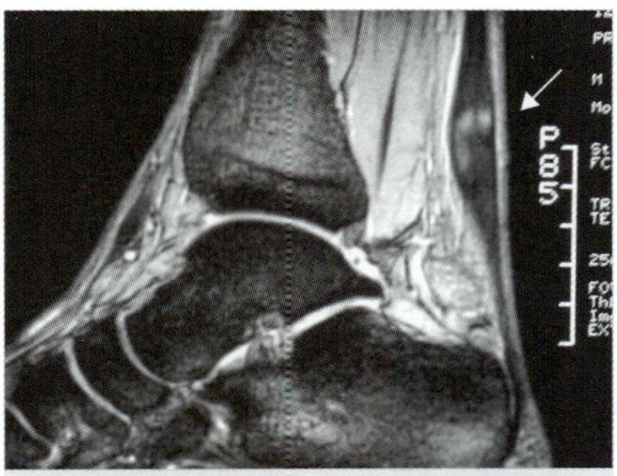

Fig. 14.3 Noninsertional Achilles tendinopathy. Degeneration and nodularity (*white arrow*) within the midportion of the tendon.

immobilization in neutral or plantar flexion, and protected weight bearing.[8]

- Physical therapy (PT) mainly consisting of eccentric exercise of the gastrocnemius - soleus complex and stretching is highly recommended as the first line of treatment.[6,10,11]
- Extracorporeal shock wave therapy (ESWT) is well supported as a second-line treatment.[11]
- Corticoid injections are not recommended as they have been associated with spontaneous tendon rupture and decreased tendon strength.[8]
- The use of biologics as platelet-rich plasma (PRP), bone marrow aspirate concentrate (BMAC), and adipose-derived stem cells (ADSCs) have been widely studied in recent years as a step between conservative and surgical treatment. Despite its promising initial results, their grade of recommendation in midsubstance Achilles tendinopathy is yet to be determined.[12]
- Ultrasound-guided brisement with high-volume injections with/or diluted anesthetics in cases of peritendinitis has also been described to break up adhesions of the tendon sheath.[8,9]

○ Surgical alternatives:
  - Percutaneous or tendoscopic stripping of the paratenon has been described for removing neovascularization and denervating the diseased area of the tendon with and without longitudinal tenotomies to stimulate a biologic repair response. The use of a novel ultrasonic cutting and radiofrequency devices has been recently described with comparative studies required to determine their efficacy.[11,13,14]
  - Open release of adhesions with or without resection of the paratenon, associated with excision of macroscopic areas of tendinopathy or calcifications through a central ellipse tenotomy.

- In cases of tendinosis, the surgical alternatives may depend on the degree of width of the tendon involved.[1,8]
- Width involved:
  * Less than 50%: ellipse and repair; tubularization.
  * Greater than 50% but less than 80%: ellipse and consider augment in low-demand patients. Flexor hallucis longus (FHL) or flexor digitorum longus (FDL) tendon transfer.
  * Greater than 80%: Ellipse or complete resection of the diseased tendon with augmentation with FHL or FDL. If completely resecting, consider V-Y advancement, turndown, or allograft reconstruction to avoid posterior gapping.

14.1.4 Insertional Achilles Tendinopathy

- Secondary to degeneration of the tendon at its insertion on the calcaneus.
- It may be associated with Haglund's deformity, which is a prominent posterosuperior aspect of the calcaneal tuberosity that causes both bursitis and tendinopathy (▶ Fig. 14.4).
- Symptoms:
  ◦ History of pain at the back of the calcaneus that deteriorates after exercise or climbing stairs and also with inactivity periods. Early morning stiffness.[10]
  ◦ Patients can relate pain or tenderness when using constrictive footwear in the zone (▶ Fig. 14.5).
- Physical examination:
  ◦ Patients typically have tenderness to palpation within the distal 2 cm of the Achilles tendon that aggravates with passive or active motion.

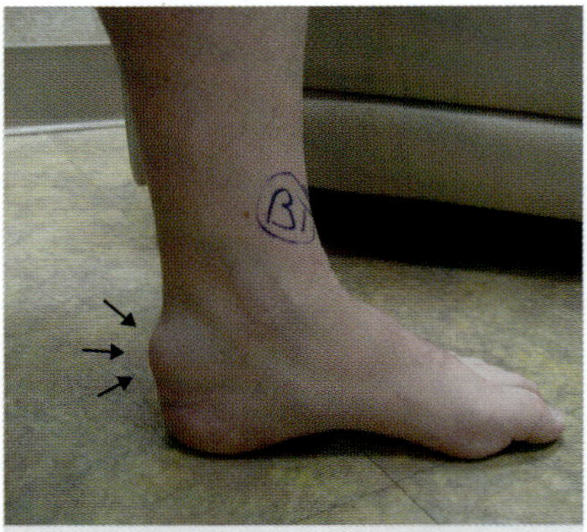

Fig. 14.4 Insertional Achilles tendinopathy. Prominence at Achilles tendon insertion (*black arrows*).

  ◦ Swelling and an enlarged posterior border of the calcaneus may be palpable.[15]
- Imaging:
  ◦ X-rays can reveal tendon insertion calcifications and Haglund's deformity (▶ Fig. 14.6).
  ◦ MRI can be useful for looking for degeneration and focal microtears of the tendon (▶ Fig. 14.7).
- Treatment:
  ◦ Conservative:
    - Same nonoperative measures as noninsertional tendinopathy.
    - Shoe modifications avoiding posterior pressure.
    - In the acute setting, a short period of immobilization can control exacerbating factors.
    - Monitored PT and stretching regimen.
    - Invasive nonsurgical treatments such as ESWT, PRP, and BMAC should be considered in cases without improvement after noninvasive therapies.[16]
  ◦ Surgical:
    - Reserved for recalcitrant disease in which conservative options have proved unsuccessful.

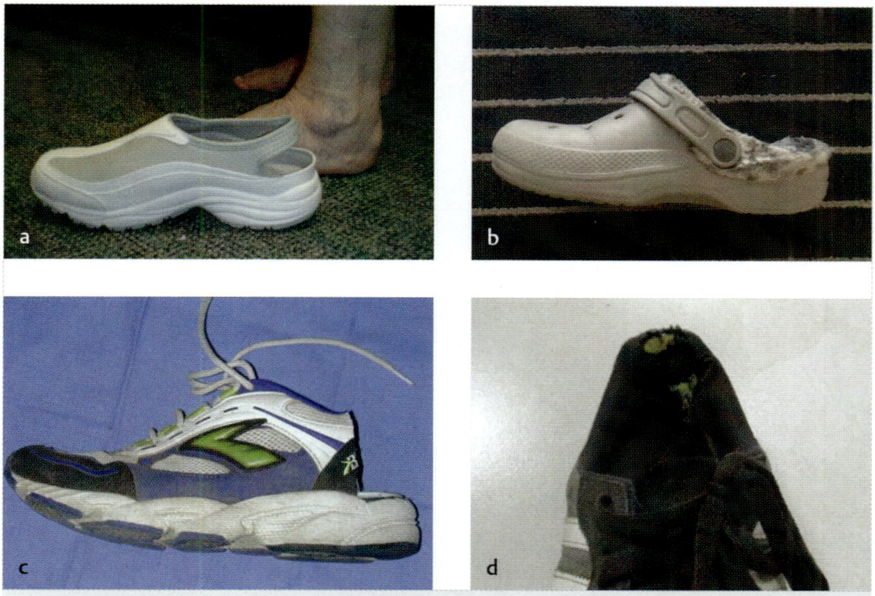

Fig. 14.5 Insertional Achilles tendinopathy. **(a,b)** Backless shoes may help reduce mechanical symptoms. **(c)** Constrictive footwear worsens symptoms and usually are modified by patients. **(d)** Heel tab wear secondary to chronic prominence in a patient with insertional Achilles tendinopathy.

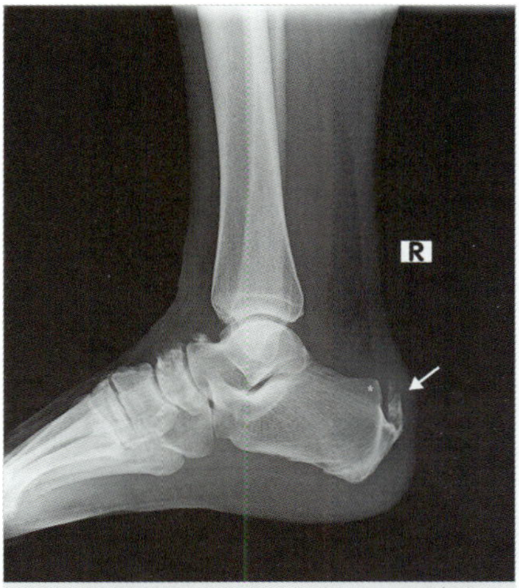

Fig. 14.6 Insertional Achilles tendinopathy. X-ray examination shows calcification of the Achilles insertion (*arrow*) and Haglund's deformity (*asterisk*).

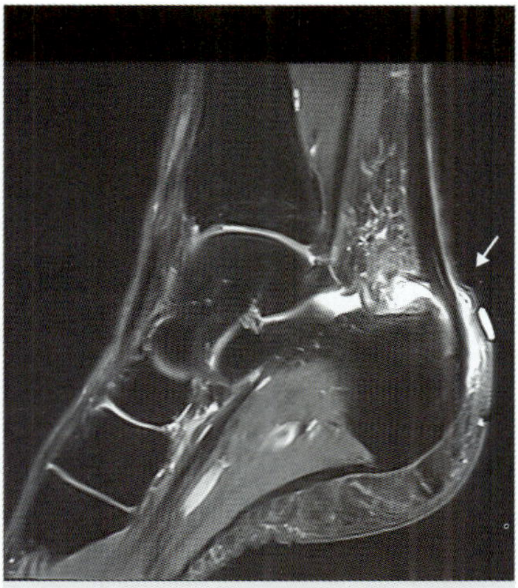

Fig. 14.7 Insertional Achilles tendinopathy. Lateral magnetic resonance imaging (MRI) T2 sequence. Note insertional edema and degeneration (*white arrow*).

- Open debridement of the degenerative insertion through a longitudinal central approach, resection of any bony prominence, reattachment of the insertion as required, and/or augmentation of the Achilles tendon using a tendon transfer or graft.[17]
- Biomechanical and clinical data suggest that 50% of the tendon attachment can be safely debrided with minimal risk of re-rupture.
- Augmentation using FHL is the most frequently used method of reconstruction. Other commonly used options are FDL and peroneus brevis (PB).[1]
- Gastrocnemius recession, in patients with associated contracture, may be performed in combination with open debridement. The effectiveness of isolated gastrocnemius recession is controversial with conflicting low-level evidence.[15]

14.1.5 Retrocalcaneal Bursitis

- Inflammation, hypertrophy, and adherence of the bursa anterior to the Achilles tendon. These changes may be associated with degenerative changes within the tendon substance.
- The bursa is compressed in the recess between the tendon and the calcaneus during ankle dorsiflexion.
- Clinically patients will present with similar symptoms as in insertional Achilles tendinopathy.
- *Two-finger squeeze:* medial and lateral pressure anterior to the Achilles tendon.
- Treatment:
  - Conservative treatment as established for insertional tendinopathy.
  - Surgical treatment includes open or tendoscopic debridement of the tendon insertion and decompression of the bursa.[10,18]

14.1.6 Acute Achilles Tendon Rupture

- Most common tendon rupture. Typically, occur in men in their 30s and 40s, with more than 75% of these injuries occurring during athletic participation, mostly recreational (weekend warrior).[19]
- Mechanism of injury involves an active, forceful, or unexpected foot plantar flexion with most of the ruptures occurring 2 to 4 cm proximal to its insertion in the calcaneus.
- Patients presenting with acute Achilles tendon rupture often report a sudden snap or popping in the heel region after pushing off. Immediate pain is present but gradually dissipates.[1,6]
- A major complaint is the difficulty to weight-bear and plantarflex the ankle with "giving way" sensation as the main symptom.
- On physical examination, acute ruptures are typically present:
  - Presence of a palpable tendon gap or divot (▶ Fig. 14.8).
  - *Positive Thompson test:* compression of the midcalf in the supine position does not elicit passive plantar flexion (▶ Fig. 14.9).
  - Decreased plantar flexion strength.
  - *Positive Matles' test:* Increased passive ankle dorsiflexion at rest in comparison with the unaffected side.

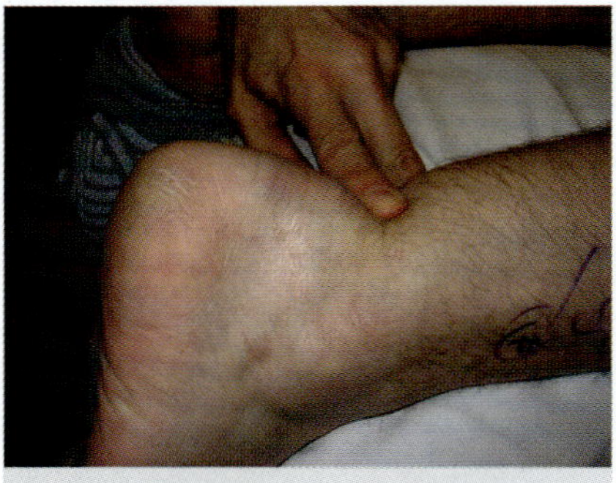

Fig. 14.8 Acute Achilles tendon rupture. Palpable tendon gap.

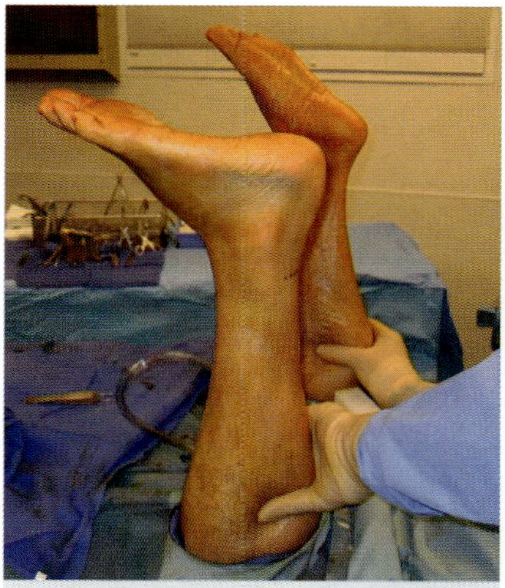

Fig. 14.9 Acute Achilles tendon rupture. Positive Thompson test. Compression of both mid-calves. There is no passive plantar flexion at the right side.

- Imaging:
  - Diagnosis is primarily clinical.
  - Radiographs should be obtained in cases of suspected Achilles tendon pathology to rule out avulsions or calcific tendon changes.
  - *Ultrasound* confirms diagnosis and estimates size of the rupture with good intraoperative correlation. It remains cheaper and more readily available than MRI but it is operator-dependent.
  - *MRI* is more accurate than ultrasound for determining the tendon cross-sectional area. Use in the acute setting may be useful for differentiating partial ruptures from focal tendinosis (▶ Fig. 14.10).[20]
- Treatment:
  - Optimal treatment remains controversial and continues to evolve. Both nonoperative and operative treatments have distinct advantages and disadvantages.[21]
  - Nonoperative treatment:
    - Conservative treatment has evolved from strict prolonged immobilization into functional bracing protocols that include limited initial non-weight-bearing and casting in equinus for 2 weeks, followed by functional bracing with an orthosis that allows progressive decreases on plantar flexion.
    - Active plantar flexion exercises are encouraged with dorsiflexion restriction for at least 6 weeks. Recent literature associates functional rehabilitation with increased range of motion, less tendon lengthening, and lower re-rupture rates (near 2%) comparable to operative treatment.[21,22]
    - Advantages:
      - No complications related to surgery (wound breakdown, infection, sural nerve paresthesias).
    - Disadvantages:
      - Adherence to functional rehabilitation protocol necessary for good outcome.

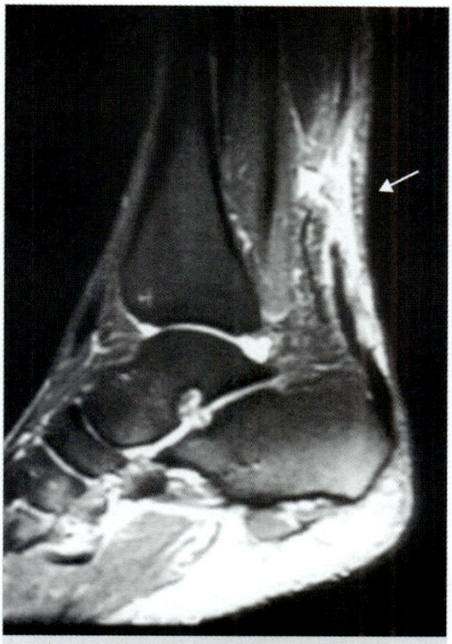

Fig. 14.10 Acute Achilles tendon rupture. Magnetic resonance imaging (MRI) showing a complete Achilles tendon rupture (*white arrow*).

    * Calf atrophy.
    * Typically, normal functioning length of the Achilles is not restored; high-demand patients may note significant muscle weakness.
- Operative treatment:
  - Several different procedures had been described for repairing acute Achilles ruptures utilizing either an open, a mini-open, or a percutaneous minimally invasive surgery (MIS) approach.
  - Open repair approach options can be midline medial (▶ Fig. 14.11) or lateral in a prone or supine position. Both tendon edges must be brought together under the appropriate tension using a nonabsorbable suture with minimal manipulation of soft tissues. Stitch patterns described include the modified Bunnell, Kessler, and Krackow techniques (▶ Fig. 14.12). Wound issues and delayed healing are the main complications reported.[1,19]
  - The mini-open repair approach involves small incisions that allow direct visualization of the ruptured tendon ends. This technique has been reported to have better outcomes concerning return to walking and sports activities in comparison to the open approach.
  - MIS percutaneous techniques are associated with less rate of re-rupture or other complications such as superficial infection and wound breakage than open techniques, but with a greater incidence of sural nerve injury. Early repair elongation has also been reported.[23,24,25]
  - Advantages:
    * Improved functional outcomes concerning return to sport and faster return to work.
  - Disadvantages:
    * Invasive procedure.
    * Complications of surgery, especially wound related.

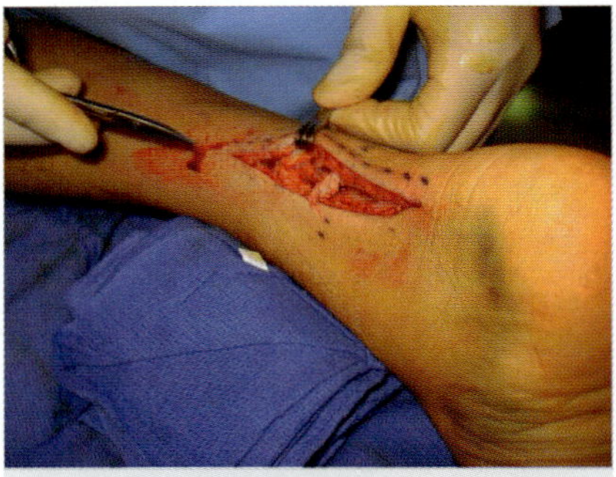

Fig. 14.11 Acute Achilles tendon rupture. Open repair through a medial approach.

14.1.7 Chronic Achilles Tendon Rupture

- Patients presenting with chronic Achilles ruptures may be the result of delay in seeking medical attention due to decrease in the level of pain after the initial period of discomfort or misdiagnosis at the initial evaluation (up to 25% of patients).[26]
- The transition from what is considered an acute to a chronic rupture is not clear in the literature. The most common classification system includes the following:
  - *Acute:* ruptures less than 2 weeks old.
  - *Subacute:* injuries from 3 to 6 weeks old.
    - Chronic: rupture exceeding 6 weeks.
- Usually disorganized fibrous tissue fills the gap between the retracted stumps. This tissue lacks any significant orientation or functionality. Contraction of the tendon and adhesions are found as early as 3 to 4 days after the injury. Occasionally, the tendon may heal in continuity in an elongated position, leading to a loss in the mechanical efficiency of the gastroc-soleus complex.[1,27]
- Symptoms may be vague and not necessarily localized at the Achilles region, such as swelling around the ankle and weakness or fatigue with ambulation.
- Physical examination:
  - Similar findings can be found respecting acute ruptures.

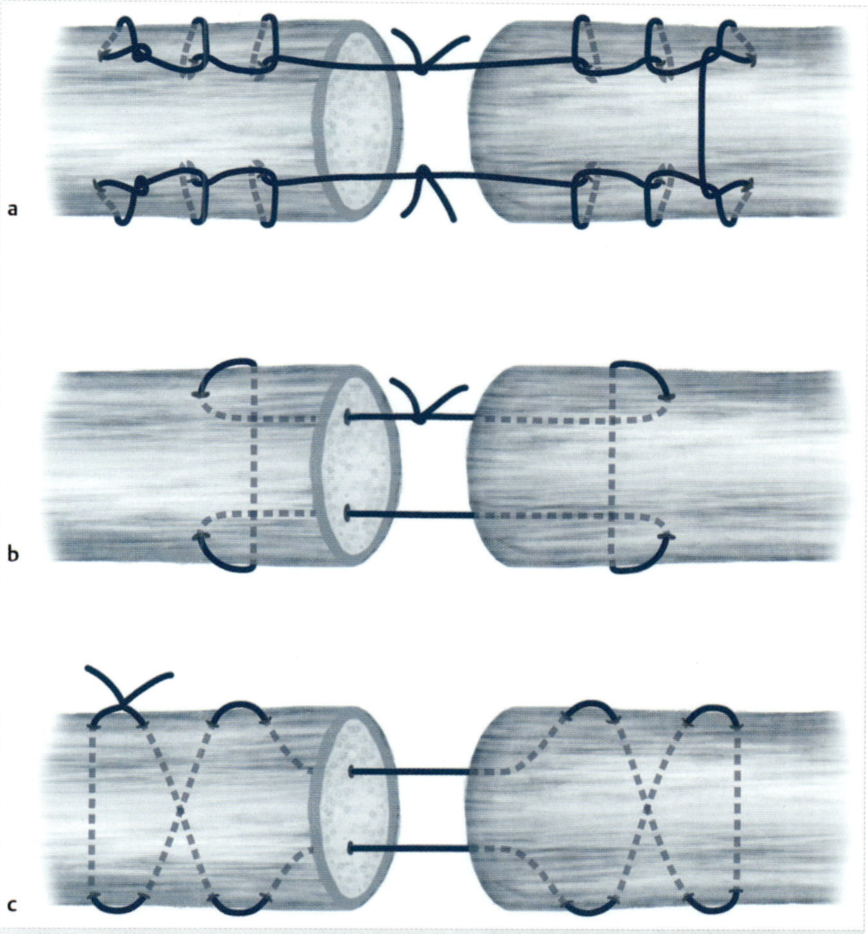

Fig. 14.12 Techniques for tendon repair. **(a)** modified Bunnell's technique. **(b)** Kessler's technique. **(c)** Krackow's technique.

- Fibrous tissue incorporation can result in a negative Thompson test and absence of palpable gap; however, some patients may have skin contracture around the rupture (► Fig. 14.13).
- Plantar flexion strength may be maintained at the expense of recruiting the posterior tibial tendon and FHL tendon, but weakened comparing to the contralateral extremity.
- Excessive dorsiflexion is noted relatively to the other side.

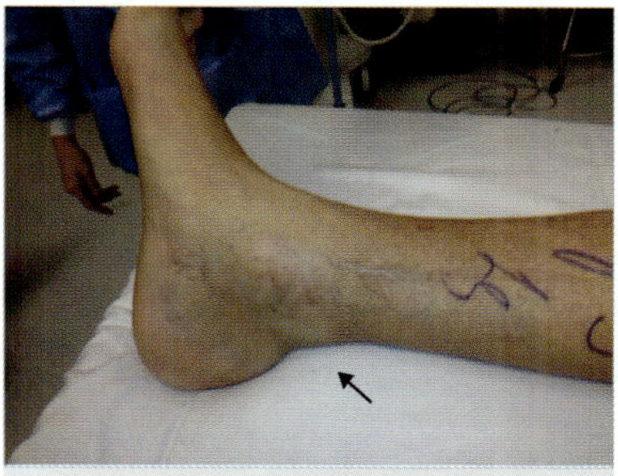

Fig. 14.13 Chronic Achilles tendon rupture. Skin contracture around the rupture (*arrow*).

- Imaging:
  - Ultrasound and MRI are useful to evaluate the size of the tendon gap and assist in surgical planning (▶ Fig. 14.14).
- Treatment:
  - Conservative:
    - Nonoperative treatment may be considered for patients with low demand and associated comorbidities, such as peripheral vascular disease as well as for patients without significant functional deficit.
    - The use of a hinged molded carbon-fiber ankle–foot orthosis (AFO) is recommended for stability improvement.[27]
  - Surgical:
    - Most of the patients with chronic Achilles tendon ruptures demonstrate poor healing potential with functional impairment requiring surgery.
    - Options for surgical treatment include the following:

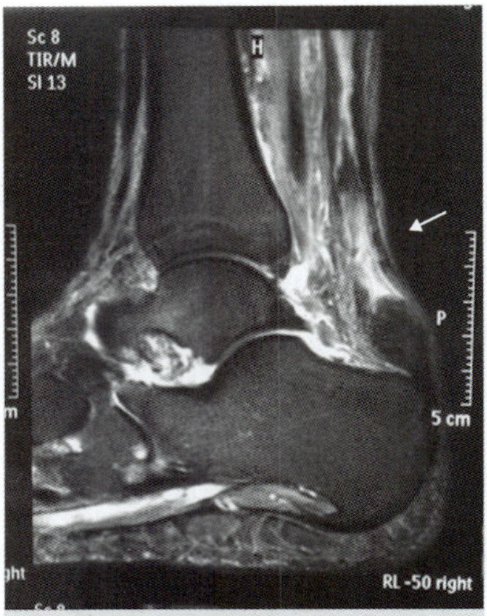

Fig. 14.14 Chronic Achilles tendon rupture. Magnetic resonance imaging (MRI) showing gap and fibrosis around both remaining tendon stumps (*white arrow*).

      * Direct repair: may be achieved for gaps less than 3 cm after debridement. Due to tissue retraction, defects of such small size are rare.
      * V-Y advancement: for gaps between 1 and 3 cm.
      * Turndown procedure with tendon augmentation for gaps between 3 and 5 cm.
      * FHL or FDL tendon transfer: for gaps larger than 5 cm. Specially in cases with preoperative atrophy of the gastrocnemius/soleus muscle.
      * *Augmentation with synthetics or allografts:* Dermal tissue matrix or Achilles tendon allografts are usually used for large defects greater than 5 cm.[26,28]

14.2 Peroneal Tendons

14.2.1 Anatomy

- The PB originates from the lower two-thirds of the fibula and intramuscular septum and runs immediately posterior to the lateral malleolus. Superficial to the calcaneofibular ligament, anterior to the peroneus longus tendon, and superior to the peroneal tubercle of the calcaneus. The PB has a flattened ovoid shape and it inserts into the base of the fifth metatarsal.
- The origin of the peroneus longus muscle is from the proximal fibula extending to the proximal two-thirds of the fibula, traveling along the posterior aspect of the PB tendon, inferior to the peroneal tubercle on the lateral wall of the calcaneus, turning medially around the lateral border of the cuboid, and inserting on the first metatarsal.[29]
- Both the PB and longus tendons traverse the posterior aspect of the fibula in the retromalleolar sulcus and the superior peroneal retinaculum (SPR). These structures form a fibro-osseous tunnel

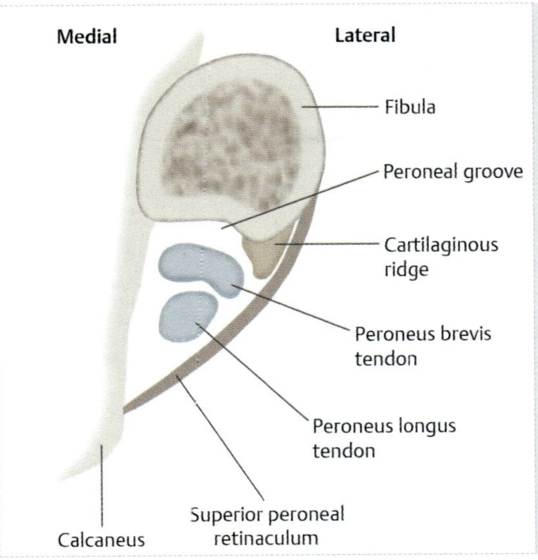

Fig. 14.15 Peroneal tendons. Note the position of the peroneus brevis anterior to the peroneus longus tendon both contained by the superior peroneal retinaculum.

(▶ Fig. 14.15). Anatomic studies have shown that most of the sulcus are concave in 82%, flat in 11%, and convex in 7%. There is no consensus whether these differences in the anatomy of the sulcus (flat or convex) have a role on the development of peroneal tendon instability.[30,31]

- The posterolateral aspect of the lateral malleolus has a fibrocartilaginous rim that deepens the retromalleolar sulcus. Both tendons share a common synovial sheath enveloping them.
- *Vascular supply:* Posterior peroneal artery, with branches of the medial tarsal artery supplying the distal part of the peroneus longus.
- The peroneus longus has two avascular zones: the region where the tendon turns around the lateral malleolus and the region where the tendon changes its direction under the cuboid. On the other hand, the PB tendon has its intratendinous blood supply discontinued at the retromalleolar sulcus. These regions with watershed zones are susceptible to chronic degenerative changes.[32]
- Peroneus quartus, an accessory muscle in the lateral compartment of the leg, with an incidence of 6.6 to 21.7% is commonly associated with peroneal tendinopathy, instability, and stenosing tenosynovitis. This tendon causes symptoms by virtue of the bulk behind the fibula contained in the retinaculum.
- The peroneus longus functions as the primary evertor of the foot, first metatarsal plantarflexor, and secondary ankle plantarflexor.
- The PB acts to evert and abduct the foot and as a secondary ankle plantarflexor.
- Both tendons serve as dynamic stabilizers for the ankle and hindfoot against inversion forces.[31,32]

14.2.2 History and Physical Examination

- Consider a peroneal tendon injury in a patient who presents with lateral ankle pain.
- Previous history of ankle sprain, ankle, or calcaneus fracture may be present.
- Ligamentous stability of the ankle should be addressed, as well as history of chronic

instability or giving way. Use of ciprofloxacin or other fluoroquinolones should be included in the history.
- Assessment of the hindfoot and forefoot should be performed due to the high association with peroneal pathology in patients with hindfoot varus and/or cavus.[33]

14.2.3 Peroneal Tenosynovitis/Tendonitis

- Etiology:
  - Tenosynovitis as well as tendonitis may be associated with peroneal subluxation/dislocation, peroneal groove abnormalities, hypertrophy of the peroneal tubercle, low-lying PB muscle belly, and peroneus quartus.
  - Trauma to the peroneal tendons is usually from a direct blow or twisting injury. Overuse injuries (repetitive microtrauma) or inflammatory arthropathies (e.g., lupus, rheumatoid arthritis) have also been described.
- Symptoms:
  - Patients usually complain of vague pain on the posterolateral aspect of the hindfoot that is increased with activity and diminished by rest (▶ Fig. 14.16). A traumatic episode as an inversion injury to the ankle may be associated with the onset of discomfort.[29,33]
- Physical examination:
  - Pain with palpation along the course of the peroneal tendons inferior to the fibula and with passive inversion of the foot or active eversion of the forefoot against resistance.
  - A palpable thickening may be present, as well as warmth and swelling on the lateral border of the ankle.
- Imaging:
  - Ultrasound is widely available and may confirm the diagnosis.
  - MRI is helpful in distinguishing tenosynovitis from other peroneal tendon pathology as complete or partial tears (▶ Fig. 14.17).[31]
- Treatment:
  - Conservative:
    - PT, changes in training techniques, and orthotics.
    - Casting or walking boot for 3 to 4 weeks may be used in severe cases.

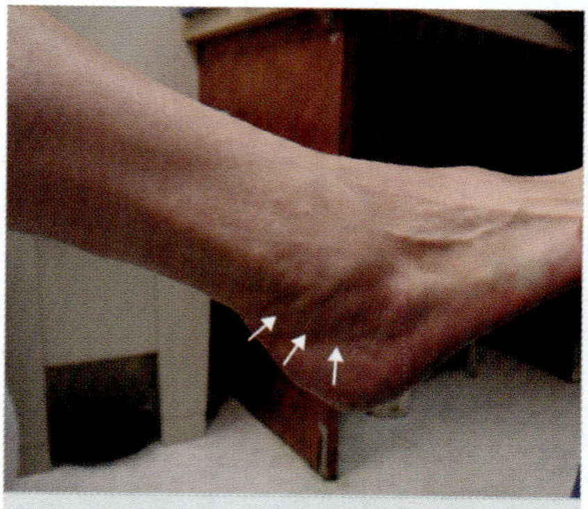

Fig. 14.16 Peroneal tendons. Patients relate pain on the posterolateral aspect of the ankle (*white arrows*).

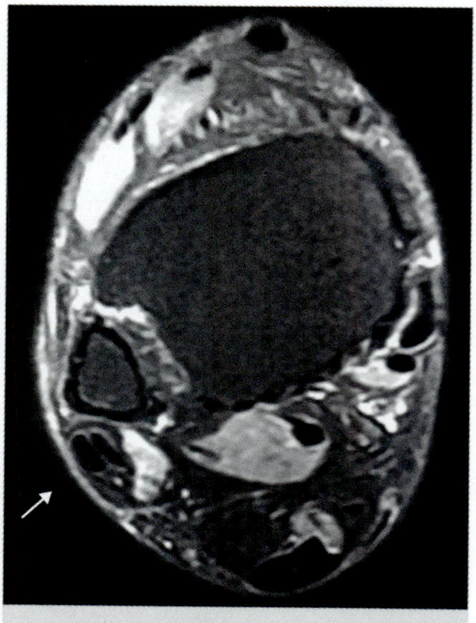

Fig. 14.17 Peroneal tendons tenosynovitis. Magnetic resonance imaging (MRI) showing excess fluid around both peroneal tendons (*arrow*).

- With continued symptoms, some authors recommend ultrasound-guided corticoid injections but with concerns regarding the risk of tendon rupture.
- PRP or bone marrow concentrate injection may be helpful in treating recalcitrant tendinopathy.[34]

◦ Surgical:
- Open tendon debridement associated synovectomy is reserved for cases in which conservative measures fail.[29,30,32]
- Peroneal tendoscopy has gained popularity and may be useful for evaluation of tendon integrity, synovectomy, and endoscopic release.[35]
- In cases of a hypertrophic peroneal tubercle, shaving or resection has showed good results in addition to retinaculum interposition between the surface of the calcaneus and peroneus longus.
- In the rare case of stenosing tenosynovitis, division of the tendon sheath roof and release of the retinaculum have proven useful.[36]

14.2.4 Peroneal Tendon Instability

- Mechanism of injury:
  - Acute peroneal tendon dislocations most commonly result from a sudden, forceful, passive dorsiflexion of an everted foot with a sudden, strong contraction of the peroneal muscles. Dislocation with the foot in inversion has also been described.
  - The strong contraction of the peroneal muscles produces the superior peroneal retinaculum (SPR) to tear off its fibular periosteal attachment. The peroneus longus is more laterally located and thus more prone for dislocation comparing to PB, although in some cases both tendons may dislocate.[30]
  - Chronic subluxation can also occur in patients with recurrent ankle sprains due to chronic stretching and elongation of the SPR allowing the tendons to roll around, predisposing the tendons to tears.[37]
  - Peroneal subluxation is commonly associated with tears of the PB tendon, especially in the cases where chronic ankle instability is present.
- History:
  - In the setting of an acute dislocation, the patient recalls a significant episode of trauma. A painful snapping sensation may be associated with the actual disruption and retromalleolar tenderness.
  - Chronic peroneal instability usually coexists with a history of "recurrent sprains." Snapping, popping, or instability is the main complaint, especially on uneven ground.
- Physical examination:
  - Acutely, a variable amount of swelling and ecchymosis may be present in the retrofibular region, which can obscure the dislocated peroneal tendons.
  - Palpable crepitus can be noted over the posterior rim of the fibula. The ankle is circumducted passively allowing the identification of subluxation. Dorsiflexion and eversion also allow dislocation to occur (▶ Fig. 14.18). Examination of the

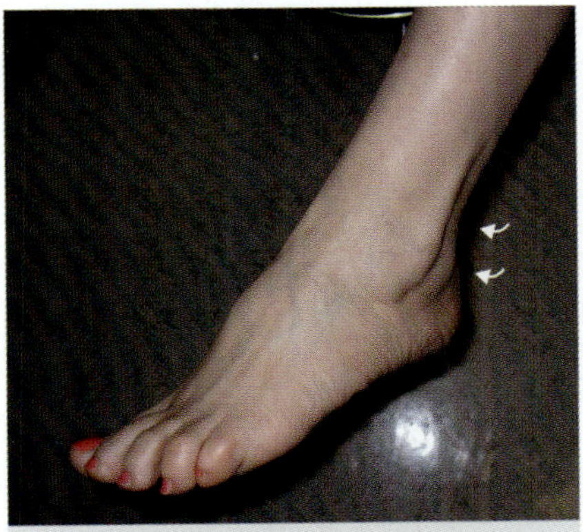

Fig. 14.18 Peroneal tendons dislocation (*white arrows*).

contralateral ankle is important to rule out normal popping of the tendons. Coexisting ankle ligament instability and peroneal tendon weakness should be identified.[30,38]

- Imaging:
  - Radiographs can demonstrate a small lateral distal fibula avulsion or cortical rim fragment.
  - Ultrasound dynamic evaluation is confirmatory in skilled hands.
  - MRI may be helpful in assessing a concomitant peroneal tendon tear (▸ Fig. 14.19).
- Treatment:
  - Conservative:
    - Nonsurgical treatment is controversial. In the acute setting, below-knee cast in mild plantar flexion for 6 weeks has been advocated for some authors recognizing a high failure rate.

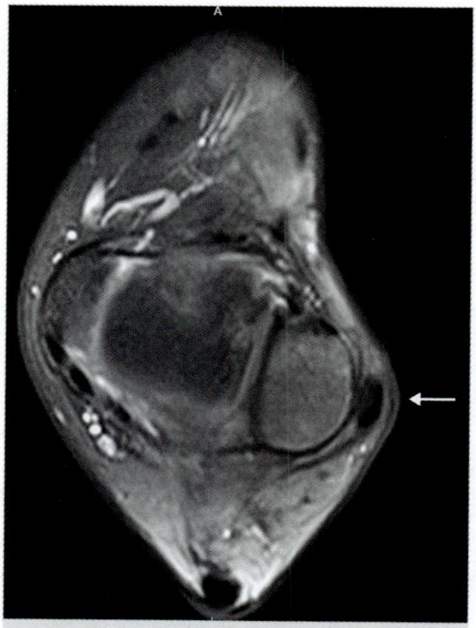

Fig. 14.19 Peroneal tendons dislocation. Magnetic resonance imaging (MRI) shows both peroneal tendons upon the lateral border of the fibula and a convex sulcus (*white arrow*).

  - Surgery:
    - Surgical reconstruction has a much higher rate of success compared with nonsurgical treatment.
    - Many different techniques have been reported to treat symptomatic peroneal tendon instability. Independently of the procedure chosen, the goals of surgery are as follows:
      * Direct repair/reconstruction of the SPR.
      * Reestablishing the fibrocartilaginous rim.
      * Groove-deepening or bone block procedures can be added specially if a flat or convex retromalleolar groove is found.[29,30,37]

14.2.5 Peroneus Brevis Tears

- Mechanism of injury:
  - Resulting often from damage caused by repeated subluxation, the true incidence of PB tears is unknown. The sharp posterolateral edge of the fibula can create a small tear in the tendon as it repeatedly subluxes over the ridge. This primary injury often extends into a longitudinal tear 2.5 to 5 cm in length.[37]
  - Tears can also result from mechanical wear at the tip of the fibula, where a relative hypovascularity and increased pressure exist.
- History and physical examination:
  - Symptoms and clinical findings are similar to those demonstrated with peroneal tenosynovitis.
  - Pain may be elicited with palpation along the course of the PB tendon posterior to the distal fibula and finishing at its insertion on the base of the fifth metatarsal.[31]
- Imaging:
  - Radiographs are usually normal.
  - MRI may be helpful in identifying longitudinal ruptures and detecting anatomic risk factors for PB tears.

- Treatment:
  - Conservative:
    - Reduced activity, shoe modifications, and lateral heel wedges.
    - Immobilization with a below-knee walking cast can diminish symptoms and allow the inflammatory process to subside.
    - Ankle or stirrup brace can diminish inversion and eversion, stopping traumatic stresses while permitting full ankle function in the sagittal plane.
    - For resistant cases with partial ruptures, PRP or bone marrow concentrate may be of help.
    - Failure of conservative treatment is common.[30,34]
  - Surgical:
    - Typically, two types of tears of the PB are identified: a single longitudinal tear or multiple longitudinal tears characterized by areas of fibrillation (▶ Fig. 14.20).
    - *Treatment options:* Repair of the tendon with resection of a major tear or defect. With degenerative fibrillation, the shredded fibers may be resected and debrided up to one half of the tendon. Tubularization of the remaining tendon should be attempted.

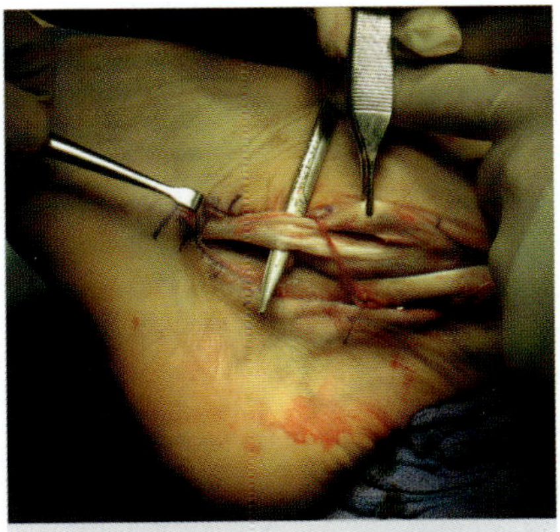

Fig. 14.20 Surgical exploration revealing a longitudinal split of the peroneus brevis.

    - Other options include turndown of the tendon proximally to bridge a gap or augment a tendon that has less than 50% remaining tendon autograft (usually FDL or FHL), allograft, or tenodesis of the PB to the peroneus longus.[29,30,39]

14.2.6 Peroneus Longus Tears

- Tears of the peroneus longus are much less common but may coexist with ruptures of the brevis. Injuries occur at the tip of the lateral malleolus, peroneal tubercle, or os peroneum.[39]
- As with the PB, injury to the peroneus longus can be acute or chronic.
- An acute injury to a healthy tendon typically is a result of a sudden inversion sprain. In the presence of an os peroneum, the tendon rupture can be caused by an avulsion fracture with diastasis and proximal retraction of the tendon or the sesamoid.
- Chronic injury to the peroneus longus usually occurs in the setting of degeneration with longitudinal splitting (▶ Fig. 14.21). Hindfoot varus and cavovarus deformity has been associated with these injuries.[37]
- Clinical findings and treatment are similar as previously presented for peroneal brevis tendon injuries.

14.2.7 Combined Peroneal Tears

- It is relatively uncommon to have combined PB and longus tears.
- Typically, a varus deformity of the hindfoot occurs that is coupled with a distinct weakness of eversion power in the forefoot.[39]
- Surgical options, depending usually on intraoperative findings and on previous tendon function, consist mainly of tendon transfers (FHL or FDL) or allograft reconstruction. Adjuvant procedures to

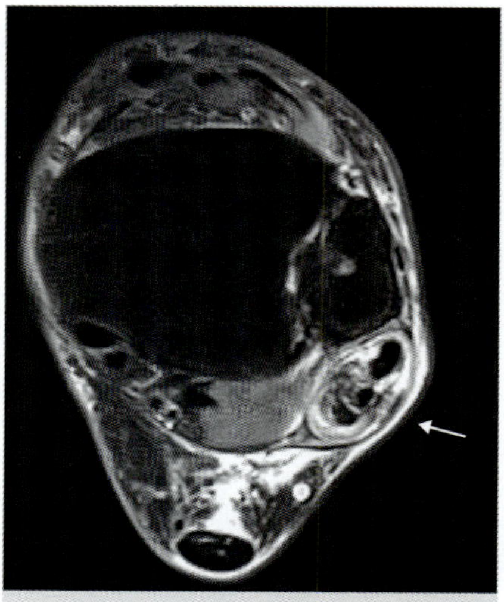

Fig. 14.21 Magnetic resonance imaging (MRI) showing chronic peroneus longus rupture and concomitant tenosynovitis (*white arrow*).

correct the hindfoot varus should be considered in order to protect the reconstructed/transferred tendons and avoid further damage to these structures.[30,33,40]

14.3 Anterior Tibial Tendon

14.3.1 Anatomy

- The anterior tibial tendon functions as the major dorsiflexor of the ankle.
- It originates from the proximal half of the anterior tibia, the lower lateral tibial condyle, lateral tibia, and the interosseous membrane, and inserts on the plantar medial aspect of the first cuneiform and the plantar base of the first metatarsal.[41]
- At the level of the lower and middle thirds of the tibia, it becomes tendinous and is surrounded by the synovial sheath.
- Innervated by the deep peroneal nerve, the anterior tibial tendon functions to dorsiflex and invert the foot and provides controlled plantar flexion at the heel strike.[37]
- The tendon passes beneath the superior extensor retinaculum and the upper and lower limbs of the inferior extensor retinaculum.
- Despite being a relatively well-vascularized structure, an avascular zone is found where the tendon runs under the superior and inferior retinaculum. This results in an area 1 to 2 cm from the insertion that is at risk of tendinopathy or rupture.[37]

14.3.2 Anterior Tibial Tendinopathy

- Anterior tibial tendon tendinopathy is an uncommon pathology.
- Symptoms include swelling and tenderness at the distal insertion on the medial cuneiform.
- It most commonly occurs in overweight female patients aged 50 to 70 years and also in young active athletes developing anterior ankle pain at the level of the extensor retinaculum secondary to overuse.[42]
- Conservative treatment includes nonsteroidal anti-inflammatories, PT, longitudinal arch support, and night splints.
- Operative treatment strategies are reserved for cases with poor response to conservative measures. Debridement of the diseased tendon with or without reinsertion as well as gastrocnemius recession had been described as surgical options with acceptable outcomes.[42,43]

14.3.3 Anterior Tibial Tendon Rupture

- Anterior tibial tendon can rupture in the acute or chronic degenerative setting.
- An acute disruption of the tendon can occur with trauma at any age from fractures of the tibia or lacerations.

- A spontaneous rupture can occur from an underlying degenerative process contributed in some cases by inflammatory arthritis, gout, rheumatoid arthritis, extrinsic compression or impingement from an underlying exostosis of the midfoot, a local steroid injection, and diabetes.[34]
- History:
  - A patient with anterior tibial tendon rupture often complains of swelling of the anterior ankle and foot region in association with weak dorsiflexion. A foot drop may be significant or minimal.
  - Moderate pain associated with a tendon rupture usually subsides quickly.
  - In chronic disruptions, a patient's main complaint can be a vague sensation of weakness and decreased power of dorsiflexion.
- Physical examination:
  - Swelling of the anterior ankle can disguise the rupture although with time a palpable defect becomes apparent (▶ Fig. 14.22).
  - A fixed lump or mass on the anterior ankle can develop from the end of the retracted proximal tendon segment.
  - Lack of dorsiflexion power might be appreciated in comparison to the contralateral side. The patient is typically unable to walk on their heels.
  - Recruitment of the EHL and extensor digitorum longus (EDL) tendons may maintain the ability to dorsiflex the ankle, but without the anterior tibial tendon function, a gait disturbance typically occurs.
- Imaging:
  - MRI can be helpful in defining tendinopathy or an anterior tibial tendon rupture. In patients presenting late, who do not recall a traumatic or precipitating event, MRI can be helpful in making a diagnosis of rupture (▶ Fig. 14.23).
- Treatment:
  - Acute ruptures in the setting of trauma or laceration are almost certainly amenable for direct repair, which likely will improve ambulation and decrease morbidity.
  - Degenerative spontaneous ruptures, usually unnoticed in older low-demand patients, may be treated conservatively. Bracing may be prescribed in order to regain normal gait.
  - Direct repair is typically nonamenable to perform due to retraction and tendon degeneration on the chronic setting.
  - Reconstruction for chronic ruptures usually involves tendon transfer (EHL, EDL, or PB) or interposition grafting with either autograft or allograft.[39]

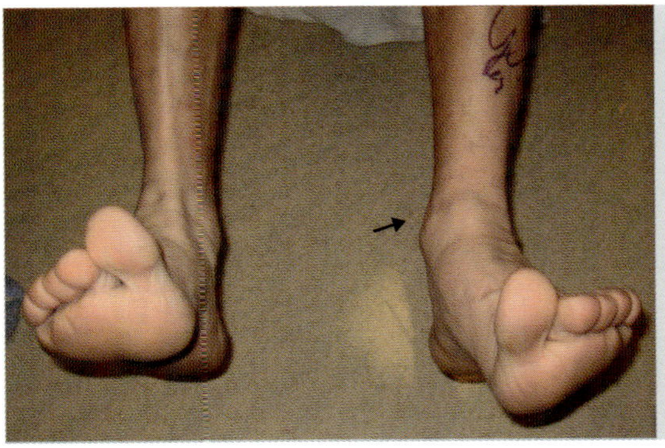

Fig. 14.22 Anterior tibial tendon rupture. Asymmetrical dorsiflexion on the left ankle in comparison to the contralateral side (*black arrow*).

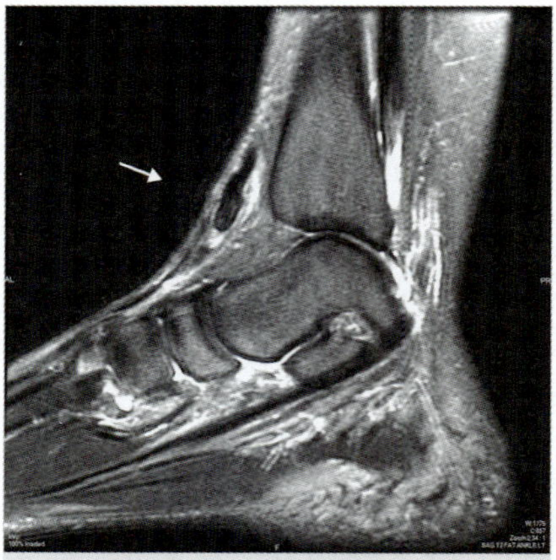

Fig. 14.23 Magnetic resonance imaging (MRI) showing anterior tibial tendon rupture (*white arrow*).

14.4 Flexor Tendons

14.4.1 Flexor Hallucis Longus

- Anatomy:
  - The FHL tendon is the major plantarflexor of the great toe. It originates from the posterior aspect of the fibula and interosseous membrane. It runs distally underneath the flexor retinaculum and within the tendon sheath, which attaches to the posterior talus and calcaneus, forming a fibro-osseous tunnel.
  - The tendon lies medial to the os trigonum in the groove between the medial and lateral tubercles of the talus. Then the FHL runs distally and medially to the groove on the plantar surface of the sustentaculum tali, and it crosses dorsal to the FDL interconnecting through the knot of Henry at the level of the first tarsometatarsal joint.
  - The tendon runs underneath the intersesamoid ligament and between both of flexor hallucis brevis (FHB) heads and then inserting in the distal phalanx of the hallux.
  - The blood supply to the FHL originates from both the posterior tibial and medial plantar arteries, and it is innervated by the tibial nerve.
- FHL tenosynovitis:
  - The most common location is proximally at the level of the sustentaculum tali as the tendon enters the fibro-osseous tunnel.
  - It may be associated with an os trigonum.
  - Other locations have been noted at the knot of Henry, where it is usually confused with plantar fasciitis and in the intersesamoid ligament producing a functional hallux rigidus manifestation.[44]
  - History and physical examination:
    - Patients often complain of pain in the area of stenosis, a catching sensation, and weakness during running, jumping, or rising on the ball of the foot.
    - Pain along the medial aspect of the ankle and subtalar joint is usually noted (▶ Fig. 14.24). However, it may be present in the midfoot or distally on the tendon insertion depending on the location of the disease. Triggering of the hallux may be also present. Crepitus on motion along the posterior medial ankle may be noted.
    - *Tomasen Sign*: with the ankle in dorsiflexion, metatarsophalangeal (MTP) joint dorsiflexion is lost because of tightness of the FHL tendons as it courses through the fibro-osseous tunnel.[45]
  - Imaging:
    - X-rays can show a hypertrophic os trigonum.
    - MRI is useful for assessment and location of the disease.
  - Treatment:
    - Conservative:
    - Restricted activity, change in dancing or training technique, ice, and NSAIDs have proven to diminish symptoms.
    - Bracing and casting may relieve acute inflammation.
    - PT consisting of icing, massage ultrasound, and FHL stretching.

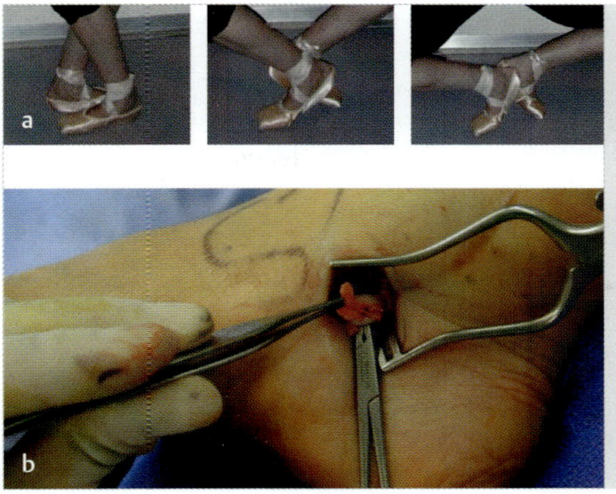

Fig. 14.24 Flexor hallucis longus (FHL) tenosynovitis in a professional dancer. **(a)** Preoperative swelling of the tendon sheath while performing a grand plié. **(b)** Intraoperative photograph of tendon sheath release. A flap tear of the tendon is identified and resected.

    - Steroid injections are not recommended as they can contribute to spontaneous rupture.
  - Surgery:
    - Operative treatment may be considered if conservative treatment is unsuccessful.
    - Open FHL debridement and fibro-osseous tunnel release are associated with resection of a prominent large os trigonum.
    - Arthroscopic removal of the os trigonum has been advocated, but a complete FHL release and debridement through this approach is challenging, due to the limited access to the FHL sheath.[45,46]
- FHL rupture:
  - Usually secondary to lacerations of the foot, although isolated spontaneous ruptures have been reported in the literature.
  - Injury to the FHL has been reported during harvesting of the FDL tendon during reconstruction surgery and hallux valgus surgery.[47]
  - The site of disruption can be divided into the following zones:
    - *Zone 1:* distal to the sesamoids in the area just proximal to the FHL insertion.
    - *Zone 2:* between the sesamoids and the knot of Henry.
    - *Zone 3:* proximal to the knot of Henry.
  - Zones 1 and 2 are not characterized by retraction of the proximal segment because of fibrous slip connecting the FHL and FDL tendons. Zone 3 injuries lead to proximal retraction of the tendon.[48]
  - History and physical examination:
    - Subjective loss of push-off and a feeling of giving way.
    - Normal active extension of the hallux interphalangeal (IP) joint but with no active plantar flexion.
    - Swelling or tenderness at the MTP joint and sesamoid region can denote distal rupture.
    - Pain and swelling of the posteromedial aspect of the ankle can develop with a proximal FHL tendon rupture.
  - Imaging:
    - As with FHL tenosynovitis, MRI is useful to evaluate tendon continuity.
  - Treatment:
    - The authors recommend repairing the FHL tendon in cases of lacerations or ruptures in young active patients.
    - In neglected ruptures without loss of IP joint plantar flexion or loss of push-off strength, the real necessity to perform surgery must be evaluated.
    - Surgical options include direct end-to-end repair, free graft

reconstruction, tenodesis to the FDL and split tendon lengthening.[37,47,48]

14.4.2 Flexor Digitorum Longus

- Anatomy:
  - The FDL tendon is the primary plantarflexor of the lesser toes and secondary plantarflex and inverts the foot. Innervated by the tibial nerve, it originates on the posterior tibia below the soleal line, it courses on the plantar aspect of the tarsus in the deep midfoot before inserting on the distal phalanx of the lateral four toes.
  - It is at risk of laceration in the toes as well as more proximally in the ball of the foot or arch with penetrating injuries.[49]
- History and physical examination:
  - Spontaneous FDL tendon rupture has not been reported, but some cases have been noted after cortisone injections for interdigital neuromas.
  - FDL tenosynovitis can occur in patients with posterior tibial tendon dysfunction caused by overcompensation for the inversion weakness by flexing their toes.
  - Septic FDL tenosynovitis can occur when a toe or metatarsal ulcer tracks into the FDL sheath. A mid-arch or ankle abscess can develop.
  - Besides this, FDL tendon rupture is almost always associated with penetrating laceration. The patient usually describes a history of stepping on a piece of glass or sharp object.
  - Lacerations distal to the knot of Henry is associated with weakness or absence of plantar flexion of the lesser toes. Because most patients have poor functional control of flexion or extension of the lesser toes, this may be unnoticed. Stabilizing the MTP joint and asking the patient to plantarflex the tip of the toe may demonstrate the tendon disruption.
  - Proximal to the knot of Henry (due to the connecting slips from the FHL), flexion of the distal interphalangeal (DIP) joint can be maintained. At the ankle level, FDL injury is often associated with tibial nerve symptoms and in the midfoot with medial plantar nerve symptoms.
- Treatment:
  - *Wound and laceration exploration*: Primarily repair of the tendon when possible, using a Bunnell, Kessler, or Krackow technique. Postoperative below-knee splint immobilization for 4 to 6 weeks with protected weight bearing.
  - Remaining function can obviate the need for surgery, especially in lacerations proximal to the knot of Henry.[37]

14.5 Extensor Tendons

14.5.1 Extensor Digitorum Longus

- The EDL is relatively superficial and easily lacerated with open or closed trauma.
- Anatomy:
  - The EDL originates from the lateral tibial condyle, the anterior crest of the fibula, and the interosseous membrane. It inserts on the base of the terminal phalanges of the lesser toes.
  - Innervated by the deep peroneal nerve, the EDL functions to extend the toes at the DIP joint and to dorsiflex and evert the foot.
- Physical examination:
  - Absence of extension of the lesser toes at the MTP joint.
  - Associated with weakness of eversion and dorsiflexion of the foot.
  - Diagnosis is difficult because of the ability of the EDB to partially substitute the function of the EDL in some cases.
  - On palpation, a gap may be noted after tendon disruption.

- Status of the superficial and deep peroneal nerves should be evaluated.
- Treatment:
  - Surgical exploration is mandatory after a laceration. Careful and comprehensive wound management is important.
  - The EDL can be primarily treated with end-to-end repair in acute injuries. In spontaneous/chronic ruptures, reconstruction with tendon transfers or free tendon grafting has been proposed.[50]

14.5.2 Extensor Hallucis Longus

- Anatomy:
  - The EHL originates on the midportion of the anterior fibula and the interosseous membrane. It inserts on the base of the distal phalanx of the hallux.
  - Innervated by the deep peroneal nerve, it extends the hallux and everts the foot.[51]
- History and physical examination:
  - Spontaneous ruptures of the EHL tendon occur, but lacerations are more common.
  - Patients might experience a sudden pop in cases of subcutaneous rupture of the EHL.
  - Ecchymosis and tenderness to palpation.
  - Inability to dorsiflex the great toe and a gap may be noted.
- Treatment:
  - Lacerations affecting the EHL should be approximated and repaired with a nonabsorbable suture with a modified Kessler or Krakow technique.
  - In cases of delayed repair and retracted tendon, a more proximal incision may be necessary in the area of the anterior ankle to recover the proximal retracted stump. A tendon graft (autograft or allograft) or tendon transfer (EDB or EDL) may be necessary in the cases where a direct repair is not possible.[52]

14.6 Posterior Tibial Tendon

14.6.1 Subluxation Dislocation

- Traumatic dislocation of the posterior tibial tendon occurs rarely.
- Often, these cases have a delay diagnosis, having been treated for a variety of diagnoses including ankle sprains, tendinitis, subtalar joint injury, or any traumatic event.
- Clinically characterized by severe medial and posteromedial pain with features of tibial neuralgia.
- Delay in diagnosis and treatment has not appeared to have deleterious effect outcomes in reported cases in the literature.[53]
- Mechanism of injury:
  - Most commonly, a traumatic injury is characterized by inversion of the foot with either forced dorsiflexion or plantar flexion associated with a violent contraction of the posterior tibial tendon.
- Surgical exploration findings include elevation of the retinacular periosteal sleeve, tears or avulsion of the retinaculum, a lax retinaculum, or a shallow retromalleolar groove.
- Treatment:
  - Conservative care has been noted to be uniformly unsuccessful.
  - Operative treatment has proved to be effective in returning patients to full activity.
  - Surgical stabilization is performed by relocating the posterior tibial tendon and repairing or reconstructing the flexor retinaculum with or without a groove-deepening procedure.[54]

14.7 Key Testing Facts

	Clinical features	Physical examination	Imaging findings	Treatment
Noninsertional Achilles tendinopathy	Pain at the midportion of the tendon, usually occurring during exercise *Peritendinitis:* paratenon inflammation only. Normal tendon *Peritendinitis with tendinosis*: further inflammation with intratendinous degeneration *Tendinosis*: associated with normal aging and overuse. Tendon calcification and nodularity	Pain elicited in the midportion of the tendon *Peritendinitis:* tenderness remains in one location throughout the range of motion (ROM) *Tendinosis:* tenderness moves as the ankle dorsiflex or plantarflex	MRI and ultrasound (US) are useful to locate degeneration within the tendon or incomplete tendon ruptures	*Conservative:* PT, orthotics, heel lifts, ESWT, PRP, and BMAC *Operative:* Ellipse and repair. Consider augmentation in cases with > 50% width or > 5 cm resection. FHL or FDL transfer
Insertional Achilles tendinopathy	Pain and stiffness at the back of the calcaneus Tenderness when using constrictive footwear	Insertional pain at the posterior aspect of the calcaneus. Prominent enlarged posterior border may be palpable	*X-ray:* Haglund's deformity (commonly associated). Tendon calcifications *MRI:* degeneration and focal microtears within the tendon	*Conservative:* same measures as noninsertional tendinopathy ***Operative:*** **open debridement, resection of bony prominences, reattachment of the tendon (< 50% debrided) or augmentation with FHL, FDL, or PB (> 50% debrided)**
Acute Achilles tendon rupture	Most common tendon rupture Usually men in their 30s and 40s, with 75% occurring in athletic participation Patients relate a sudden snap or popping at the posterior ankle with immediate pain	Palpable tendon gap Positive Thompson's and Matles' tests Decreased plantar flexion strength	*X-ray:* useful to rule out avulsions or calcifications *US:* confirms diagnosis and estimates size of the ruptures *MRI:* may have a role in detecting partial ruptures	Controversial. Good outcomes have been reported with conservative and operative treatment *Conservative:* multiple functional bracing protocols *Operative:* direct repair using either an open, mini-open, or percutaneous technique

	Clinical features	Physical examination	Imaging findings	Treatment
Chronic Achilles tendon rupture	May be the result of delay in seeking medical attention or misdiagnosis at initial evaluation Initial discomfort and tenderness, followed by vague symptoms and weakness or fatigue with ambulation	Similar findings respecting acute ruptures **Palpable gap may be absent due to fibrous tissue incorporation. Skin contracture around the rupture**	US and MRI to evaluate the size of the tendon gap and assist in surgical planning	*Conservative:* low-demand patients without significant functional deficit ***Operative:*** **direct repair** in **gaps** **<3 cm; V-Y advancement** in **gaps between 1** and **3 cm; turn-down procedure** in **gaps between 3** and **5 cm;** and **FHL or FDL transfer for gaps > 5 cm**
Peroneal tenosynovitis/ tendonitis	Posterolateral ankle pain that increases with activity Previous history of ankle sprain or direct trauma may be present Peroneal pathology is related to the presence of the following: peroneus quartus, low-lying PB muscle belly, hypertrophic peroneal tubercle, and peroneal groove abnormalities	Pain on palpation of the peroneal tendons and with active eversion of the forefoot against resistance **Swelling among the lateral border of the ankle**	Both US and MRI are helpful in distinguishing tenosynovitis from other peroneal tendon pathology	***Conservative:*** PT, orthotics, walking boot, PRP, and BMAC ***Operative***: open debridement with tenosynovectomy Tendoscopy may be useful for release and assessment of tendon integrity
Peroneal tendons instability	Acute dislocation: sudden strong contraction of the peroneal muscles in dorsiflexed and everted foot produces tearing of the SPR *Chronic subluxation*: patients with recurrent ankle sprains stretch and elongate the SPR allowing tendons to roll Dislocation/subluxation predisposes to tendon tears	*Acute:* Painful snapping with retromalleolar swelling and tenderness. Palpable thickening may be present *Chronic:* Atraumatic snapping and popping of the peroneals, especially on uneven ground. Associated with ankle instability and recurrent sprains	*US:* dynamic evaluation is confirmatory *MRI:* assessment for concomitant tears	*Conservative* treatment has a high failure rate *Operative:* SPR repair/ reattachment. Groove-deepening or bone block procedures

	Clinical features	Physical examination	Imaging findings	Treatment
Peroneal tendons tears	Posterolateral ankle pain similar to peroneal tenosynovitis/tendonitis. *PB:* most commonly injured as it passes through the SPR or at the tip of the fibula *Peroneus longus:* m**uch less common injury, occurring at the level of the tip of the fibula, peroneal tubercle, or os peroneum**	Similar finding as peroneal tenosynovitis/tendonitis Retromalleolar swelling Assessment of hindfoot varus and/or cavus	MRI is the gold standard for diagnosis of peroneal tears	*Conservative:* bracing, PT, immobilization with below-knee casting or walking boot, PRP, and BMAC Failure of conservative treatment is common. *Operative:* Debridement and resection of major tears up to one half of the tendon width. Tubularization. Irreparable tears may need turndown procedures, free tendon transfers (FDL or FHL), or tenodesis
Anterior tibial tendon rupture	*Acute disruption:* typically, after trauma or lacerations on the anterior ankle *Spontaneous rupture:* secondary to an underlying degenerative process The patient usually relates swelling of the anterior ankle and vague sensation of weakness	Foot drop and loss of dorsiflexion power in comparison to the contralateral side Palpable defect on the anterior ankle. Swelling may disguise the gap in the acute setting Recruiting of the EHL and EDL may maintain the ability to dorsiflex the ankle	MRI can define an anterior tendon rupture, especially in patients who do not recall a traumatic event	*Conservative:* low-demand older patients may achieve normal gait with bracing *Operative:* Acute ruptures may be amenable to direct repair. Chronic ruptures require tendon transfer (EHL, EDL, or PB) or reconstruction using autograft or allograft
FHL tenosynovitis	**Most common location at the level of the sustentaculum tali as the tendon enters the fibro-osseous tunnel. Associated with a prominent os trigonum.** Other locations include the knot of Henry and the intersesamoid ligament Pain along the medial aspect of the ankle. Complaints of catching sensation and weakness of the hallux	Pain and crepitation on motion along the posterior medial ankle, the midfoot, or hallux depending on the location of the disease Positive Tomasen's sign	MRI is useful for assessment and location of the disease X-ray can show a hypertrophic os trigonum	*Conservative:* restricted activity, change in training technique, PT, and bracing *Operative:* open or arthroscopic FHL debridement and fibro-osseous tunnel release, resection of prominent os trigonum

References

[1] Clanton TO, Mullens JH, Schon LC, Tartaglione JP. Achilles tendon disorders including tendinopathies and ruptures. In: Porter D, Schon LC, eds. Baxter's the Foot and Ankle in Sport. 3rd ed. Philadelphia, PA: Elsevier; 2020:163–205.e1

[2] Chiodo CP. Understanding the anatomy and biomechanics of ankle tendons. Foot Ankle Clin. 2017; 22(4):657–664

[3] Winnicki K, Ochała-Kłos A, Rutowicz B, Pękala PA, Tomaszewski KA. Functional anatomy, histology and biomechanics of the human Achilles tendon: a comprehensive review. Ann Anat. 2020; 229: 151461

[4] Dederer KM, Tennant JN. Anatomical and functional considerations in Achilles tendon lesions. Foot Ankle Clin. 2019; 24(3):371–385

[5] Dalmau-Pastor M, Fargues-Polo B, Jr, Casanova-Martínez D, Jr, Vega J, Golanó P. Anatomy of the triceps surae: a pictorial essay. Foot Ankle Clin. 2014; 19(4):603–635

[6] Egger AC, Berkowitz MJ. Achilles tendon injuries. Curr Rev Musculoskelet Med. 2017; 10(1):72–80

[7] Yang X, Meng H, Quan Q, Peng J, Lu S, Wang A. Management of acute Achilles tendon ruptures: a review. Bone Joint Res. 2018; 7(10):561–569

[8] Singh A, Calafi A, Diefenbach C, Kreulen C, Giza E. Noninsertional Tendinopathy of the Achilles. Foot Ankle Clin. 2017; 22(4):745–760

[9] Pearce CJ, Tan A. Non-insertional Achilles tendinopathy. EFORT Open Rev. 2017; 1(11):383–390

[10] Maffulli N, Longo UG, Kadakia A, Spiezia F. Achilles tendinopathy. Foot Ankle Surg. 2020; 26(3):240–249

[11] Jarin I, Bäcker HC, Vosseller JT. Meta-analysis of noninsertional Achilles tendinopathy. Foot Ankle Int. 2020; 41(6):744–754

[12] Indino C, D'Ambrosi R, Usuelli FG. Biologics in the treatment of Achilles tendon pathologies. Foot Ankle Clin. 2019; 24(3):471–493

[13] Sanchez PJ, Grady JF, Saxena A. Percutaneous ultrasonic tenotomy for Achilles tendinopathy is a surgical procedure with similar complications. J Foot Ankle Surg. 2017; 56(5):982–984

[14] Wagner P, Wagner E, Ortiz C, Zanolli D, Keller A, Maffulli N. Achilles tendoscopy for non insertional Achilles tendinopathy. A case series study. Foot Ankle Surg. 2020; 26(4):421–424

[15] Chimenti RL, Cychosz CC, Hall MM, Phisitkul P. Current concepts review update: insertional Achilles tendinopathy. Foot Ankle Int. 2017; 38 (10):1160–1169

[16] Dilger CP, Chimenti RL. Nonsurgical treatment options for insertional Achilles tendinopathy. Foot Ankle Clin. 2019; 24(3):505–513

[17] Barg A, Ludwig T. Surgical strategies for the treatment of insertional Achilles tendinopathy. Foot Ankle Clin. 2019; 24(3):533–559

[18] Uquillas CA, Guss MS, Ryan DJ, Jazrawi LM, Strauss EJ. Everything Achilles: knowledge update and current concepts in management: AAOS exhibit selection. J Bone Joint Surg Am. 2015; 97(14): 1187–1195

[19] Schipper O, Cohen B. The acute injury of the achilles: surgical options (open treatment, and, minimally invasive surgery). Foot Ankle Clin. 2017; 22(4):689–714

[20] Ernat JJ, Johnson JD, Anderson CD, Ryan PM, Yim DG. Does clinical exam and ultrasound compare with MRI findings when assessing tendon approximation in acute Achilles tendon tears? A clinical study. J Foot Ankle Surg. 2019; 58(1):161–164

[21] Kadakia AR, Dekker RG, II, Ho BS. Acute Achilles tendon ruptures: an update on treatment. J Am Acad Orthop Surg. 2017; 25(1):23–31

[22] Lerch TD, Schwinghammer A, Schmaranzer F, et al. Return to sport and patient satisfaction at 5-year follow-up after nonoperative treatment for acute Achilles tendon rupture. Foot Ankle Int. 2020; 41 (7):784–792

[23] Gatz M, Driessen A, Eschweiler J, Tingart M, Migliorini F. Open versus minimally-invasive surgery for Achilles tendon rupture: a meta-analysis study. Arch Orthop Trauma Surg. 2021; 141(3):383–401

[24] Hsu AR, Jones CP, Cohen BE, Davis WH, Ellington JK, Anderson RB. Clinical outcomes and complications of percutaneous achilles repair system versus open technique for acute Achilles tendon ruptures. Foot Ankle Int. 2015; 36(11):1279–1286

[25] Alcelik I, Saeed ZM, Haughton BA, et al. Achillon versus open surgery in acute Achilles tendon repair. Foot Ankle Surg. 2018; 24(5):427–434

[26] Kraeutler MJ, Purcell JM, Hunt KJ. Chronic Achilles tendon ruptures. Foot Ankle Int. 2017; 38(8):921–929

[27] Chen C, Hunt KJ. Open reconstructive strategies for chronic Achilles tendon ruptures. Foot Ankle Clin. 2019; 24(3):425–437

[28] Song Y-J, Hua Y-H. Tendon allograft for treatment of chronic Achilles tendon rupture: a systematic review. Foot Ankle Surg. 2019; 25(3):252–257

[29] Davda K, Malhotra K, O'Donnell P, Singh D, Cullen N. Peroneal tendon disorders. EFORT Open Rev. 2017; 2(6):281–292

[30] van Dijk PAD, Kerkhoffs GMMJ, Chiodo C, DiGiovanni CW. Chronic disorders of the peroneal tendons: current concepts review of the literature. J Am Acad Orthop Surg. 2019; 27(16):590–598

[31] Bahad SR, Kane JM. Peroneal tendon pathology: treatment and reconstruction of peroneal tears and instability. Orthop Clin North Am. 2020; 51(1): 121–130

[32] Brodsky JW, Zide JR, Kane JM. Acute peroneal injury. Foot Ankle Clin. 2017; 22(4):833–841

[33] Hamid KS, Amendola A. Chronic rupture of the peroneal tendons. Foot Ankle Clin. 2017; 22(4): 843–850

[34] Pedowitz D, Beck D. Presentation, diagnosis, and nonsurgical treatment options of the anterior tibial

tendon, posterior tibial tendon, peroneals, and Achilles. Foot Ankle Clin. 2017; 22(4):677–687
[35] Bernasconi A, Sadile F, Smeraglia F, Mehdi N, Laborde J, Lintz F. Tendoscopy of Achilles, peroneal and tibialis posterior tendons: an evidence-based update. Foot Ankle Surg. 2018; 24(5):374–382
[36] Watson GI, Karnovsky SC, Levine DS, Drakos MC. Surgical treatment for stenosing peroneal tenosynovitis. Foot Ankle Int. 2019; 40(3):282–286
[37] Coughlin MJ, Schon LC. Disorder of the tendons. In: Coughlin MJ, Saltzman CL, eds. Mann's Surgery of the Foot and Ankle. 9th ed. Philadelphia, PA: Elsevier Saunders; 2014:1188–1291
[38] Espinosa N, Maurer MA. Peroneal tendon dislocation. Eur J Trauma Emerg Surg. 2015; 41(6): 631–637
[39] Myerson M, Li S, Porter DA. Rupture of the anterior tibial and peroneal tendons. In: Porter D, Schon LC, eds. Baxter's the Foot and Ankle in Sport. 3rd ed. Philadelphia, PA: Elsevier; 2020:144–162
[40] Sherman TI, Koury K, Orapin J, Schon LC. Lateral transfer of the flexor digitorum longus for peroneal tendinopathy. Foot Ankle Int. 2019; 40 (9):1012–1017
[41] Karauda P, Podgórski M, Paulsen F, Polguj M, Olewnik Ł. Anatomical variations of the tibialis anterior tendon. Clin Anat. 2021; 34(3):397–404
[42] Gossett L, Gossett PC, Roberts J, Anderson J. Gastrocnemius recession for the treatment of tibialis anterior tendinopathy. Foot Ankle Orthop. 2019; 4(3):2473011419852940
[43] Lemmens L, van Beek N, Verfaillie S. Postoperative results of distal tibialis anterior tendinosis. Foot Ankle Surg. 2020; 26(8):851–854
[44] Sharpe BD, Steginsky BD, Suhling M, Vora A. Posterior ankle impingement and flexor hallucis longus pathology. Clin Sports Med. 2020; 39(4): 911–930
[45] Vosseller JT, Dennis ER, Bronner S. Ankle injuries in dancers. J Am Acad Orthop Surg. 2019; 27(16): 582–589
[46] Rungprai C, Tennant JN, Phisitkul P. Disorders of the flexor hallucis longus and os trigonum. Clin Sports Med. 2015; 34(4):741–759
[47] Park JY, Wang C, Kim HD, Kim HN. Tendon split lengthening technique for flexor hallucis longus tendon rupture. J Orthop Surg Res. 2017; 12(1):165
[48] Anastasopoulos N, Paraskevas G, Lazaridis N, Natsis K. Reconstruction of neglected flexor hallucis longus tendon rupture: a case report. J Foot Ankle Surg. 2018; 57(6):1256–1258
[49] Lui TH. Flexor digitorum longus tendoscopy. J Foot Ankle Surg. 2012; 51(5):690–692
[50] Hamaoka K, Watanabe K, Kamiya T, Teramoto A, Yamashita T. Nontraumatic chronic subcutaneous extensor digitorum longus tendon rupture in a recreational runner: a case report. JBJS Case Connect. 2020; 10(2):e0058
[51] Al-Qattan MM. Surgical treatment and results in 17 cases of open lacerations of the extensor hallucis longus tendon. J Plast Reconstr Aesthet Surg. 2007; 60(4):360–367
[52] Bastías GF, Cuchacovich N, Schiff A, Carcuro G, Pellegrini MJ. Technique tip: EDL-to-EHL double loop transfer for extensor hallucis longus reconstruction. Foot Ankle Surg. 2019; 25(3):272–277
[53] Goucher NR, Coughlin MJ, Kristensen RM. Dislocation of the posterior tibial tendon: a literature review and presentation of two cases. Iowa Orthop J. 2006; 26:122–126
[54] Mullens J, Whiteside W, Nilssen E, Kennedy C. Dislocated posterior tibial tendon treated with plate buttress fixation in a collegiate gymnast: a case report and review of the literature. Foot Ankle Spec. 2016; 9(4):361–366

15 Athletic Injuries of the Foot and Ankle

Brian C. Lau and Annunziato Amendola

Abstract

Foot and ankle injuries are common in sports. History and physical examination are important to diagnose injuries and guide treatment planning for injuries such as ankle fractures, turf toe, ankle instability, syndesmotic injuries, Achilles tendon ruptures, metatarsal fractures, fracture of the base of the fifth metatarsal, navicular fractures, and Lisfranc injuries. Imaging may help supplement treatment planning. Care and treatment should be guided by long-term care and outcomes of the athlete and not be compromised by pressure to return to play.

Keywords: arthroscopy for ankle fracture, turf toe, ankle instability, syndesmosis, Achilles, stress fractures, Lisfranc

15.1 Overview

- General information:
  - Foot and ankle injuries are common among athletes with an annual incidence of up to 39% in collegiate football players.[1]
- Evaluation:
  - Most of these entities present with a spectrum of severity. A through history and physical examination, with appropriate diagnostic tests, and a high index of suspicion can guide a physician through diagnosis and treatment plan.[2]

15.2 Ankle Fracture in Athletes

- Etiology and pathophysiology:
  - The most common surgical indication for foot and ankle injuries in collegiate athletes[3]:
  - Presents status post inversion or eversion injury or direct blow.
- Symptoms:
  - Pain, inability to bear weight, gross deformity, tenderness, or crepitus along medial or lateral malleolus.
  - Evaluate for any open lesions, neurovascular status, and ipsilateral lower extremity injury.
- Diagnostics and classification:
  - X-rays are indicated with Ottawa ankle rules (see ▶ Table 15.1).[4]
  - *Stress view:* gravity stress or external rotation for Weber B fractures.
  - Greater than 4 to 5 mm medial widening consistent with unstable bimalleolar equivalent.
  - Weber ankle fracture classification (see ▶ Fig. 15.1a) (also refer to chapter 20).

Table 15.1 Ottawa foot and ankle rules

Ottawa ankle rules	Ottawa foot rules
Ankle radiographs (anteroposterior, lateral, and mortise) are required if there is malleolar zone pain and any of the following:	Foot radiographs (anteroposterior, lateral, and mortise) are required if there is midfoot zone pain and any of the following:
1. Inability to weight bear immediately after injury and in the emergency department	1. Inability to weight bear immediately after injury and in the emergency department
2. Pain to palpation over the posterior edge or tip of the medial or lateral malleoli to 6 cm above	2. Bony tenderness over the base of the 5th metatarsal
	3. Bony tenderness over the navicular

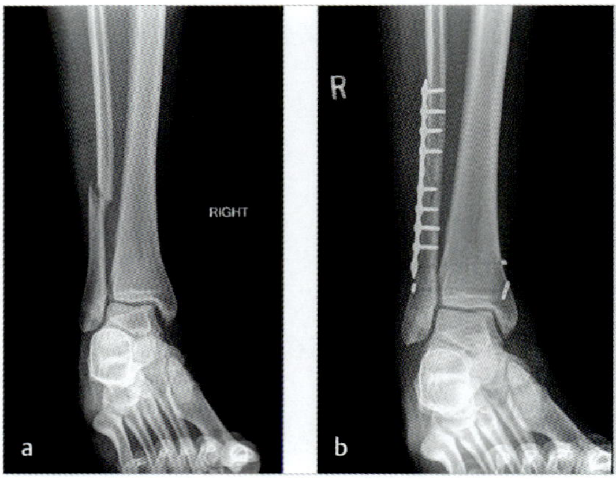

Fig. 15.1 A 20-year-old male lineman with a Weber C ankle fracture during a game. **(a)** Injury films. **(b)** Postoperative films.

- Conservative management:
  - Indications:
    - Weber A.
    - Weber B with normal mortise when stressed and no medial deltoid tenderness.
  - Walking boot with limited weight bearing for 6 to 8 weeks.
- Surgical intervention:
  - Indications:
    - Unstable Weber B, Weber C ankle fractures.
    - Weber B with medial deltoid tenderness.[5,6,7]
  - Procedure:
    - Ankle arthroscopy to evaluate for syndesmotic and chondral injury (see ▶ Fig. 15.2):
      - Removal of loose bodies, debridement to stable border.
      - No acute chondral reconstruction.
      - Assessment of the syndesmosis and deltoid.
    - Open reduction and internal fixation (ORIF) of the lateral malleolus (see ▶ Fig. 15.1b).
    - Syndesmotic sssessment[8]:
      - External rotation test and/or Cotton tests (along with arthroscopic assessment of the syndesmotic drive-through sign and medial drive-through sign with a 3.5-mm shaver):
        - If negative: splint.
        - If syndesmotic drive-through or Cotton tests are positive, syndesmotic fixation with suture tapes.
          - Two divergent suture button devices:
            - If it remains unstable:
              - Direct deltoid repair.
        - If medial drive-through sign is positive:
          - Direct deltoid repair
- Rehabilitation:
  - Non-weight-bearing × 4 weeks in a boot.
  - Early range of motion 3 to 4 weeks post-op.
  - Weight bearing at 6 weeks. May consider physical therapy if there is difficulty with regaining range of motion or gait.
  - Return to sport in 3 to 6 months.

15.3 Turf Toe

- Etiology and pathophysiology:
  - Planted foot in equinus, dorsiflexion of the first metatarsophalangeal (MTP) joint with axial load:
    - Common with tackles with the foot planted in equinus with load onto the heel resulting in forced dorsal flexion of the hallux MTP joint.
  - Plantar plate injury of the first MTP joint.

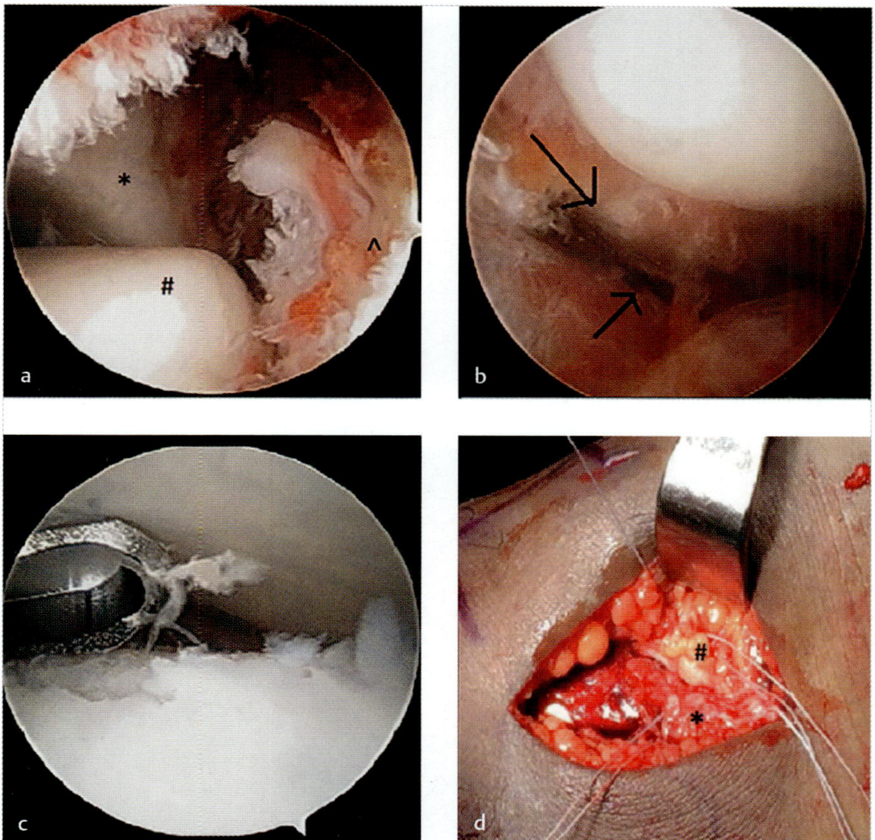

Fig. 15.2 Arthroscopic evaluation of a fracture. **(a)** Anterior inferior tibiofibular ligament disruption: talus (#), tibia (*), and fibula (^). **(b)** Deep deltoid injury (*arrows*). **(c)** Medial talar shoulder cartilage injury. **(d)** Curvilinear incision along the anterior aspect of the medial malleolus for fixation of the deep deltoid (*) and superficial deltoid (#).

    - May be associated with sesamoid injury or osteochondral lesions of the MTP joint.
    - May be associated with a late traumatic hallux valgus.
- Symptoms:
    - Pain and swelling of the MTP joint.
    - Decreased push-off strength and difficulty with cutting activities.
- Diagnostics and classification:
    - Hallux swelling and alignment.
    - MTP Lachman test (stabilization of the metatarsal head with one hand and vertical force applied to the proximal phalanx; increased translation compared to contralateral uninjured side), valgus instability.
    - Flexor hallucis longus (FHL) strength:
    - First toe radiographs:
        - Evaluate for proximal migration of sesamoids; may observe small fleck of bone from proximal phalanx or distal sesamoid that indicates a capsular avulsion (see ▶ Fig. 15.3).
        - *Stress view:* forced hallux MTP dorsiflexion view.
            - Helps with assessment of distance from distal sesamoid to the base of

    the phalanx (normal average: 8 mm).
  - Contralateral comparison radiographs (see ▶ Fig. 15.3).
  - Live fluoroscopy can be helpful to evaluate instability.
- Magnetic resonance imaging (MRI) to detect subtle capsular or plantar plate injuries.
- Turf toe grading scale (see ▶ Table 15.2).

- Conservative management:
  - Indications:
    - Grade I and II turf toe.
    - Nonsteroidal anti-inflammatory drugs (NSAIDs), ice, and elevation. Hallux immobilized in plantarflexed position in walking boot, crutches as needed for comfort, return to play when able to run and cut at full speed without discomfort. Taping, toe spica, or turf toe plate orthotic may assist with return to play, 4 to 6 weeks.
- Surgical intervention:
  - Indications:
    - Grade III turf toe (early within 2 weeks); or failure of conservative management (4–6 weeks), proximal migration of sesamoid, progressive hallux malalignment, or clawing after immobilization.
  - Procedure:
    - Medial L-shaped incision or dual plantar incision (medial and plantar) to protect plantar medial cutaneous nerve, and improve lateral exposure (see ▶ Fig. 15.4).
      * Single L-shaped incision extends medial at the junction of the dorsal skin and plantar skin distally and then transversely at the interphalangeal plantar skin crease.

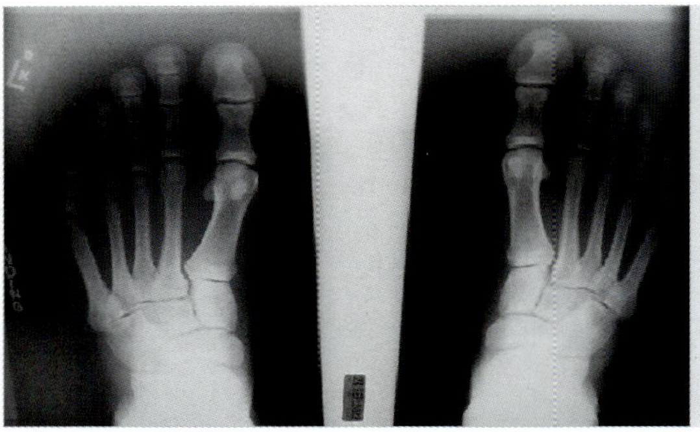

Fig. 15.3 Radiographs of the left foot turf toe with comparison the right foot. Note the retracted position of the sesamoids compared to the contralateral side.

Table 15.2 Turf toe grading scale and management

Grade	Description	Return to play
I	Attenuation of the plantar structures, localized swelling, and minimal ecchymosis	As tolerated
II	Partial tear of the plantar structures, moderate welling, and restricted motion due to pain	Walking boot, crutches as needed for comfort, taping, or shank orthotic may assist return to play as pain subsides
III	Complete disruption of the plantar structures, significant swelling/ ecchymosis; hallux flexion weakness, frank instability of the hallux metatarsophalangeal (MTP)	Initial immobilization in boot up to 6 wk depending on the sport and the position, taping, toe spica, turf toe plate orthotic, or bracing likely needed to return to play; generally consider for surgical management

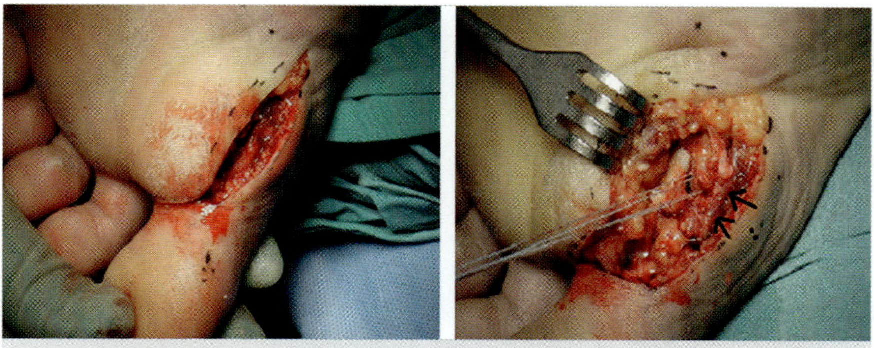

Fig. 15.4 The L-shaped incision extends medial at the junction of the dorsal skin and plantar skin distally and transversely at the interphalangeal skin crease. The plantar medial cutaneous nerve (*arrows*) is identified and protected. The plantar plate is advanced with nonabsorbable sutures.

    * Medial incision extends from the metatarsal neck to the midphalanx to provide complete visualization of the sesamoid complex.
    * Plantar incision along the lateral border of the hallux–MTP–sesamoid complex and plantar lateral cutaneous nerve carefully dissected and retracted. Suture fixation of the plantar capsule and plantar plate from lateral to medial.
    * Soft-tissue defect closed distal to sesamoids, followed by advancement of the plantar plate to the proximal phalanx in a distal to proximal fashion with advancement of the medial capsule.
    * If tear cannot be primarily repaired, it can be done with suture anchors.
    * Fluoroscopy to verify proper alignment and motion of sesamoids.
    * Evaluation of valgus stress of the hallux to test medial collateral ligament.
        ◇ May require the modified McBride bunionectomy with adductor tenotomy and direct repair of medial soft-tissue defect.
- Rehabilitation:
    ○ Non-weight-bearing in cast for 7 to 10 days followed by passive hallux plantar flexion to mobilize sesamoids (no dorsiflexion).
    ○ Active plantar flexion at 4 weeks and active dorsiflexion at 6 weeks.
    ○ Stiff hallux (turf toe plate) at 6 weeks with weight bearing.

15.4 Ankle Instability (Low Ankle Sprain)

- Etiology and pathophysiology[9,10,11,12,13,14]:
    ○ Inversion ankle injury ("rolling" ankle).
    ○ Majority of injuries to the anterior talofibular ligament (ATFL) but commonly include the calcaneofibular ligament (CFL).
        – CFL involved in 50 to 75% of injuries.
    ○ Be suspicious of medial deltoid injury.
- Symptoms:
    ○ Pain, swelling, ecchymosis, and discomfort with ambulation.
- Diagnostics and classification:
    ○ Pain along the lateral aspect of the ankle, at the ATFL or CFL.
    ○ Acutely anterior drawer and talar tilt have limited value. Diagnosis largely due to history and tenderness along the ATFL/CFL or the peroneals.
        – Check syndesmotic ligaments.
    ○ Follow Ottawa rules regarding the need for radiographs (▶ Table 15.1).

- Conservative management:
  - Indications:
    - Majority of ankle sprains.
  - Short period of immobilization (< 7 days), NSAIDs, physical therapy, and functional, proprioception training resulted in good outcomes and improvement in self-reported function.[14]
- Surgical intervention:
  - Indications:
    - Failure of conservative treatment lasting greater than 3 months.
    - Relative indications:
      - Pathologic instability as defined by greater than 10 degrees of varus tilt or 10 mm of anterior translation or by 5 degrees or 5 mm more than the contralateral side.
      - Associated osteochondral fracture of the talus.
  - Procedure:
    - If planning for surgery, evaluate hindfoot/forefoot alignment. Varus hindfoot or dropped first ray (valgus forefoot) alignment is a risk factor for chronic ankle instability and poorer surgical outcomes if not addressed at time of surgery.
    - Preoperative MRI to evaluate for other sources of persistent pain.
  - Procedure:
    - Ankle arthroscopy to evaluate for chondral injuries.
    - Oblique incision along the distal aspect of the lateral malleolus.
    - Sharp incision through the fascia and peroneal sheath.
    - Evaluation of concomitant peroneal tendon injury.
    - Repair/imbrication of the ATFL/CFL with suture anchors to bone.
    - vest-over-pants technique with the inferior extensor retinaculum to further support repair.
    - If it remains unstable to retesting of stability (anterior drawer and talar tilt)
      - Then consider allograft or perform augmentation with suture tape (Internal brace, Arthrex, Naples. FL).
    - Consider direct deltoid repair if clearly injured in high-level athletes or persistent instability.
- Rehabilitation:
  - Immobilization in boot or cast for 4 weeks.
  - Range of motion and strengthening out of boot at 4 weeks and into a lace-up ankle brace for walking and activities of daily living.
  - Functional sport-specific rehabilitation for 4 weeks.
  - Return to sports after 3 months in brace.

15.5 Syndesmotic Injury (High Ankle Sprain)

- Etiology and pathophysiology:
  - More commonly associated with external rotation and pronation injury mechanism.
  - Disruption of syndesmosis occurs in up to 24% of all ankle sprains and must be evaluated in all suspected ankle sprains.
    - Anterior inferior tibiofibular ligament (AITFL) most commonly disrupted.
    - Intraosseous component also commonly disrupted.
    - Need to evaluate for Maisonneuve variants.
      - Proximal fibular pain should prompt radiographs of the proximal fibula.
- Symptoms:
  - Pain, swelling, discomfort with ambulation. Difficulty with cutting, turning, or sprinting.
- Diagnostics and classification:
  - Squeeze test (26% sensitive and 88% specific).[8]
    - Squeeze of the midcalf elicits pain at syndesmosis.
  - Tenderness along the AITFL or the intraosseous syndesmosis (92% sensitive, 29% specific).

- Dorsiflexion–external rotation tests (71% sensitive, 63% specific).
  - Stabilize knee at 90 degrees and maximal dorsiflexion with an external rotation stress to reproduce pain at syndesmosis.
- Combination of all tests should be used; obtain as much information as possible.
- Standard radiographs may demonstrate associated malleolar fractures or proximal fibular fracture (Maisonneuve variant):
  - Stress views (gravity or external rotation stress) may demonstrate medial clear space widening (> 4–5 mm).
- Normal X-rays do not mean the syndesmosis is not injured or stable/CT scan may be obtained in revision cases.

- Conservative management:
  - Indications:
    - Most isolated stable syndesmotic injuries.
  - NSAIDs, rest, ice, and a short period of immobilization (1 week) remain the mainstay of treatment, then progressive weight bearing to full weight bearing by 2 weeks.
  - Duration to return to play is longer than low ankle sprain, often twice as long.
  - Functional and proprioception rehabilitation initiated early.
- Surgical intervention:
  - Indications:
    - Associated malleolar fractures.
    - Clear demonstration of syndesmosis instability on examination and imaging modalities.
    - If pain or instability remains at 4 to 6 weeks postinjury.
  - Procedure:
    - Preoperative MRI to evaluate syndesmosis and for associated injuries.
    - Ankle arthroscopy to probe syndesmosis and deltoid under direct visualization.
    - Dynamic stabilization with two knotless suture button construct.
    - In divergent pattern to allow more physiologic motion (see ▶ Fig. 15.1a for suture button construct; may be performed with a two- to three-hole plate if no associated fractures).
      * Placed at 15 mm above the tibial plafond angled 30 degrees posterior to anterior.
        ◇ No clamp reduction.
      * A two- to three-hole lateral fibular buttress plate with suture button through holes if an athlete is returning to contact activity.
    - Repeat stress testing intraoperatively and direct repair or suture anchor repair of the deltoid ligament.
- Rehabilitation:
  - Non-weight-bearing in cast or boot for 6 weeks.
  - At 6 weeks, begin strengthening and mobility and as tolerated, then move on to sport-specific training.
  - May return to sport as early as 12 weeks if the patient progressed well during sport-specific training.
  - Should return to sport with lace-up ankle brace.

15.6 Achilles Ruptures

- Etiology and pathophysiology[15]:
  - *Eccentric contraction:* push-off/forced plantar flexion; tend to be midsubstance (4–5 cm) above insertion of the Achilles.
  - Evaluate for exposure to anabolic steroids, fluoroquinolones
- Symptoms:
  - Acute sharp pain/pop in the heel with forced plantar flexion and difficulty with gait.
  - Patients generally do not have persistent pain after an acute event.
- Diagnostics and classification:
  - Place the patient prone and evaluate:
    - Palpable defect (sensitivity 73% and specificity 89%).

    - *Matles' test:* observe for greater resting dorsiflexion of injured side (sensitivity 88% and specificity 85%).
    - *Thompson's test:* lack of plantar flexion with squeeze of the gastrocsoleus muscle belly (sensitivity 96% and specificity 93%)
    - One hundred percent sensitivity when all three examination findings are positive.
  - Lateral radiograph to evaluate for bony avulsion or calcium deposits indicating chronic disease.
  - Advanced imaging/MRI: not needed for acute injury but may be helpful in chronic situation.[16]
  - Ultrasound evaluation becoming more commonplace.
- Conservative management[17]:
  - *Initial management:* Placement in the boot with heel lifts or splint to maintain 20-degree ankle plantar flexion.
  - There is controversy in the literature between operative and conservative management.
    - *Operative:* Increased risk of wound healing issues; decreased risk of rerupture.
    - *Nonoperative:* Increased risk of rerupture; no risk of wound healing complications.
    - Wound healing issues may be decreased with percutaneous repairs or placing knots away from the zone of injury.
  - Nonoperative management:
    - Weight bearing as tolerated in the boot with a 2-inch heel lift; must keep the boot on for first 4 weeks.
    - Boot with heel lifts with progressive reduction in heel lift size after 4 weeks.
    - Progressive/functional rehabilitation after 6 to 8 weeks.
- Surgical intervention:
  - Indications:
    - In elite athletes, generally operative management is recommended.
  - Zone of injury assists in decision-making between open and percutaneous fixation.
    - Larger zone of injury (≥ 5 cm as determined by ultrasound or MRI), recommend open treatment:
      * Place knots away from the zone of injury (▶ Fig. 15.4).
    - In smaller zone of injury (< 5 cm), percutaneous fixation is recommended:
      * The PARS Achilles Jig System, Arthrex.
    - Use two nonabsorbable sutures to oppose tear ends; use contralateral extremity as guide for restoration of proper tendon length, but it is difficult to over tension.
    - Repair paratenon with absorbable sutures.
    - Boot with heel lifts or splint in 20-degree resting plantar flexion.
- Rehabilitation:
  - Operative or nonoperative.
    - Accelerated functional rehabilitation:
      * Full weight bearing with 20-degree (2-cm heel lift) plantar flexion at 3 to 5 days in the nonoperative group and at 8 to 10 days in the operative group.
      * *Nonoperative:* functional boot for 8 weeks with decrease in heel lift weekly.
      * *Operative:* functional boot with heel lift for 3 weeks; may return to exercises at 4 weeks (also refer to chapter 14).

15.7 Metatarsal Fractures

- Etiology and pathophysiology:
  - Most common bony injury of the foot; up to 88.5% of all fractures of the foot.
  - Stress fractures common in the second and third metatarsal ray.
  - Acute fractures with twisting, direct trauma, or crush injuries.

- Symptoms:
  - Swelling, pain, and ecchymosis of the midfoot.
  - Difficulty and/or pain with ambulation.
- Diagnostics and classification:
  - Standard radiographs of the foot (anteroposterior [AP], lateral, oblique):
    - Stress fractures may be negative early but will demonstrate callus later.
    - MRI if high clinical suspicion.
- Conservative management:
  - Indications:
    - Majority of metatarsal fractures.
  - Elevation, icing, weight bearing with hard-sole shoe (post-op shoe, walker boot).
  - If significant pain or swelling, then may splint or short duration of immobilization (7–10 days).
- Surgical intervention:
  - Indications:
    - More than 3 to 4 mm or greater than 10 degrees of dorsal or plantar translation or angulation.
    - May fix with plate or Kirshner's wires.
- Rehabilitation:
  - *Nonoperative management:* limited activity for 6 to 8 weeks with protected weight bearing.
  - *Operative management:* Non-weight-bearing × 2 weeks in controlled ankle motion (CAM) boot. At 3 weeks may begin weight bearing and gentle exercises. At 4 weeks, if there is no pain, then may return to sport-specific activity.

15.8 Base of the Fifth Metatarsal Fractures

- Etiology and pathophysiology:
  - Seventy percent of metatarsal fractures occur at the base of the fifth metatarsal.
  - Acute fractures with twisting, direct trauma.
- Symptoms:
  - Swelling, pain, and ecchymosis over the lateral foot.
  - Difficulty and/or pain with ambulation.
- Diagnostics and classification:
  - Standard radiographs of the foot (AP, lateral, and oblique):
    - Stress fractures may be negative early but will demonstrate callus later.
    - MRI if high clinical suspicion.
    - Scrutinize the base of the fifth metatarsal:
      - Zone classification:
        - *Zone 1 (avulsion):* tuberosity avulsion.
        - *Zone 2 (Jones):* the metaphysis–diaphysis junction with extension into the fourth–fifth intermetatarsal articulation.
        - *Zone 3 (Dancers'):* diaphyseal fracture
- Conservative management:
  - Indications:
    - Zone 1 (avulsion) or zone 3 nondisplaced.
  - Elevation, icing, weight bearing with hard-sole shoe (post-op shoe, walker boot).
  - If significant pain or swelling, then may splint or short duration of immobilization (7–10 days).
- Surgical intervention:
  - Indications:
    - Zone 2 (Jones) or zone 3 (stress fracture), base of the fifth fracture due to tenuous blood supply.[18]
      - Delayed union rates of 25 to 66% and nonunion rates of 7 to 28%.
    - More than 3 to 4 mm or > 10 degrees of dorsal or plantar translation or angulation.
  - Technique (▶ Fig. 15.5):
    - Percutaneous screw fixation; ≥ 4.5 mm diameter and ≥ 40 mm in length; fluoroscopic guidance.
    - Maintain "high and inside" starting position.

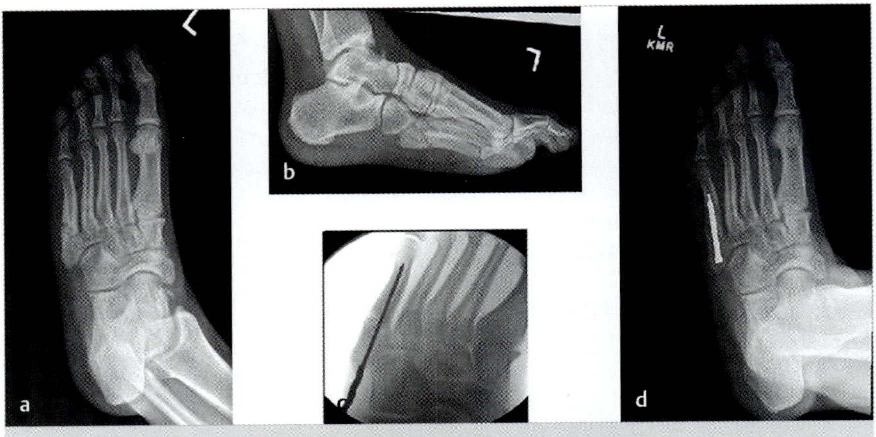

Fig. 15.5 Jones' fracture. **(a)** Oblique and **(b)** lateral radiographs demonstrating a zone 2 fracture. **(c)** Intraoperative fluoroscopy with guidewire and cannulated drill in place. **(d)** Postoperative radiograph demonstrating final construct with screws distal to the fragment site and interval healing.

- *Cannulated instrumentation:* guidewire, drill, cannulated tap to determine screw diameter.
- Screw threads must cross the fracture site and have good fixation distally.
- In elite athletes, consider augmentation with bone marrow aspirate concentrate.

- Rehabilitation:
  - *Nonoperative management:* limited activity for 6 to 8 weeks with protected weight bearing.
  - *Operative management:* non-weight-bearing × 2 weeks in CAM boot. At 3 weeks, may begin weight bearing and gentle exercises. At 4 weeks, if no pain, then may return to sports-specific activity.

15.9 Stress Fractures of the Navicular

- Etiology and pathophysiology:
  - Overuse injury.
  - Poor nutrition.
  - Poor conditioning/training.
  - Runners and basketball players.
- Symptoms:
  - Gradual onset of pain and swelling of the midfoot.
  - Initially pain only with sporting activities, but as it becomes more chronic will affect function of activities of daily living.
- Diagnostics and classification:
  - Point tenderness over the "N" spot between the anterior tibialis and the extensor hallucis longus along the dorsum of the navicular.
  - Pain when on tiptoes or when performing single-leg hop on the affected leg.
  - Imaging:
    - Radiographs may be negative.
    - MRI/CT/bone scan if high index of suspicion (see ▶ Fig. 15.6).
      - Classification:
        - *Type 1:* dorsal cortical fracture.
        - *Type 2:* dorsal fracture that propagates into the body of the navicular.
        - *Type 3:* fracture propagates to the second cortex either in plantar direction, medially, or laterally.

- Conservative management:
  - Indications:
    - Type 1:
      - Non-weight-bearing for 6 weeks in the boot or splint.
- Surgical intervention:
  - Indications:
    - Type 2 or 3; or failure of conservative management of type 1 (see ▸ Fig. 15.7):

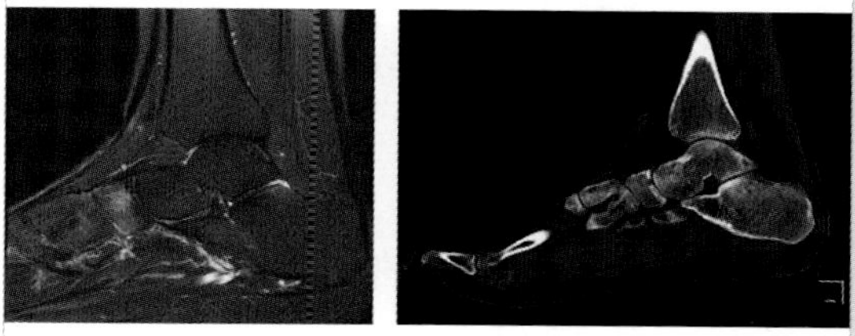

Fig. 15.6 Navicular stress fracture radiographs are typically normal. Magnetic resonance imaging (MRI) fluid-sensitive sequence will demonstrate increased signal and computed tomography (CT) scan may demonstrate cortical defect. A high index of suspicion is required to order advanced imaging.

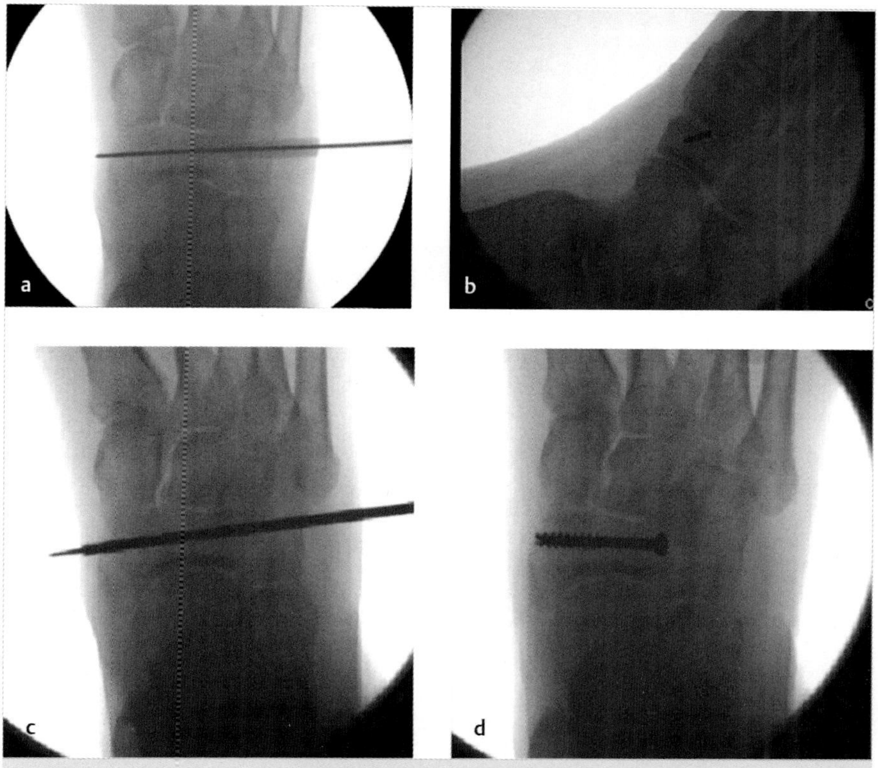

Fig. 15.7 Navicular stress fracture fixation. **(a,b)** Guidewire placed and confirmed in proper location in sagittal and coronal planes and **(c)** cannulated drill. **(d)** Partially threaded screw placed.

        * Percutaneous screw fixation: cannulated partially threaded 3.5-mm screws ± bone grafting or bone marrow aspirate concentrate.
- Rehabilitation:
    - At 6 weeks of nonoperative treatment: perform CT scan:
        - If pain is resolving and repeat CT scan shows evidence of healing, then initiate progressive weight bearing.
        - If no healing at 6 weeks on CT scan, bone stimulation initiated with continued non-weight-bearing.

15.10 Lisfranc Injuries

- Etiology and pathophysiology:
    - Classically axial loading of a fixed, plantarflexed foot.
    - May also be noncontact twisting injuries in high-level athletes resulting in ligamentous injury.
    - Proximal-medial column Lisfranc injury variant common in football players:
        - Force extends through the intercuneiform joint and exits through the naviculocuneiform joint leading to unstable first ray and instability at multiple joints.
- Symptoms:
    - Painful weight bearing; difficulty with heel rise.
    - Plantar ecchymosis, swelling, and point tenderness across the bases of the first and second metatarsals.
- Diagnostics and classification:
    - Radiographs:
        - Weight bearing radiographs of the foot (AP, lateral, and oblique):
            * Contralateral side for comparison.
            * *AP view:* disruption of continuity of line from the medial base of the second metatarsal to the medial side of the middle cuneiform; widening of distance between the first and second rays.
            * *Oblique view:* disruption of continuity line from the medial side of the base of the fourth metatarsal with the medial side of the cuboid.
            * *Lateral view:* dorsal subluxation of the first ray.
            * "Fleck" sign of bony injury at the base of the second metatarsal.
            * Stress testing under fluoroscopy: pronation and adduction of the foot.
            * MRI if high index of suspicion of ligamentous injury; consider CT scan if higher energy or with other bony fractures.
            * *Proximal-medial column Lisfranc:* May have negative radiographs or stress views but edema in the naviculocuneiform joint.
- Conservative management:
    - Indications:
        - MRI edema or increased signal in Lisfranc region, no displacement.
        - Protected weight bearing for 4 weeks with progressive increase in activity.
- Surgical intervention:
    - Indications:
        - Any bony injury or ligamentous injury with displacement.
        - ORIF preferred over fusion in high-level athletes.
    - Procedure:
        - ORIF with dorsal incision at the first intermetatarsal webspace.
            * "Homerun" screw from the proximal aspect of the medial cuneiform to the distal-lateral aspect of the second metatarsal base.
            * Bridge plate preferred over transarticular screws to avoid articular cartilage damage.
            * Proximal-medial column Lisfranc injury variant.
            * Requires intercuneiform screw.
- Rehabilitation:
    - Non-weight-bearing for 3 to 4 weeks.
    - Progressive weight bearing and range of motion at 4 to 8 weeks.
    - Removal of hardware at 4 to 6 months.
- The key testing points are listed in.

15.11 Key Testing Facts

Topics	Key points
Ankle fracture in athletes	• Arthroscopic assessment of acute chondral injuries • Suture button repair of syndesmosis to allow physiologic motion • Direct deltoid repair as necessary
Turf toe	• Contralateral comparison radiographs ± forced dorsiflexion MTP radiograph • Evaluate for valgus instability of the MTP; may require modified McBride • Most turf toe can be treated nonoperatively. Surgical management for complete ruptures indicated by proximally migrated sesamoids, grossly unstable, or failure of conservative management
Ankle instability	• Early functional rehabilitation for nonoperative or operative management • Ankle arthroscopy to evaluate for concomitant injury • Use of suture tape may expedite return to play in high-level athletes
Syndesmotic injury	• Syndesmotic injury should be tested in all suspected ankle sprains • Syndesmotic injury leads to a longer duration of time until return to play • Dynamic suture button fixation allows physiologic motion and decrease the need for reoperation to remove hardware • Evaluation and direct repair of the deltoid may be necessary
Achilles ruptures	• Operative vs. nonoperative management is a patient-driven decision • Operative management has increased risk of wound healing complications • Nonoperative management has increased risk of rerupture and slight decrease of plantar flexion strength
Metatarsal fractures	• Majority of metatarsal fractures can be treated nonoperatively • May consider operative treatment in cases of > 3–4 mm or > 10 degrees of dorsal or plantar translation or angulation
Base of the 5th metatarsal fractures	• Scrutinize the base of the 5th metatarsal fractures • Percutaneous screw fixation of zone 2 (Jones') fractures with screw ≥ 4.5 and ≥ 40 mm in length
Stress fractures of the navicular	• High index of suspicion as navicular stress fractures are difficult to diagnose • High rate of delayed union or nonunion; must closely monitor
Lisfranc injuries	• Beware of the proximal-medial column Lisfranc injury variant • Use of bridge plates over transarticular screws to avoid articular cartilage damage in high-level athletes

References

[1] Westermann RW, Kerr ZY, Wehr P, Amendola A. Increasing lower extremity injury rates across the 2009–2010 to 2014–2015 seasons of National Collegiate Athletic Association football: an unintended consequence of the "targeting" rule used to prevent concussions? Am J Sports Med. 2016; 44(12):3230–3236

[2] Hong CC, Pearce CJ, Ballal MS, Calder JDF. Management of sports injuries of the foot and ankle: an update. Bone Joint J. 2016; 98-B(10): 1299–1311

[3] Hunt KJ, Hurwit D, Robell K, Gatewood C, Botser IB, Matheson G. Incidence and epidemiology of foot and ankle injuries in elite collegiate athletes. Am J Sports Med. 2017; 45(2):426–433

[4] Stiell IG, McKnight RD, Greenberg GH, et al. Implementation of the Ottawa ankle rules. JAMA. 1994; 271(11):827–832

[5] Hsu AR, Lareau CR, Anderson RB. Repair of acute superficial deltoid complex avulsion during ankle fracture fixation in national football league players. Foot Ankle Int. 2015; 36(11):1272–1278

[6] Chan KB, Lui TH. Role of ankle arthroscopy in management of acute ankle fracture. Arthroscopy. 2016; 32(11):2373–2380

[7] Takao M, Uchio Y, Naito K, Fukazawa I, Kakimaru T, Ochi M. Diagnosis and treatment of combined intra-articular disorders in acute distal fibular fractures. J Trauma. 2004; 57(6):1303–1307

[8] Sman AD, Hiller CE, Rae K, et al. Diagnostic accuracy of clinical tests for ankle syndesmosis injury. Br J Sports Med. 2015; 49(5):323–329

[9] Anderson RB, Hunt KJ, McCormick JJ. Management of common sports-related injuries about the foot and ankle. J Am Acad Orthop Surg. 2010; 18(9): 546–556

[10] Hsu AR, Anderson RB. Foot and ankle injuries in American football. Am J Orthop. 2016; 45(6): 358–367

[11] Lau BC, Moore LK, Thuillier DU. Evaluation and management of lateral ankle pain following injury. JBJS Rev. 2018; 6(8):e7

[12] Ferran NA, Maffulli N. Epidemiology of sprains of the lateral ankle ligament complex. Foot Ankle Clin. 2006; 11(3):659–662

[13] Amendola A, Drosdewech D. Tendon and ligament disorders of the foot and ankle. In: Bulstrode C, Buckwalter J, Carr AJ, et al, eds. Oxford Textbook of Orthopedics and Trauma. Vol. 2. New York, NY: Oxford University Press; 2002:1305–1314

[14] Jones MH, Amendola AS. Acute treatment of inversion ankle sprains: immobilization versus functional treatment. Clin Orthop Relat Res. 2007; 455(455):169–172

[15] Willits K, Amendola A, Bryant D, et al. Operative versus nonoperative treatment of acute Achilles tendon ruptures: a multicenter randomized trial using accelerated functional rehabilitation. J Bone Joint Surg Am. 2010; 92(17):2767–2775

[16] Garras DN, Raikin SM, Bhat SB, Taweel N, Karanjia H. MRI is unnecessary for diagnosing acute Achilles tendon ruptures: clinical diagnostic criteria. Clin Orthop Relat Res. 2012; 470(8):2268–2273

[17] Amendola A. Outcomes of open surgery versus nonoperative management of acute Achilles tendon rupture. Clin J Sport Med. 2014; 24(1):90–91

[18] Smith JW, Arnoczky SP, Hersh A. The intraosseous blood supply of the fifth metatarsal: implications for proximal fracture healing. Foot Ankle. 1992; 13 (3):143–152

16 Arthroscopy

Augustine M. Saiz Jr., Christopher D. Kreulen, and Eric Giza

Abstract

Arthroscopy of the ankle is a proven and valuable technique for both diagnosis and treatment of ankle pathology. Arthroscopy is a minimally invasive approach to the ankle joint and permits structures in addition to a magnified, clean view. Detailed anatomical knowledge allows access to the joint and surrounding structures while minimizing complications. A variety of pathologic conditions ranging temporally from acute to chronic, or structurally from osseous to soft tissues, can be addressed via arthroscopy. Different portals for access can be established based on the different indications for arthroscope; therefore, establishing a sound differential diagnosis is critical before proceeding with the procedure.

Keywords: ankle arthroscopy, portal placement, impingement, osteochondral defect, ankle instability, subtalar

16.1 Introduction

Ankle arthroscopy has developed over the last 40 years to become a standard diagnostic and therapeutic technique for a variety of ankle pathologies.[1,2,3,4,5,6] The greatest benefit of the advent of ankle arthroscopy has been the ability to provide a minimally invasive approach to the joint compared to previous open techniques. Arthroscopic approaches have the advantages of direct visualization of structures, improved assessment of articular cartilage, less postoperative morbidity, faster rehabilitation, earlier resumption of sports, and outpatient treatment.[1,2,3,4,5,6] Furthermore, with detailed anatomical knowledge, complications from ankle arthroscopy are minimal.[1,2,3,4,5,6] The overall result has been improved diagnosis and therapeutic capability with less risk and improved recovery.

16.2 Anterior Ankle Arthroscopy

- **Anatomy**
  - Extensive knowledge of the gross anatomy and open approaches to the ankle are of paramount importance as the surgeon needs to understand the relationship of intra-articular landmarks with the adjacent extra-articular structures. Failure to do so could lead to complications if conversion to open procedures is necessary.
  - The tibialis anterior tendon serves as a landmark for the anteromedial portal at the level of the anterior ankle joint line.[7,8] The anteromedial portal is located medial to the tibialis anterior tendon (▶ Fig. 16.1).
    - The long saphenous vein and saphenous nerve are usually located medial to this portal and care should be taken to avoid these structures.
  - The anterolateral portal location is on the anterior ankle joint line and lies lateral to the peroneus tertius tendon or alternatively lateral to the extensor digitorum longus tendons.
    - The intermediate cutaneous branch of the superficial peroneal nerve is within proximity and should be avoided.[9] Marking of this structure in the preoperative holding area is recommended. This structure can be palpated by inverting the foot and running hand over the lateral ankle/dorsum of the foot.
  - The posteromedial and posterolateral coaxial portals are located in parallel with the bimalleolar axis.[10]
  - The posterolateral coaxial portal is located posterior to the peroneus longus tendon.

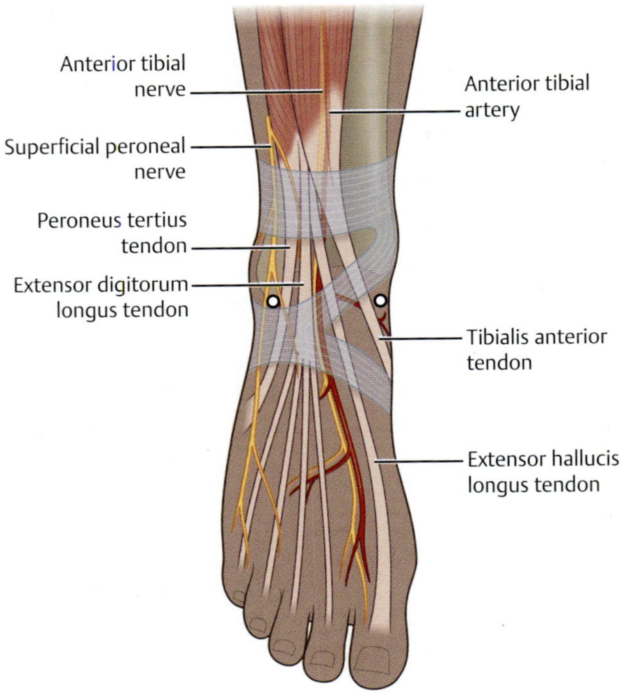

Fig. 16.1 Anterior anatomy of the ankle. The *circles* demonstrate anteromedial and anterolateral portals.

    - The sural nerve on average is located 6.6 mm from the posterolateral coaxial portal.[10]
  - The posteromedial coaxial portal is located between the posterior colliculus of the medial malleolus and the posterior tibial tendon.
    - Alternatively, it may be placed between the flexor digitorum longus and the posterior tibial tendon.
    - The posterior tibial nerve is on average located 5.7 mm from the posteromedial coaxial portal.
  - An anatomic safe zone exists between the intermediate branch of the superficial peroneal nerve and the sural nerve (▶ Fig. 16.2).
- **Indications**:
  - Soft tissue and bony impingement, synovitis, loose bodies, distal tibial and talus osteophytes, osteochondral defects, and synovial chondromatosis[11,12,13,14] (▶ Fig. 16.3).
  - Ankle fractures such as Weber type B or C distal fibular fractures or Tillaux fractures may benefit from arthroscopy-assisted open reduction and internal fixation.[15,16]
  - Arthroscopy-assisted ankle arthrodesis.[15]
    - verification of lateral ligament or syndesmotic instability.

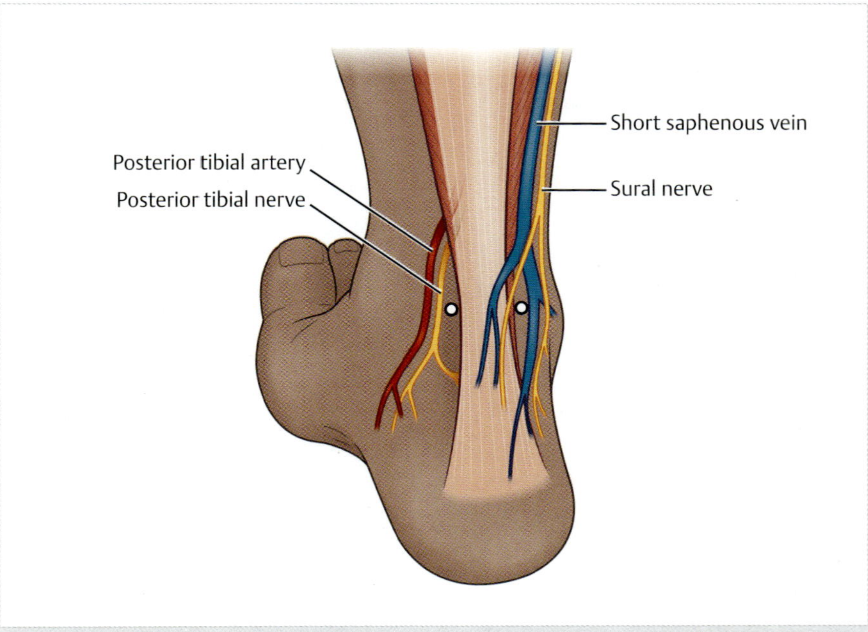

Fig. 16.2 Posterior ankle anatomy. The *circles* represent potential portals.

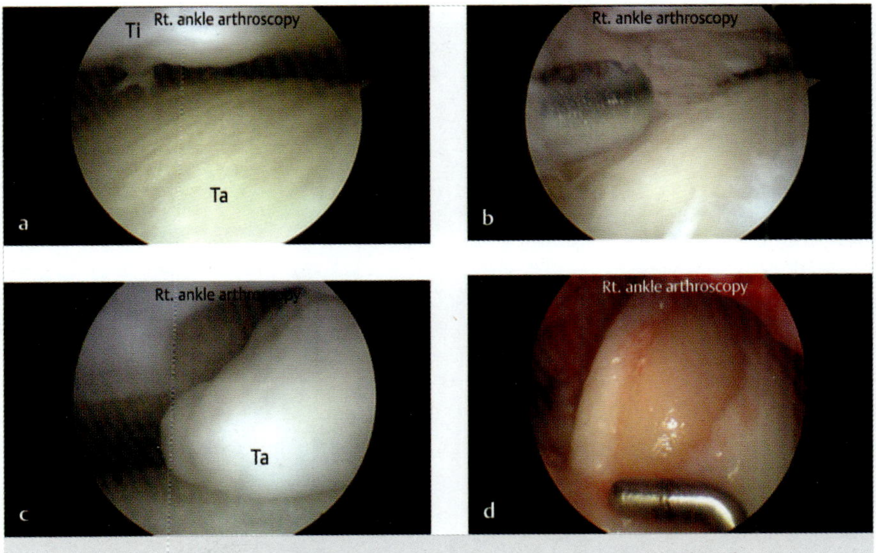

Fig. 16.3 Arthroscopic images of the ankle with anterior impingement. **(a)** Tibiotalar joint. **(b)** Chondromalacia of the tibiotalar joint. **(c)** Loose body in joint. **(d)** Grade IV chondromalacia of the talar dome due to impingement. L, loose body; Ta, talus; Ti, tibia.

- **Contraindications**:
  - Absolute contraindications are infection and severe degenerative change of the tibia and talus if not performing a fusion.
  - Relative contraindications are vascular disease and severe edema.
- **Diagnosis**:
  - The need for establishing an accurate preoperative diagnosis is important as a purely diagnostic ankle arthroscopy is of limited value with only 26 to 43% of patients benefitting from the procedure.
  - For cases of soft-tissue ankle impingement or internal derangement without a definitive radiographic or physical examination finding, a diagnostic injection is necessary:
    - A 3-mL mixture of bupivacaine, lidocaine, and ketorolac/corticosteroid are injected into the ankle medial to the tibialis anterior tendon.
      - If performed, ankle arthroscopy and/or open surgical procedures should be delayed 3 months to decrease risk of infection.
      - The patient returns to the office in 3 to 4 weeks.
      - A temporary alleviation of symptoms after the injection are indicative of an internal ankle impingement, which would benefit from arthroscopy.
      - No relief from symptoms may indicate that further workup of the ankle symptoms is necessary prior to proceeding with surgical intervention.
- **Conservative management**:
  - Trial of activity modification, immobilization with brace, nonsteroidal anti-inflammatory drugs (NSAIDs), physical therapy with modality treatments, range-of-motion exercises, neuromuscular coordination training, and strengthening depending on the condition.
- **Surgical intervention**
  - *Preoperative planning*:
    - Review of imaging studies to determine the port placement.
    - Standard anteromedial and anterolateral portals are sufficient to access the anterior and central tibiotalar pathology.
    - The posterior portals are required when it is necessary to address pathology in the posterior capsule or the posterior talar lesions:[17]
      - This typically requires prone positioning.
    - Preoperative popliteal block or epidural anesthesia.
    - Marking of the tibialis anterior tendon, tertius tendon, and superficial peroneal nerve intermediate branch (▶ Fig. 16.4).
    - Examination under anesthesia including anterior drawer test and talar tilt.
  - *Positioning*:
    - Ankle arthroscopy with distraction may be used (▶ Fig. 16.5).
      - Distraction may result in tightening of the anterior capsule leading to reduction of the anterior working space where loose bodies and osteophytes are usually located.

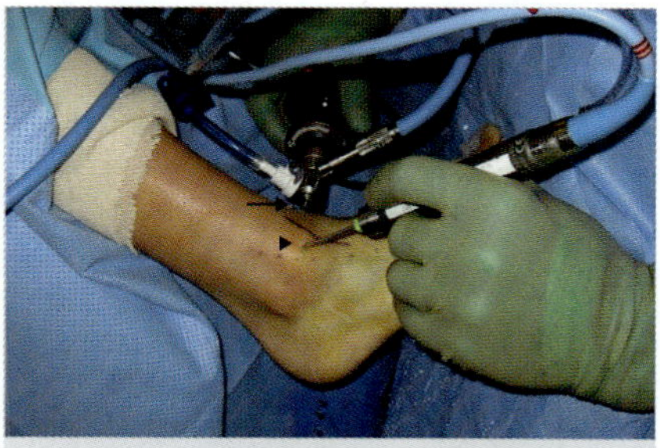

Fig. 16.4 Anterior ankle arthroscopic portals established. The *arrowhead* indicates the anterior lateral portal, the *arrow* indicates the anteromedial portal, and the *dotted line* on the skin indicates the intermediate dorsal cutaneous nerve mapped out.

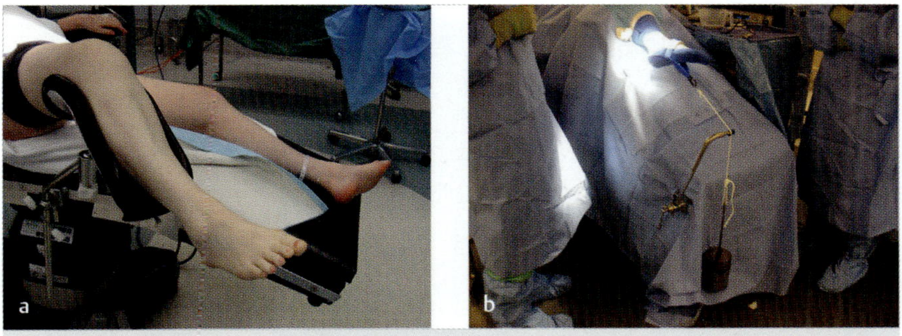

Fig. 16.5 Positioning. **(a)** Leg holder. **(b)** Distraction setup.

    * Dorsiflexion increases the size of the anterior working area, and additionally, the talar articular cartilage becomes concealed from iatrogenic damage.
    * Distraction may be useful in the treatment of ossicles or loose bodies caught in the syndesmotic area or for posterior ankle pathologies without use of the posterior portals.
- *Placement of the anterior portals*:
  - Inject the ankle with 10 mL of sterile saline via the anteromedial ankle in a similar fashion to arthrocentesis with needle placement medial to the tibialis anterior tendon.
    * This allows for identification and correct orientation for the anteromedial arthroscopy portal.
  - Make a 5-mm longitudinal skin incision and spread subcutaneous tissue down and then through the capsule with a small hemostat; fluid gush confirms intra-articular location.
  - Use a blunt-tip trocar with an arthroscopic cannula to enter the joint and insert the arthroscope, a 2.9-mm 30-degree instrument depending on preference, and start water flow. Also have a 2.9-mm 70-degree and 1.9-mm arthroscope available.
    * When necessary, the 1.9-mm scope can improve access to difficult locations within the ankle.
    * Water flow pressure is typically 35 to 40 mm Hg using a machine pump.
  - Under arthroscopic control, the anterolateral portal is made by inserting a spinal needle or an 18-gauge needle lateral to the peroneus tertius tendon while respecting the superficial peroneal nerve.
    * The needle allows for water flow through the needle for better visualization and confirms the correct location for the anterolateral portal.
  - In a similar fashion, a 5-mm longitudinal incision is made at the anterolateral portal position and dissection with a hemostat is performed and a trocar followed by an arthroscopic cannula is introduced.
  - The anteromedial inferior portal is an accessory portal that can be helpful when there is pathology of the deltoid ligament insertion.
    * Through the anteromedial portal, the medial gutter is visualized.
    * Again an 18-gauge needle is introduced into the inferior medial gutter, usually about 10 mm inferior to the anteromedial portal.
    * An incision is made and the portal established as previously described.
    * This allows access to the far inferomedial ankle joint and deltoid insertion.

- *Posterior coaxial portals*:
  - Arthroscope and inflow in the anterolateral portal.
  - Vertical skin incision made posterior to the peroneal tendon sheath and 1.5 cm proximal to the tip of the fibula.[18]
  - Keep the ankle in neutral dorsiflexion and insert the trocar and arthroscopic sheath anterior and slightly inferior on a plane parallel to the bimalleolar axis.
    - Confirm the intracapsular placement by briefly inserting arthroscope.
  - Insert a long switching rod through the cannula and direct it toward the medial malleolus using the rod to palpate the posterior colliculus and penetrate just anterior to the posterior tibial tendon.
  - Incise over the tented skin and a cannula can be passed over the switching rod into the posterior ankle recess.
    - Alternatively, the medial portal can be made directly using a small, vertical incision posterior to the medial malleolus posterior colliculus.
- *Arthroscopic examination*:
  - Start in the lateral "safe zone," which is at the 2 to 4 o'clock position to see the tibia, fibula, and talus (▶ Fig. 16.6).
  - Transition to the medial "safe zone" at the 8 to 10 o'clock position to see the medial malleolus, tibia, and talus.
  - Then examine the talar neck, for anterior impingement, medial and lateral gutters, central and medial and lateral talus, and posterior ankle.
- *Complications*:
  - Injury to the neurovascular structures, instrument breakage, articular surface damage, neuroma formation, infection, and reflex sympathetic dystrophy.
    - Complication rate ranges from 0.7 to 17%, with neurologic injury being the most common.

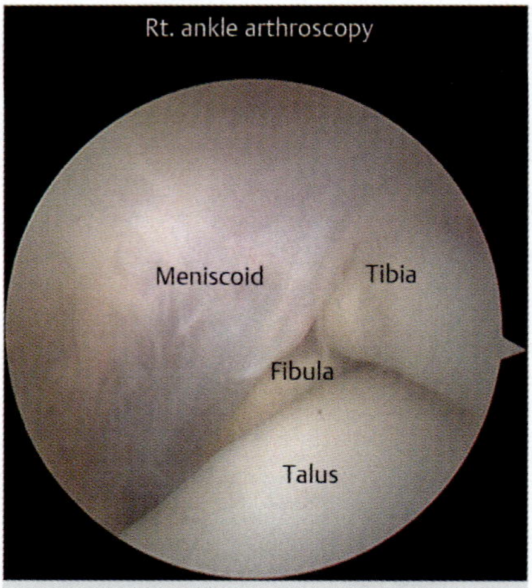

Fig. 16.6 Lateral view in the "safe zone."

  - The superficial peroneal nerve is at highest risk and injury associated with the anterolateral portal, followed by the sural nerve and then the saphenous nerve.[19]
- *Wound care*:
  - Closure with 3–0 nylon to prevent sinus formation.
  - Sterile dressing applied.
  - Sutures out in 2 weeks.

- **Rehabilitation**:
  - Depends on the condition being treated.
  - Most conditions treated with 5 to 7 days of postoperative, well-padded splint and then weight bearing as tolerated afterward.
  - If treating osteochondritis dissecans (OCD), often a period of non-weight-bearing is required.
  - Early range of motion encouraged except in case of fusion.

16.3 Posterior Ankle Arthroscopy

- **Anatomy**:
  - The deep location of the hindfoot structures can make direct access

difficult due to the shape of the ankle joint.
   - Historically, the hindfoot is approached with a three-portal technique consisting of the anteromedial, anterolateral, and posterolateral portals with the patient in the supine position.
   - Risked injury with the posterolateral portal to the tibial nerve, posterior tibial artery, and local tendons; additionally, pericapsular or extracapsular posterior pathologic conditions not accessible.[20]
- ◦ Posterior ankle arthroscopy and endoscopy enable visualization and allow accessibility to the posterior half of the tibiotalar joint, subtalar joint, and extra-articular structures such as the os trigonum, flexor hallucis longus tendon, and posterior syndesmotic ligaments[21] (▶ Fig. 16.7).
- ◦ The flexor hallucis longus tendon runs within a tendon sheath that begins 1 cm proximal to the subtalar joint and binds the tendon to the posterior talus and calcaneus, forming a fibro-osseous tunnel.[21]
- ◦ The posteromedial neurovascular bundle is consistently medial to the flexor hallucis longus tendon.
   - Instruments introduced from the posteromedial portal do not risk injury to the neurovascular bundle as long as they remain lateral to the flexor hallucis longus tendon.

- **Indications**:
   - ◦ Posteriorly located OCDs, ossicles, loose bodies, posttraumatic calcifications or avulsion fragments, posterior tibial rim osteophytes, chronic synovitis, flexor hallucis longus tendinopathy, intraosseous talar ganglion, subtalar arthrodesis, deep portion of the deltoid ligament pathology, symptomatic os trigonum, and posterior ankle impingement[22,23] (▶ Fig. 16.8).
- **Contraindications**:
   - ◦ Acute infection or severe degenerative changes.
- **Diagnosis**:
   - ◦ The patient usually has deep pain in the posterior aspect of the ankle joint.
   - ◦ Pain with palpation of the posterior aspect of the talus.

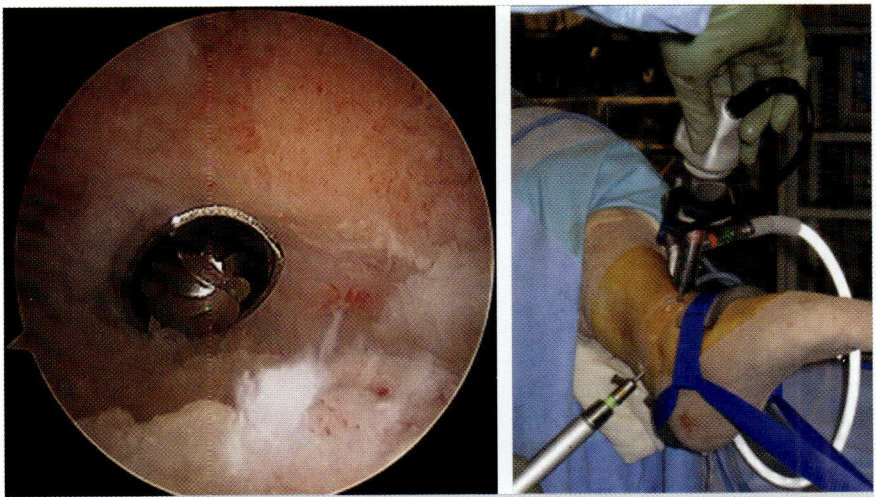

Fig. 16.7 Establishment of the posterior ankle portal. View of the instrument entering the posterior portal.

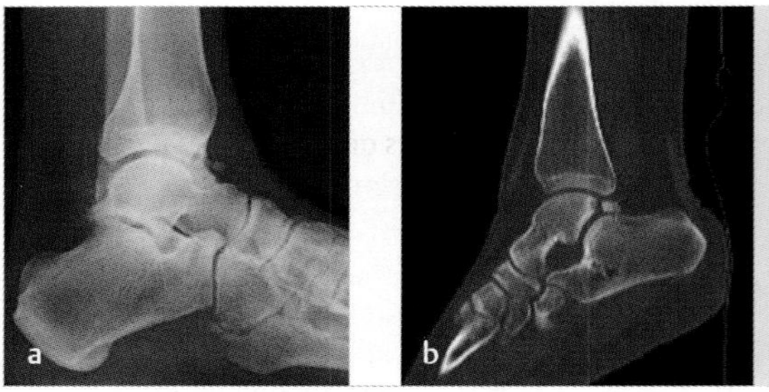

Fig. 16.8 **(a)** X-ray showing calcifications in the Achilles tendon and os trigonum. **(b)** Computed tomography (CT) scan demonstrating the os trigonum.

- Pain with passive forced plantarflexion.
- Tender over the flexor hallucis longus tendon.
- Confirmation of pathology on imaging including possibly computed tomography (CT) or magnetic resonance imaging (MRI).

- **Conservative management**:
  - Rest, ice, anti-inflammatory medication, possible ankle immobilization, corticosteroid injection, and physical therapy depending on the pathology.
- **Surgical intervention**:
  - *Preoperative planning*:
    - Outpatient procedure under general or epidural anesthesia.
    - Images reviewed and examination performed under anesthesia assessing the stability of the ankle joint.
  - *Positioning*:
    - A 4.0-mm 30-degree arthroscope is routinely used.
    - The foot is placed at the end of the table so that the ankle can be fully dorsiflexed.
  - *Approach*:
    - Landmarks are the lateral malleolus, medial and lateral borders of the Achilles tendon, and the sole of the foot.
      * Reference line is drawn from the tip of the lateral malleolus to the Achilles tendon parallel to the sole of the foot, and the portals are placed just above this line at the same level in the horizontal plane just medial and lateral to the Achilles tendon.
  - *Posterolateral portal*:
    - Vertical stab incision made for the posterolateral portal just lateral to the Achilles tendon.
    - The subcutaneous layer is split with a small hemostat directed anteriorly in the direction of the interdigital webspace between the first and second toes.
    - Once the hemostat touches bone, it is exchanged for a blunt trocar and the arthroscope is introduced.
    - The direction of view is 30 degrees to the lateral side.
  - *Posteromedial portal*:
    - A vertical stab incision is made for the posteromedial portal just medial to the Achilles tendon.
    - A small hemostat is introduced and directed toward the arthroscope at a 90-degree angle.
    - Once the hemostat touches the arthroscope shaft, it is moved anteriorly in the direction of the ankle joint, all the way down, touching the arthroscope shaft until it touches bone.
    - The arthroscope is pulled slightly back until the tip of the hemostat visualized.
    - The hemostat is used to spread the extra-articular soft tissue in front of the tip of the lens.
    - The hemostat can be exchanged for a cannula or an arthroscopic instrument.

- *Working in the posterior ankle*:
  - Adipose tissue can be removed and with it the thin joint capsule revealing the subtalar joint and the posterior talofibular ligament.
  - At the level of the ankle joint, the posterior tibiofibular and talofibular ligaments are identified and the posterior ankle can be visualized.
  - The posterior talar process can be identified as can the flexor hallucis longus tendon medially.
    - * Never place the shaver medial to flexor hallucis longus tendon as there is risk of injury to the neurovascular structures.
  - With the arthroscope, the tip of the medial malleolus and deep portion of the deltoid ligament can be visualized.
  - It can open the joint capsule from inside out at the level of the medial malleolus to open the posterior tibial tendon sheath.
  - With manual distraction of the os calcis, the posterior aspect of the ankle can be opened to allow instrument access.
- *Wound care*:
  - Closure is done with 3–0 nylon to prevent sinus formation.
  - Sterile dressing is applied.
  - Sutures are removed in 2 weeks.
- *Complications*:
- Tibial nerve and vascular injury, flexor hallucis longus tendon injury, and sural nerve injury.

• **Rehabilitation**:
  - Immediate range-of-motion exercises and weight bearing as tolerated.

16.4 Subtalar Arthroscopy

• **Anatomy**
  - The subtalar joint is formed between the talus and the calcaneus (► Fig. 16.9).
  - In terms of arthroscopy, the joint is divided into the anterior (talocalcaneonavicular) and posterior (talocalcaneal) articulations.[24]

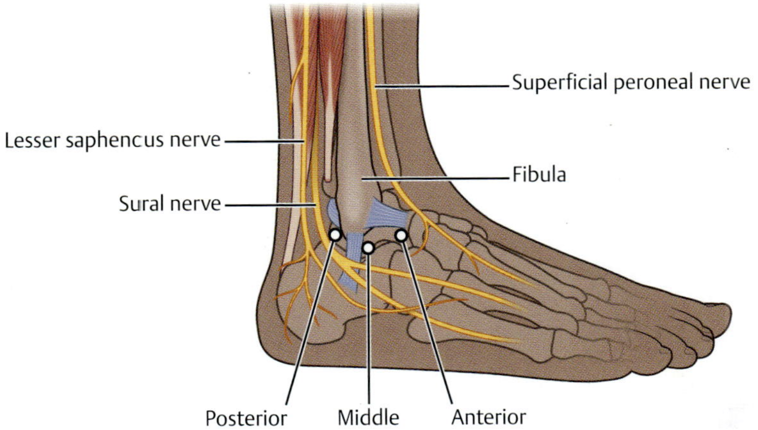

Fig. 16.9 Anatomy of the structures surrounding the subtalar joint. The *circles* demonstrate the potential port sites.

- The tarsal canal separates the anterior and posterior articulations; the sinus tarsi is a large lateral opening in the tarsal tunnel.
- Within the tarsal canal and sinus tarsi are the interosseous talocalcaneal ligament, inferior extensor retinaculum roots, the cervical ligament, fatty tissue, and blood vessels.
- The posterior subtalar joint has a synovial lining with a posterior capsular pouch with lateral, medial, and anterior recesses.

- **Indications**:
  - Sinus tarsi syndrome, loose bodies, lateral talar osteophyte or nonunion, fusion, and diagnostic.[24]
- **Contraindications**:
  - Severe arthritis if not planning fusion.
- **Diagnosis**:
  - Patients with subtalar pathology often present with feeling of instability when walking on uneven terrain.
    - This can be differentiated on physical examination from lateral ankle instability by holding the ankle in place and solely manipulating the subtalar joint by cupping the heel and shucking medial to lateral, back and forth. This will recreate discomfort and feelings of instability isolated to the subtalar joint.
  - Restricted and/or painful motion with inversion and eversion.
  - Tender over the sinus tarsi.
  - X-rays, especially Broden's views, may show loose bodies; CT can show intra-articular pathology; MRI may detect chronic inflammation or fibrosis within the subtalar joint, OCD lesions, chondral injuries, or ligamentous pathology.
- **Conservative management**:
  - Injection of corticosteroid, foot orthosis, NSAIDs, ankle brace, and therapy especially to focus on peroneal tendon strengthening.
- **Surgical intervention**:
  - *Preoperative planning*:
    - Outpatient procedure under general or epidural anesthesia.
    - Images reviewed and examination performed under anesthesia assessing the stability of the ankle joint.
  - *Positioning*:
    - Semilateral position with distraction with easy access to the posterolateral portal.
      - Prone positioning is also an option.
  - *Approach*:
    - Three portals: central, posterolateral, and anterolateral (▶ Fig. 16.10).
    - Distend the joint first with a needle and 20-mL saline from the posterolateral portal.

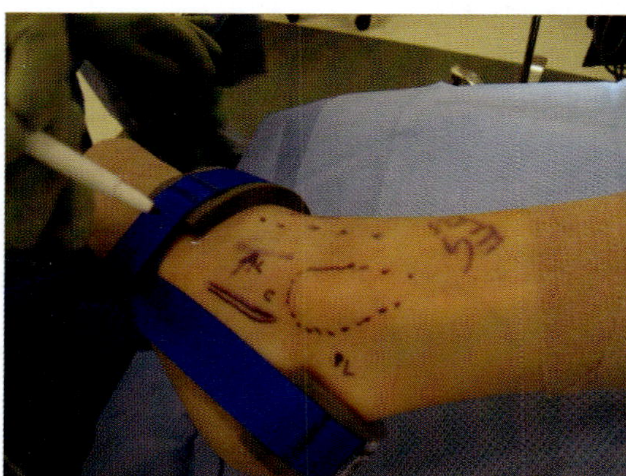

Fig. 16.10 Preoperative marking and distraction for subtalar arthroscopy. AL, anterolateral portal; C, central portal; PL, posterolateral portal. The *dashed oval* area marks the fibula.

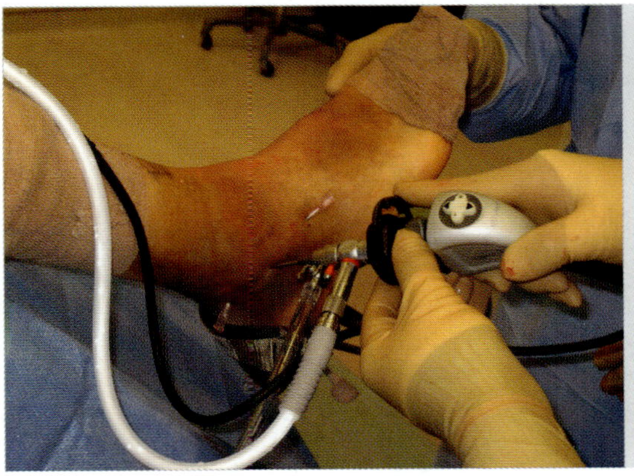

Fig. 16.11 Establishment of the posterolateral portal for inflow and central portal with an arthroscope. Calcaneal traction in place.

- *Portal placement*:
  - The first portal established is the center portal, one thumb breadth beneath the center of the fibula directed toward the anterior plafond.
  - Then the posterolateral portal is made under direct visualization at the level of the distal fibula between the posterior fibula and the Achilles tendon with care taken to avoid sural nerve (▶ Fig. 16.11).
  - Finally, the anterolateral portal is established under direct visualization with the entrance being about 1 cm distal and 2 cm anterior to the distal fibular tip.
- *Wound care*:
  - Closure with 3–0 nylon to prevent sinus formation.
  - Sterile dressing applied.
  - Sutures are removed in 2 weeks.
- *Complications*:
  - Neurovascular injury, especially sural nerve and superficial peroneal nerve, is rare, but is the most common complication of ankle arthroscopy.

16.5 Key Testing Facts

- Many pathologic conditions ranging from OCDs to fractures can be treated by ankle arthroscopy.
- The tibialis anterior tendon serves as a landmark for the anteromedial portal on the ankle joint line. The peroneus tertius serves as a landmark for the anterolateral portal.
- The superficial peroneal nerve is at highest risk and injury associated with the anterolateral portal, followed by the sural nerve and then the saphenous nerve.
- The posterior ankle arthroscopy enables visualization and accessibility to the posterior half of the tibiotalar joint, subtalar joint, and extra-articular structures.
- The subtalar arthroscopy is an excellent method for the treatment of various subtalar pathology; the portals are central, posterolateral, and anterolateral; the sural nerve and small saphenous vein are at greatest risk.

References

[1] Burman MS. Arthroscopy or the direct visualization of joints. J Bone Joint Surg Am. 1931; 13(4):669–695

[2] van Dijk CN, Scholte D. Arthroscopy of the ankle joint. Arthroscopy. 1997; 13(1):90–96

[3] van Dijk CN, van Bergen CJ. Advancements in ankle arthroscopy. J Am Acad Orthop Surg. 2008; 16(11): 635–646

[4] Ferkel RD, Small HN, Gittins JE. Complications in foot and ankle arthroscopy. Clin Orthop Relat Res. 2001(391):89–104

[5] Guhl JF, Boynton MD, Parisien JS, eds. Foot and Ankle Arthroscopy. Berlin: Springer Science & Business Media; 2004

[6] Ferkel RD, Scranton PE, Jr. Arthroscopy of the ankle and foot. J Bone Joint Surg Am. 1993; 75 (8):1233–1242

[7] van Dijk CN, Scholten PE, Krips R. A 2-portal endoscopic approach for diagnosis and treatment of posterior ankle pathology. Arthroscopy. 2000; 16(8):871–876

[8] Golanó P, Vega J, Pérez-Carro L, Götzens V. Ankle anatomy for the arthroscopist. Part I: The portals. Foot Ankle Clin. 2006; 11(2):253–273, v

[9] Ferkel RD, Heath DD, Guhl JF. Neurological complications of ankle arthroscopy. Arthroscopy. 1996; 12(2):200–208

[10] Smyth NA, Zwiers R, Wiegerinck JI, et al. Posterior hindfoot arthroscopy: a review. Am J Sports Med. 2014; 42(1):225–234

[11] Zengerink M, Szerb I, Hangody L, Dopirak RM, Ferkel RD, van Dijk CN. Current concepts: treatment of osteochondral ankle defects. Foot Ankle Clin. 2006; 11(2):331–359, vi

[12] Schuman L, Struijs PA, van Dijk CN. Arthroscopic treatment for osteochondral defects of the talus. Results at follow-up at 2 to 11 years. J Bone Joint Surg Br. 2002; 84(3):364–368

[13] Biedert R. Anterior ankle pain in sports medicine: aetiology and indications for arthroscopy. Arch Orthop Trauma Surg. 1991; 110(6):293–297

[14] Niek van Dijk C. Anterior and posterior ankle impingement. Foot Ankle Clin. 2006; 11(3):663–683

[15] Hsu AR, Gross CE, Lee S, Carreira DS. Extended indications for foot and ankle arthroscopy. J Am Acad Orthop Surg. 2014; 22(1):10–19

[16] Drez D, Jr, Guhl JF, Gollehon DL. Ankle arthroscopy: technique and indications. Foot Ankle. 1981; 2(3): 138–143

[17] Lijoi F, Lughi M, Baccarani G. Posterior arthroscopic approach to the ankle: an anatomic study. Arthroscopy. 2003; 19(1):62–67

[18] Acevedo JI, Busch MT, Ganey TM, Hutton WC, Ogden JA. Coaxial portals for posterior ankle arthroscopy: An anatomic study with clinical correlation on 29 patients. Arthroscopy. 2000; 16 (8):836–842

[19] Drakos M, Behrens SB, Mulcahey MK, Paller D, Hoffman E, DiGiovanni CW. Proximity of arthroscopic ankle stabilization procedures to surrounding structures: an anatomic study. Arthroscopy. 2013; 29(6): 1089–1094

[20] Nickisch F, Barg A, Saltzman CL, et al. Postoperative complications of posterior ankle and hindfoot arthroscopy. J Bone Joint Surg Am. 2012; 94(5): 439–446

[21] Golanò P, Mariani PP, Rodríguez-Niedenfuhr M, Mariani PF, Ruano-Gil D. Arthroscopic anatomy of the posterior ankle ligaments. Arthroscopy. 2002; 18(4):353–358

[22] Ogut T, Ayhan E, Irgit K, Sarikaya AI. Endoscopic treatment of posterior ankle pain. Knee Surg Sports Traumatol Arthrosc. 2011; 19(8):1355–1361

[23] Sitler DF, Amendola A, Bailey CS, Thain LM, Spouge A. Posterior ankle arthroscopy: an anatomic study. J Bone Joint Surg Am. 2002; 84(5):763–769

[24] Frey C, Gasser S, Feder K. Arthroscopy of the subtalar joint. Foot Ankle Int. 1994; 15(8):424–428

17 Neurologic Disorders

Emily C. Vafek, Christopher E. Gross, and Simon Lee

Abstract
Entrapment neuropathies of the lower extremities can be a source of pain in the foot and ankle. Essential to the diagnosis and treatment of these syndromes is an understanding of peripheral nerve anatomy and common sites of compression.

Keywords: Morton's neuroma, tarsal tunnel syndrome, jogger's foot, Baxter's neuritis, anterior tarsal tunnel syndrome

17.1 Interdigital Neuroma (Morton's Neuroma)

- Interdigital neuroma (IDN) is an entrapment neuropathy of the c digit nerve as it passes between the metatarsal heads and beneath the transverse metatarsal ligament.

17.1.1 Etiology and Pathophysiology

- It is not a neoplastic lesion or inflammatory process.
- Histopathology: perineural fibrosis and neural degeneration.[1]
- Its pathophysiology is poorly understood and it is believed to be the result of compression of the nerve under the transverse metatarsal ligament.
- Other theories: Repetitive microtrauma of the tethered nerve between the metatarsal heads related to tight shoes and high heels and inflammation of the distal metatarsophalangeal (MTP) bursa leading to secondary fibrosis in the digital nerves.[2]

Anatomy

- Anatomic considerations may play a role in the development of IDN.
- The *medial plantar nerve* (MPN) has four digital branches including the proper digital nerve to the great toe as well as the first, second, and third common digital nerves.
- The *lateral plantar nerve* (LPN) branches into the proper digital nerve of the small toe as well as the fourth common digital nerve, which has a communicating branch that passes to the third common digital nerve.
- This contribution from both the medial and LPNs to the third common digital nerve is thought to result in a relatively increased size of the nerve with greater risk of developing IDN.[3]
  - An anatomic dissection study revealed the presence of this communicating branch in 27% of specimens leading the authors to question this as a contributing factor.[4]
- IDNs are seen most commonly in the third webspace, between the third and fourth metatarsal heads, and occasionally occur in the second webspace.
- The second and third webspaces have relatively less distance between the metatarsal heads than the first and fourth webspaces.
- The mobility between the relatively rigid medial three rays and the more mobile lateral two rays may also contribute to the increased incidence of IDN in the third webspace.[3]

17.1.2 Symptoms

- Symptoms present as pain localized to the plantar aspect of the forefoot between the metatarsal heads.[3]

- Patients frequently describe the pain as burning, tingling, or electric with pain radiating into the effected toes.
- Patients may also report the sensation of walking on a lump.[1]
- The symptoms are made worse by high-heeled or tight-fitting shoes and are relieved by shoe removal or walking barefoot.
- Women are more often affected than men, which is thought to be secondary to wearing narrow-toe box shoes, which increases the pressure in the forefoot.[1]
- IDNs are typically unilateral.

17.1.3 Diagnostics

- It is based on a patient's history and physical examination.
- Palpation of the involved webspace reproduces the pain and can cause pain radiating to the affected toes.
- *Mulder's click*: Simultaneous dorsally directed pressure in the webspace with medial and lateral compression of the metatarsal heads may elicit a palpable bursa click, which reproduces the patient's symptoms.[2]
- Palpation of the adjacent MTP joints can rule out synovitis as the source of pain.
- *Radiographs*: Evaluate for underlying osseous abnormalities such as subluxation, deformity, or MTP arthritis.
- Magnetic resonance imaging (MRI) can be obtained to rule out other pathologies but is typically not necessary to establish a diagnosis.[3]
- Ultrasonography has also been described in the diagnosis of IDN, but it is operator dependent and difficult to image the small-caliber digital nerves limiting its diagnostic utility.[2]
- Electrodiagnostic studies are not used in diagnosing an IDN but may be used to rule out peripheral neuropathy or radiculopathy as a source of pain.
- The clinical diagnosis may be verified with an injection of 1 to 2 mL of lidocaine into the webspace plantar to the intermetatarsal ligament. Resolution of the patient's symptoms confirms the diagnosis.[1]

17.1.4 Conservative Management

- Shoe wear modification is the mainstay of nonoperative treatment and includes wide, soft, and low-heeled shoes.
- Metatarsal pads may also be utilized to relieve pressure in the forefoot.
  - The pad is placed just proximal to the metatarsal heads resulting in increased space between the heads and decompression of the nerve with weight bearing.[3]
- Corticosteroid injections can provide short-term relief but show limited long-term improvement.[1]
  - Repeat corticosteroid injections into the forefoot may also lead to adverse outcomes such as fat pad atrophy or plantar plate rupture and damage to the MTP joint capsule resulting in lesser toe deformity.

17.1.5 Surgical Intervention

- Operative treatment consists of surgical excision of the neuroma, most often through a dorsal approach, with good clinical outcomes.[1]
- A dorsal incision is made in the midline of the affected webspace, approximately 3 cm in length.
- Dissection is carried down through the subcutaneous tissue with care taken to protect the dorsal digital nerves.
- The metatarsal heads are exposed and a laminar spreader is positioned between the heads to place the transverse metatarsal ligament on tension.
- A Freer elevator is used to dissect the interspace and is placed just plantar to the intermetatarsal ligament to protect

the digital nerves as the ligament is sharply transected.
- The common digital nerve is identified and resected 2 to 3 cm proximal to the metatarsal heads, which allows the stump to retract proximally into the intrinsic musculature while the distal portion is removed.[3]
- Outcomes have varied with Giannini et al[5] reporting 78% good or excellent results, Womack et al[6] reporting 51% good or excellent results, and more recently Bucknall et al[7] reporting 79% good or excellent results.

17.2 Recurrent Interdigital Neuroma

- It presents as persistent or recurrent pain following neuroma excision.

17.2.1 Etiology and Pathophysiology

- Recurrent IDN can be the result of inadequate resection of the neuroma at the time of the primary procedure.
- Plantar nerve branches can tether the common digital nerve resulting in a failure of the stump to retract adequately.[3]
- Recurrent IDN can also occur with the formation of a bulb neuroma at the neural stump, which can be adhered to the soft tissues or against the metatarsal head or bone leading to pain.[2]

17.2.2 Symptoms

- Similar to primary IDN, patients with recurrent neuromas present with plantar forefoot pain.
- The pain can be described as electric or burning and is typically worse with weight bearing and activities.
- The pain may also be localized to a specific area of tenderness near the metatarsal head.[3]

17.2.3 Diagnostics

- A physical examination in combination with the clinical history is the basis for making this diagnosis.
- The forefoot is examined in a manner similar to the evaluation of a primary neuroma.
- Particular care should be taken to identify a localized area of tenderness, which may exhibit electriclike pain on palpation (a positive Tinel's sign).[3]
- The examiner should also evaluate for potential differential diagnoses of pain including MTP joint synovitis or tarsal tunnel syndrome.

17.2.4 Conservative Management

- Nonoperative treatment of recurrent IDN is similar to that of primary neuromas.
- Shoe wear modifications, including soft wide-toed shoes, can be used to relieve pressure in the metatarsal heads and webspaces.
- Additional medications to treat neuropathic type pain, such as tricyclic antidepressants or antiseizure medications, such as gabapentin or pregabalin, may be considered.[3]

17.2.5 Surgical Intervention

- Revision excision of a recurrent IDN may be approached through a dorsal incision or a plantar incision.
- The plantar approach allows for improved access to the proximal stump but can result in a painful plantar scar.
- A plantar transverse or longitudinal incision is made approximately 1 cm proximal to the weight-bearing surface of the metatarsal heads.[3]
- The dissection is made through the subcutaneous tissue and the plantar fascia to expose the interdigital nerve.
- Nerve branches are identified and the nerve is transected proximally.

- The nerve can then be transposed into muscle to help prevent recurrent neuroma symptoms.
- A compressive dressing is placed to the forefoot at the conclusion of the procedure and remains in place for 2 to 3 weeks.
- Sutures are removed at 2 weeks and the plantar incision is protected in a postoperative shoe until the incision is healed.
- Satisfactory results can be achieved in 60 to 80% of cases.[3]

17.3 Tarsal Tunnel Syndrome

Tarsal tunnel syndrome is an entrapment neuropathy of the tibial nerve as it passes posterior and inferior to the medial malleolus.[8]

17.3.1 Etiology and Pathophysiology

- The tarsal tunnel is a fibro-osseous space created by the tibia forming the anterior wall, the talus, and calcaneus forming the lateral wall and the flexor retinaculum forming the roof.[1]
- Contents: posterior tibialis tendon, flexor digitorum longus tendon, flexor hallucis longus tendon, tibia nerve, and posterior tibial artery and vein.
- The tibial nerve divides into three terminal branches within the tarsal tunnel: the medial calcaneal nerve, LPN, and MPN.[3]
- The causes of tarsal tunnel syndrome are varied and can be identified in up to 80% of patients.[9]
- Causes include the following:
    - A specific injury or trauma (severe ankle sprain, crush injury, ankle fracture or dislocation, calcaneus fracture, etc.).
    - Space-occupying lesions (ganglion cyst, lipoma, neurilemmoma, varicosities, tenosynovitis, exostoses, etc.).
    - Hindfoot deformity (varus leading to compression and valgus leading to traction).[9]

17.3.2 Symptoms

- Patients present with pain in the medial ankle and plantar foot which, is often exacerbated by activity and relieved with rest.
- Pain can be diffuse and difficult for the patient to describe and is often reported variously as burning, electric, shooting, numb, and tingling.[3]

17.3.3 Diagnostics

- Physical examination begins with assessment of posture and foot alignment while standing, particularly noting hindfoot varus or valgus.
- The motion of the ankle and subtalar joints is assessed looking for potential underlying injury or arthritic condition.
- The course of the tibial nerve is palpated to assess for any sites of point tenderness or irritability as well as any palpable masses indicating a space-occupying lesion.[1,3]
- Part of the diagnostic evaluation includes obtaining plain radiographs and an MRI to identify bony or soft-tissue etiologies.[1]
- Electrodiagnostic studies are obtained to evaluate for areas of compression, potential double crush syndrome with a more proximal lesion, or underlying peripheral neuropathy.[10]

17.3.4 Conservative Management

- Nonoperative treatment is based on the etiology of the tarsal tunnel syndrome.
- Patients with identified space-occupying lesions should undergo excision.
- For patients without space-occupying lesions, conservative modalities include

administration of mediations such as anti-inflammatories, tricyclic antidepressants, gabapentin, or pregabalin.
- Topical medications, such as lidocaine patches, may be used.[3]
- Bracing or orthotics can be used to correct hindfoot deformity, and activity modification can be utilized if there is a functional component to the symptoms:[1]
  - A varus-producing heel wedge can help.

17.3.5 Surgical Intervention

- Surgical treatment is customized to the identifiable cause of the tarsal tunnel syndrome.
- Space-occupying lesions should be resected and structural alignment deformity should be corrected.
- If no underlying structure cause is found and the patient continues to have pain despite conservative care, tibial nerve release can be performed.[3]
- The entire flexor retinaculum is incised to release the tarsal tunnel and neurolysis of the tibial nerve is carried proximally and distally to the three terminal branches.[1]

17.4 Lateral Plantar Nerve Entrapment (Baxter's Neuropathy)

Entrapment of the first branch of the LPN (Baxter's nerve) can be a source of chronic plantar medial heel pain.

17.4.1 Etiology and Pathophysiology

- The LPN is a branch of the tibial nerve that provides sensation to the plantar lateral aspect of the foot.
- The first branch of the LPN runs between the abductor hallucis muscle and the quadratus plantae where it can become compressed by the deep fascia.[3]
- Hypertrophy of these muscles may also contribute to nerve compression.
- The syndrome is often found in long-distance runners, but it can also be seen in other athletes such as those who participate in soccer, tennis, or dance.[3]
- The LPN can also be injured iatrogenically such as during the plantar approach to insert an intramedullary nail for a tibiotalocalcaneal arthrodesis.

17.4.2 Symptoms

- Patients present with plantar medial heel pain that is worse with activity.
- The location of the symptoms can cause plantar fasciitis to be mistaken as the cause of pain.
- Patients may describe pain radiating proximally to the medial ankle as well as distally across the lateral plantar foot.[1]

17.4.3 Diagnostics

- Physical examination of the patient presenting with suspected Baxter's neuropathy includes thorough evaluation of the entire course of the tibial nerve and its branches.
- Pain may be elicited with palpation of the first branch of the LPN deep to the abductor hallucis muscle reproducing pain radiating proximally and distally.[3]
- Imaging, such as radiographs and MRI, can be used to look for underlying bony abnormalities that may be contributing to compression.
- Electrodiagnostic studies can be used to evaluate compression of the tibial nerve and localize the site of compression.[1]

17.4.4 Conservative Management

- Nonoperative management focuses on minimizing external pressure and includes activity modification, gel heel cups, heel cord stretching, and the use of anti-inflammatory medications.

17.4.5 Surgical Intervention

- Operative treatment involves neurolysis of the LPN through an oblique incision over the medial aspect of the heel.
- The superficial and deep fascia of the abductor hallucis muscle is divided, and the course of the nerve is followed distally releasing any potential sites of compression.[3]
- A small portion of a calcaneus osteophyte may be resected if bony impingement is present in addition to a partial release of the medial plantar fascia with good reported outcomes.[11]

17.5 Medial Plantar Nerve Entrapment (Jogger's foot)

Jogger's foot is an entrapment neuropathy of the MPN typically occurring at the knot of Henry.

17.5.1 Etiology and Pathophysiology

- MPN provides sensation to the medial sole and the plantar first, second, and third and medial half of the fourth toes.
- It provides motor innervation to the abductor hallucis, flexor hallucis brevis, flexor digitorum brevis, and the first lumbrical mucsles.[3]
- After branching off of the tibial nerve, the MPN travels under the flexor retinaculum and deep to the abductor hallucis muscle.
- It runs along the plantar surface of the flexor digitorum longus, passes through the knot of Henry, and continues along the medial border of the foot.[3]
- The MPN can become compressed by the abductor hallucis fascia, within the abductor hallucis muscle belly or at the knot of Henry (the junction of the flexor digitorum longus tendon and the flexor hallucis longus tendon).[12]
- Orthotics that have a built-up medial arch support cause external compression of the nerve resulting in this clinical entity.

17.5.2 Symptoms

- Patients present with exercise-induced pain localized to the medial plantar arch and foot.
- It is often described as a deep ache or shooting pain into the medial three toes.[3]
- It typically occurs in long-distance runners with hindfoot valgus and may be connected to a new pair of orthotics or shoes.[1]

17.5.3 Diagnostics

- Physical examination includes an assessment of the patient's weight-bearing hindfoot alignment as well as observation of potential areas of compression within their shoes or as the patient stands on their orthotics.[1]
- Percussion of the MPN can reveal a positive Tinel's sign.
- Plain radiographs may be used to rule out underlying bony abnormalities and assess for alignment deformities.
- MRI can be used to evaluate for potential underlying space-occupying lesions.[12]

17.5.4 Conservative Management

- Nonoperative management includes activity modification, discontinuation of orthotics causing external compression, and the use of anti-inflammatory medications.[1]

17.5.5 Surgical Intervention

- Operative treatment of MPN entrapment that has failed conservative management involves surgical release of the nerve.

- A 7- to 8-cm longitudinal incision is made inferior to the talonavicular joint and dissection is performed through the subcutaneous tissue to expose the superficial abductor fascia.
- The superficial fascia is released followed by release of the deep fascia to the level of the knot of Henry.[3]

17.6 Anterior Tarsal Tunnel Syndrome

Anterior tarsal tunnel syndrome occurs with entrapment of the deep peroneal nerve (DPN) under the inferior extensor retinaculum.

17.6.1 Etiology and Pathophysiology

- The DPN is located between the extensor hallucis longus and extensor digitorum longus muscles as it crosses under the superior extensor retinaculum 3 to 5 cm proximal to the ankle joint.
- The DPN then travels beneath the **Y**-shaped oblique superior band of the inferior extensor retinaculum and divides approximately 1 cm proximal to the ankle joint.
- The lateral branch provides motor innervation to the extensor digitorum brevis muscle and sensory to the ankle joint.
- The medial branch continues together with the dorsalis pedis artery under the oblique inferior band of the inferior extensor retinaculum at the level of the talonavicular joint and provides sensation to the first webspace.[1,3]
- Each crossing point under a band of the extensor retinaculum can be a potential site of entrapment.
- Additionally, dorsal osteophytes at the talonavicular joint or in the first or second tarsometatarsal joints can cause compression of the nerve.
- Other causes leading to this syndrome include trauma, such as repetitive ankle sprains causing a neuropraxic injury, and external compression (e.g., jogger's key tightly laced into their running shoe).[3]

17.6.2 Symptoms

- Patients with entrapment of the DPN present with pain in the dorsum of the foot radiating to the first webspace.
- Symptoms may be worsened with certain shoe wear that places increased pressure across the anterior ankle, such as ski boots, or with specific athletic activities, such as sit-ups with the ankles held under a rigid restraint.[3]
- Symptoms can be worse at night because the ankle is in a prolonged plantarflexed position.
- If the patient describes pain occurring with exercise, exertional compartment syndrome should be considered as a possible cause of symptoms.

17.6.3 Diagnostics

- A physical examination should evaluate the entire course of the DPN in an effort to identify the site of compression.
- Plain radiographs are obtained to evaluate for the presence of osteophytes around the midfoot.[13]
- Electrodiagnostic studies can be helpful in differentiating distal lesions from proximal compression or peripheral neuropathy.[14]
- A local nerve block can also be used as a diagnostic tool to confirm a specific site of compression.[3]

17.6.4 Conservative Management

- Nonoperative treatments include anti-inflammatory medication, shoe wear modification to minimize external compression, and activity modification to avoid exacerbating symptoms.

- If ankle laxity and repetitive sprains are a contributing feature, ankle braces and physical therapy may be beneficial.
- Night splints may be employed to hold the foot in neutral dorsiflexion and decrease the tension on the DPN.[1]

17.6.5 Surgical Intervention

- For patients who fail to improve with conservative measures, surgical release of the DPN may be performed.
- A 5- to 7-cm anterior incision is made to explore the area.
- The specific area of compression is identified preoperatively and the extensor retinacular release is focused to that site to minimize the risk of tendon bowstringing postoperatively.
- Additional contributing causes are addressed based on specific etiology including excision of dorsal talonavicular osteophytes and ankle ligament reconstruction in the setting of instability.[3]
- In a series of 20 patients who underwent surgical release, Dellon reported 80% achieved satisfactory outcomes.[13]

17.7 Superficial Peroneal Nerve Entrapment

Entrapment of the superficial peroneal nerve (SPN) occurs as it exits the deep fascia of the lateral compartment of the leg.

17.7.1 Etiology and Pathophysiology

- The SPN courses through the lateral compartment of the leg, innervating the peroneus longus and peroneus brevis muscles, exits the deep fascia 8 to 12.5 cm proximal to the tip of the lateral malleolus, and then travels subcutaneously across the ankle and provides sensation to the dorsal ankle and foot.[3]
- Entrapment of the nerve can be caused by thickening of the fascial tunnel, herniation of the muscle through the fascial defect as the SPN exits the fascia or by the mass effect of a soft-tissue mass such as a lipoma or ganglion.
- Neuropraxic injuries can also be observed with trauma or repetitive ankle instability.[1]
- Iatrogenic nerve injury can be seen with placement of the anterolateral portal during ankle arthroscopy.

17.7.2 Symptoms

- Patients present with pain localized to the dorsal ankle and foot, which can be burning in nature.
- Associate symptoms include tingling and numbness.
- Pain is typically worse with activities, particularly those that place the foot in maximal inversion and plantar flexion.[1]

17.7.3 Diagnostics

- Physical examination may elicit point tenderness at the site where the SPN exits the deep fascia and a palpable fascial defect may be appreciated.
- Percussion at the defect may be associated with a positive Tinel's sign.[3]
- An MRI can be useful in the setting of a suspected soft mass.
- Electrodiagnostic studies are typically unreliable and do not aid in diagnosis or treatment.[15]
- A local anesthetic injection can also be used to confirm the diagnosis.[1]

17.7.4 Conservative Management

- Initial treatment is directed at preventing repetitive stretching of the SPN during ankle inversion or with instability by utilizing ankle bracing or physical therapy.[1]

- Sources of external compression are eliminated and anti-inflammatories may be used.

17.7.5 Surgical Intervention

- Surgical treatment involves decompression of the SPN by release of the deep fascia in the area where the nerve exits the lateral compartment.
- An approximately 7-cm incision is made over the course of the SPN in the area of maximal symptoms.
- The fascia is incised proximally and distally to the exit point of the nerve.
- Styf and Morberg reported 80% success rate with resolution of symptoms following decompression of the SPN in 17 patients.[15]

17.8 Sural and Saphenous Nerve Entrapment

Entrapment of the sural and saphenous nerves is a rare clinical entity that can occur as a result of trauma or iatrogenic injury.

17.8.1 Etiology and Pathophysiology

- Within the lower leg, the sural nerve courses midline in the posterior calf and then crosses the lateral border of the Achilles tendon approximately 9.8 cm proximal to the calcaneus and runs next to the short saphenous veins as it travels into the lateral aspect of the heel.[9]
- Within the foot, the sural nerve runs inferior to the peroneal tendon sheath and gives off branches providing sensation to the lateral heel and the lateral aspect of the fifth ray.[3]
- The sural nerve can become compressed along the lateral ankle, the lateral aspect of the calcaneus or the fifth metatarsal often secondary to trauma resulting in bony overgrowth, or following surgery with the development of scar tissue.[1]
- The saphenous nerve travels along the medial border of the tibia along with the greater saphenous vein and provides sensation to the medial aspect of the ankle and foot.
- It is most commonly entrapped proximally at the level of the knee as it penetrates the subsartorial fascia, just proximal to the medial femoral condyle but within the ankle.
  - Entrapment can occur secondary to trauma or surgical procedures, such as saphenous vein harvesting for coronary bypass.[3]

17.8.2 Symptoms

- Patients may present with burning pain or dysesthesias in the sensory distribution of the effected nerve.
- For the sural nerve, that includes pain in the posterolateral leg, lateral ankle, and lateral foot.
- For the saphenous nerve, pain can present in the medial ankle and foot.[1]

17.8.3 Diagnostics

- The diagnosis of sural or saphenous nerve entrapment is typically made clinically through the history and physical examination.
- A careful history is taken looking for past direct trauma along the course of the nerve or a history of surgical procedures.[3]
- A physical examination is performed palpating along the course of nerve to evaluate for any specific sites of tenderness or tenderness over previous surgical incisions.
- Plain radiographs and MRI can be obtained to evaluate for bony or soft-tissue mass compression.
- Similar to other nerve entrapments, electrodiagnostic studies are used to rule out more proximal impingement or underlying peripheral neuropathy.[1]

17.8.4 Conservative Management

- If symptoms are exacerbated by specific motions, activity modification may be recommended.
- Anti-inflammatories and topical analgesic medications can provide relief particularly if the nerve entrapment is in a superficial location.
- For sural nerve pain generated by chronic lateral ankle instability, bracing and physical therapy may alleviate symptoms.[3]

17.8.5 Surgical Intervention

- Surgical treatment involves local decompression and neurolysis of the nerve at the site of entrapment.
- If pain persists following neurolysis, neurectomy with transection of the nerve and burial into adjacent muscle or bone may be performed with the understanding that this leads to permanent sensory deficits.[1]

17.9 Key Testing Facts

Interdigital neuroma	• Entrapment neuropathy of the common digital nerve. • The pathophysiology is incompletely understood and it is believed to be caused by increased pressure between the metatarsal heads with tethering of the nerve as it travels beneath the transverse intermetatarsal ligament. • It is most commonly seen in the third webspace, unilateral, and in women. • Patients report burning and tingling pain in the plantar aspect of the forefoot in the affected webspace.
Recurrent interdigital neuroma	• It occurs as the result of incomplete resection of a primary IDN or the formation of a painful bulbous neural stump. • Patients present with localized plantar tenderness, and palpation of the affected area can reproduce electriclike symptoms. • Conservative treatment is similar to primary neuromas and includes shoe wear modification. • Surgical treatment involves revision excision of the neuroma, often through a plantar approach, with transposition of the stump into the adjacent muscle tissue.
Tarsal tunnel syndrome	• Entrapment neuropathy of the tibial nerve as it passes posterior and inferior to the medial malleolus. • Causes of tarsal tunnel syndrome vary and include trauma, space-occupying lesions, and hindfoot malalignment. • Space-occupying lesions should be addressed surgically while neuropraxic, alignment, and idiopathic cases can be managed initially with conservative measures including medications and bracing.
Baxter's neuritis	• Entrapment of the first branch of the LPN. • Patients present with chronic plantar medial heel pain that radiates proximally to the medial ankle and distally to the plantar lateral foot. • Surgical treatment involves neurolysis of the LPN including release of the superficial and deep abductor hallucis muscle fascia.
Jogger's foot	• Entrapment of the MPN often from external compression from orthotics. • Patients present with exercise-induced pain in the medial longitudinal arch radiating to the medial three toes. • Conservative management is often successful and includes relieving the compression by avoiding orthotics. • Surgical treatment of the MPN involves release of the superficial and deep fascia of the abductor hallucis muscle.

Anterior tarsal tunnel syndrome	• Entrapment of the DPN under the inferior extensor retinaculum. • Causes include external compression from tightly laced shoes and impingement from dorsal talonavicular osteophytes. • Patients present with dorsal foot pain radiating to the first webspace. • Conservative management includes anti-inflammatory medication, bracing, night splints, and shoe wear modification. • Surgical release includes incising the extensor retinaculum at the site of compression as well as excising osteophytes and addressing laxity as needed.
Superficial nerve entrapment	• Entrapment of the SPN occurs as it exits the deep fascia of the lateral compartment. • Patients present with pain, numbness, and tingling to the dorsal ankle and foot, which is exacerbated by ankle plantar flexion and inversion. • Conservative management includes anti-inflammatories, bracing, and physical therapy. • Surgical treatment involves decompression of the SPN by a local fasciotomy.
Sural and saphenous nerve entrapment	• Sural and saphenous nerve entrapments are rare clinical entities and can be caused by direct trauma or iatrogenic injury during a surgical procedure. • Patients present with pain along the sensory distribution of the effected nerves. • Conservative management includes topical analgesic medication, while surgical treatment focuses on local neurolysis versus neurectomy.

References

[1] Pomeroy G, Wilton J, Anthony S. Entrapment neuropathy about the foot and ankle: an update. J Am Acad Orthop Surg. 2015; 23(1):58–66

[2] Weinfeld SB, Myerson MS. Interdigital neuritis: diagnosis and treatment. J Am Acad Orthop Surg. 1996; 4(6):328–335

[3] Schon LC, Reed MA. Disorders of the nerves. In: Coughlin MJ, Saltzman CL, Anderson RB, eds. Mann's Surgery of the Foot and Ankle. 9th ed. Philadelphia, PA: Saunders; 2014:621–682

[4] Levitsky KA, Alman BA, Jevsevar DS, Morehead J. Digital nerves of the foot: anatomic variations and implications regarding the pathogenesis of interdigital neuroma. Foot Ankle. 1993; 14(4): 208–214

[5] Giannini S, Bacchini P, Ceccarelli F, Vannini F. Interdigital neuroma: clinical examination and histopathologic results in 63 cases treated with excision. Foot Ankle Int. 2004; 25(2):79–84

[6] Womack JW, Richardson DR, Murphy GA, Richardson EG, Ishikawa SN. Long-term evaluation of interdigital neuroma treated by surgical excision. Foot Ankle Int. 2008; 29(6):574–577

[7] Bucknall V, Rutherford D, MacDonald D, Shalaby H, McKinley J, Breusch SJ. Outcomes following excision of Morton's interdigital neuroma: a prospective study. Bone Joint J. 2016; 98-B(10): 1376–1381

[8] Cimino WR. Tarsal tunnel syndrome: review of the literature. Foot Ankle. 1990; 11(1):47–52

[9] Webb J, Moorjani N, Radford M. Anatomy of the sural nerve and its relation to the Achilles tendon. Foot Ankle Int. 2000; 21(6):475–477

[10] Schon LC, Glennon TP, Baxter DE. Heel pain syndrome: electrodiagnostic support for nerve entrapment. Foot Ankle. 1993; 14(3):129–135

[11] Sinnaeve F, Vandeputte G. Clinical outcome of surgical intervention for recalcitrant infero-medial heel pain. Acta Orthop Belg. 2008; 74(4):483–488

[12] Donovan A, Rosenberg ZS, Cavalcanti CF. MR imaging of entrapment neuropathies of the lower extremity. Part 2. The knee, leg, ankle, and foot. Radiographics. 2010; 30(4):1001–1019

[13] Dellon AL. Deep peroneal nerve entrapment on the dorsum of the foot. Foot Ankle. 1990; 11(2):73–80

[14] Akyüz G, Us O, Türan B, Kayhan O, Canbulat N, Yilmar IT. Anterior tarsal tunnel syndrome. Electromyogr Clin Neurophysiol. 2000; 40(2): 123–128

[15] Styf J, Morberg P. The superficial peroneal tunnel syndrome. Results of treatment by decompression. J Bone Joint Surg Br. 1997; 79(5):801–803

18 Diabetes and Charcot

D. Anthony Barcel and Carroll P. Jones

Abstract

Charcot arthropathy is a progressive, destructive, noninfectious bone and joint disease that occurs in patients with peripheral neuropathy. Early recognition and treatment are the key for a successful outcome. The goal is to obtain and maintain a plantigrade foot. Early treatment consists of casting and protected weight bearing. In the long term, bracing and/or shoe wear modification are recommended. If left untreated, progressive deformity, ulceration, and deep infection may occur. Surgery is reserved for cases that are not treatable in a cast or brace, develop recurrent ulceration, and/or present with active infection. Aggressive bone resection for deformity correction and arthrodesis are important surgical principles for Charcot reconstruction. Optimizing nutrition, blood sugar control, and patient compliance are critical for successful outcomes. Even with the right techniques and postoperative protocols, limb salvage may only be successful 75% of the time.

Keywords: Charcot, neuroarthropathy, diabetic neuropathy, Charcot foot, Charcot ankle

18.1 Introduction

- Charcot neuroarthropathy was originally described by Jean-Martin Charcot in 1868 in patients with tertiary syphilis.[1]
- Charcot arthropathy is characterized by a noninfectious, osteolytic process caused by neurovascular and isolated or repetitive neurotraumatic injury leading to bone and joint destruction, which may result in deformity, dislocation, and ultimately ulceration and deep infection.[2]
- It is an uncommon, potentially debilitating condition that has been shown to have an adverse effect on health-related quality of life, particularly in diabetic patients.[2]
- Charcot is most common in the lower extremities because of weight-bearing forces. In the lower extremities, it is most common in the foot/ankle. The midfoot is the most commonly affected area, accounting for 50% of cases in the foot/ankle.
- The goal of treatment is to obtain and/or maintain a stable and plantigrade foot from presentation through the consolidation phase of the Charcot process. Ideally, this is accomplished nonoperatively,[2] but some cases will require surgery to achieve these goals.
- Unfortunately, even with appropriate nonoperative treatment, instability and deformity may lead to ulceration, deep infection, and limb loss,[3] and preventative or reactive surgery may be necessary.[4,5,6,7,8]

18.2 Etiology and Pathophysiology

All patients who develop Charcot have some degree of peripheral neuropathy (PN), whether recognized or not. Due to the fact that the most common cause of PN in the United States is diabetes, there is a strong relationship between diabetes and Charcot. The incidence of Charcot in the general diabetic population is approximately 0.3 to 1.4%,[9,10] but has been reported to be as high as 29% in diabetics with a diagnosis of neuropathy.[11]

18.2.1 Pathophysiology

Three main theories exist, and most cases involve a combination of all three: neurotraumatic, neurovascular, and an intense inflammatory-mediated process.

Neurotraumatic

- Acute/subacute fracture or dislocation or repetitive microtrauma occurs in the absence of protective sensation initiating a destructive inflammatory cascade.
- Persistent weight bearing without the use of conscious or reflexive defensive mechanisms such as activity modification, guarding, or offloading promotes further inflammation and further propagates the Charcot process.[2]
- Smaller nerves and muscles of the anterior compartment are affected earlier in the development of PN leading to variable denervation of the leg compartments. As a result, there may be both static and dynamic equinus, which causes pathologic overload of the midfoot during the terminal stance phase of gait.[6]
- Ultimately, damage to the joints and osseous structures of the foot will lead to loss of the structural integrity of the foot and fracture; dislocation and deformity may occur.
- The characteristic hypertrophic bone appearance is a result of a recurring destructive and reparative process due to the physiologic response of the affected bones.

Neurovascular

- The neurovascular mechanism is thought to be the result of overactive vasomotor autonomic neuropathy.
- Arteriovenous shunting accelerates local bone catabolism, preferentially stimulating the activity of osteoclasts leading to excessive resorption of bone.[2]
- Weakened bone in this setting results in progressive fracture, deformity, and dislocation.[12]
- Additionally, histologic studies have demonstrated increased osteoclast-to-osteoblast ratio in the presence of multiple cytokines that mediate bone resorption in Charcot arthropathy.[13,14,15]

Inflammatory

- Local inflammation is invariable and a hallmark of the acute phase of Charcot arthropathy. The fact that soft-tissue inflammation may occur before osseous changes are detectable on plain radiographs suggests that this may play an early role in the pathogenesis of Charcot arthropathy.
- Local insult initiates an inflammatory cascade. An increase in expression of the inflammatory cytokines interleukin 6 (IL-6) and IL-1β and tumor necrosis factor alpha (TNFα) has been observed in Charcot arthropathy.[13]
- These cytokines in turn increase the expression of receptor activator of NF-κB ligand (RANKL), which increases the expression of nuclear transcription factor κB (NF-κB).
- NF-κB is key in the maturation of osteoclasts, and with increased osteoclast activity, a resultant osteolysis may occur.[14]
- Osteolysis leads to further fracture, resulting in further inflammation creating a positive feedback loop by which progressive fragmentation and collapse may occur.
- It is not clear by what mechanism this process is terminated, but pain, nerve-derived neuropeptides, and self-limitation of activity leading to decreased blood flow may play a role.[14]

18.3 Clinical Presentation

Presentation may be variable and is often misdiagnosed as cellulitis, infection, or lymphedema. Making the diagnosis begins with a detailed history and physical examination. Delays in diagnosis can negatively affect outcomes and may be associated with excess cost and health care resources.[16]

18.3.1 History

- Patients often present with no clear history of a traumatic event.

- Because of the neuropathy, pain may be absent or minimal.
- One of the most common complaints is foot/ankle swelling, insidious in onset.
- Later in the process, patients may present with a deformity.
- In some cases, diabetes and/or PN has not previously been diagnosed. It is critical to pursue these lines of questioning during the history for any patient who presents with unexplained foot/ankle swelling and/or deformity.
- Patients who present with a noninfected Charcot will lack fever, leukocytosis, and systemic symptoms. Typically, glucose levels are baseline, with no significant change in insulin requirements.

18.3.2 Physical Examination

- Inspect both feet and ankles with socks and shoes off, both seated and in a standing posture. It is important to assess alignment, swelling, and erythema.
- The classic presentation in the acute phase of Charcot is a swollen, warm, and erythematous foot (► Fig. 18.1). The erythema and swelling characteristically *improve* with elevation of the limb above the level of the heart. This helps distinguish it from infection, which characteristically does *not* improve with elevation.
- During inspection, it is important to look for callouses, ulcerations, and any bony prominences that may reflect deformity and/or neuropathy. Erythema in the absence of skin compromise and infectious changes often suggests a neuropathic process.
- Although many patients with Charcot have normal vascularity, pedal pulses should be examined.
- Palpation of the foot may reveal warmth, a common finding in the early stages of Charcot.
- A 5.07 Semmes–Weinstein monofilament is a low-cost, simple, effective way to test for PN (► Fig. 18.2), and an important part of the physical examination.

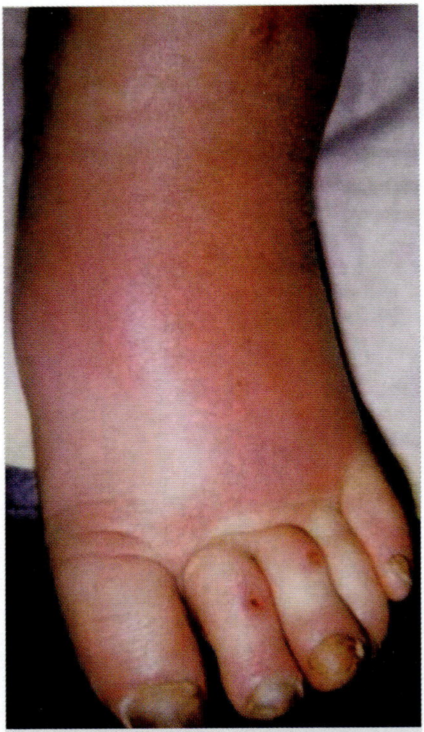

Fig. 18.1 Early in the active stage of the disease process (Eichenholtz stage I), the foot is swollen, warm, and erythematous.

- Assess all tendon/motor function, especially in the setting of deformity.
- Achilles tightness/contracture is common and should be noted.
- Depending on the timing of presentation, the foot and ankle may start to demonstrate improvement of the swelling, warmth, and erythema as the Charcot process progresses through its healing phases.

18.4 Diagnostics and Classification

18.4.1 Diagnosis

- The diagnosis of Charcot neuroarthropathy is primarily based on clinical evaluation

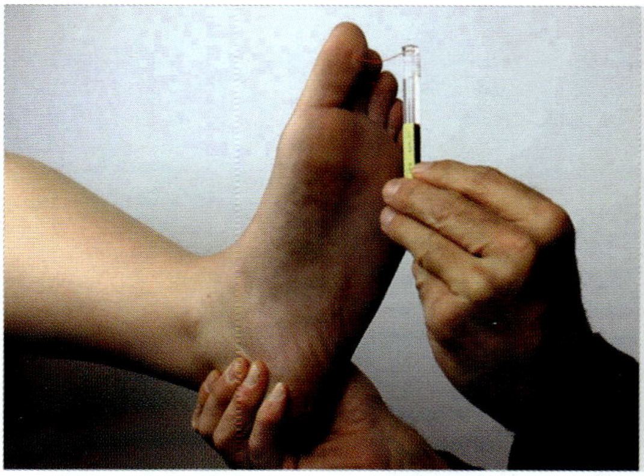

Fig. 18.2 A 5.07 (10 g) Semmes–Weinstein monofilament test is considered positive if a force substantial enough to bend the filament is applied and the patient is unable to detect the stimulus.

(as outlined earlier) and plain films. Laboratory testing is used in most cases as part of the workup but is not usually necessary to make the diagnosis.

18.4.2 Imaging

- All patients should be evaluated with weight-bearing radiographs of the foot and ankle. Serial imaging is particularly helpful for the longitudinal monitoring of structure and alignment of the foot.
- Computed tomography (CT) is rarely helpful in distinguishing Charcot arthropathy from infection or abscess and is not considered a part of the routine imaging workup. However, CT scan can be useful to analyze complex deformity for surgical planning purposes.
- The use of magnetic resonance imaging (MRI) in the early stages of Charcot arthropathy is controversial; it is not a mandatory imaging modality. The high-intensity signal observed in the bone and adjacent soft tissues on MRI of a patient with Charcot arthropathy is difficult to differentiate from the appearance of infection. MRI may be helpful when it demonstrates bony destruction adjacent to a wound/ulcer or sinus tract and may assist in identifying an abscess (consider using contrast if feasible).
- Most cases of Charcot can be diagnosed based on the clinical examination and plain films alone. Improvement with foot elevation, normal infection markers (see below), and absence of an ulcer/wound is highly unlikely to be an infected Charcot. In the cases that are difficult to determine, a three-phase tagged white blood cell (WBC) scan is the most commonly ordered study to evaluate for bone infection.

18.4.3 Additional Tests

- Complete blood count (CBC), erythrocyte sedimentation rate (ESR), and C-reactive protein (CRP; infection markers) are expected to be near normal in the setting of acute Charcot arthropathy, but should still be ordered as part of the workup.
- For diabetic patients, HgbA1C is critical to assess compliance and consistency of blood sugar control. If significantly elevated (> 8.5), surgery may be contraindicated unless there is an operative urgency (i.e., abscess).
- Vitamin D and calcium deficiencies are common and should be tested.

18.4.4 Classification

The two most commonly referenced classification systems are the Eichenholtz and Brodsky classifications. Eichenholtz[17] provided the first classification, which categorized the disease process into three stages (I–III) with stage 0 added later by Shibata et al[18,19] ▶ Fig. 18.3 (▶ Table 18.1). Brodsky[20] later introduced a classification scheme based on anatomic location of the deformity.

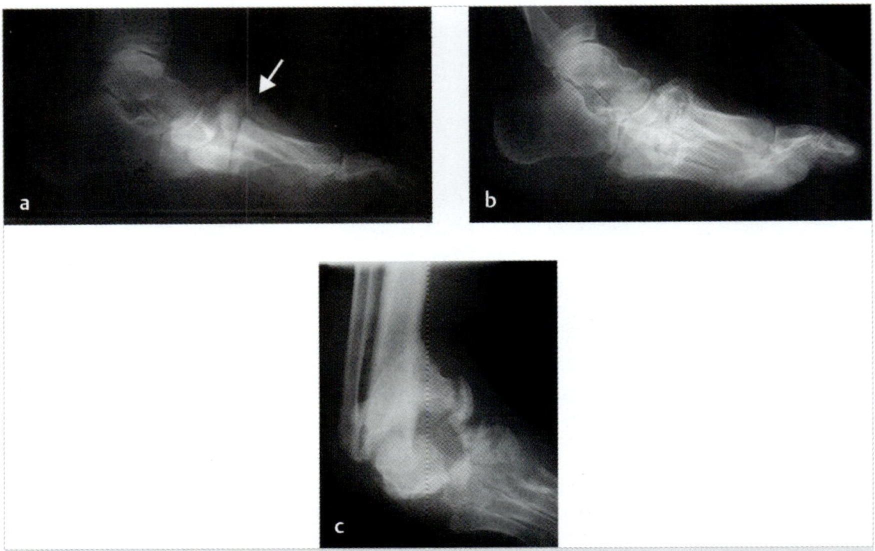

Fig. 18.3 **(a)** Lateral view of Eichenholtz stage I Charcot of the midfoot. Note extensive osteolysis, fracture, and fragmentation through the midfoot. **(b)** Lateral view of Eichenholtz stage II Charcot of the midfoot. Note the coalescence of the bone and resorption of smaller fragments at the tarsometatarsal articulations. **(c)** Anteroposterior view of Eichenholtz stage III Charcot of the ankle in a different patient. Despite the severe residual deformity, the fragmented bone has fully consolidated and matured.

Table 18.1 Modified Eichenholtz classification system and treatment summary

Stage	Symptoms	Radiographic findings	Treatment
0	Warmth, swelling, erythema	None	Immobilization, education, serial radiographs
I	Warmth, swelling, erythema, ± instability	Osteolysis, fragmentation, and joint subluxation/dislocation	TCC, serial radiographs, ± WB
II	Decreasing symptoms	Coalescence of larger fragments, resorption of bony debris	Continued TCC vs. boot or CROW
III	No warmth swelling or erythema ± deformity	Consolidation of large fragments and rounding of bony edges	Plantigrade: custom orthosis with a rocker bottom sole Nonplantigrade: CROW vs. AFO vs. surgical intervention

Abbreviations: AFO, ankle–foot orthosis; CROW, Charcot restraint orthotic walker; TCC, total contact cast; WB, weight bearing.
Source: Adapted from Rosenbaum and DiPreta.[19]

Brodsky Classification

- Type 1: Most common and involves all or portions of the tarsometatarsal and naviculocuneiform joints.
- Type 2: Injury of the transverse tarsal (talonavicular [TN] and calcaneocuboid [CC]), subtalar (ST), or all three joints of the hindfoot (TN, CC, and ST joints).
- Type 3: Involvement of the ankle (3A) and/or calcaneal tuberosity (3B). Type 3B is uncommon but may involve avulsion of the superior tuberosity.
- Type 4: Any combination of the previous three types.
- Type 5: Only the forefoot is involved.

18.5 Conservative Management

Ideally, during the course of treatment, the foot and ankle is protected until the Charcot process reaches stage III, and deformity/ulceration is avoided. Ultimately, the goal of treatment is to obtain and maintain a plantigrade (near normally aligned) foot and ankle.

18.5.1 Eichenholtz Stage 0

- Treatment of prodromal, Eichenholtz stage 0 Charcot osteoarthropathy should consist of protected weight bearing versus total contact casting depending on severity of symptoms. Patient education is paramount to setting expectations and building a relationship to foster compliance and ultimately provide the best outcome. Serial radiographs are recommended to monitor for progression throughout the course of the Charcot event.

18.5.2 Eichenholtz Stage I

- The mainstay of early Eichenholtz stage I treatment is immobilization. There is limited role for surgery in the early active phase (exceptions would include a dislocation with skin compromise).
- Traditionally, total contact casting has been used for immobilization for the first 2 to 4 months. Frequent cast removal (1–2 weeks) and skin examination should be performed until the patient has reached stage II and can be transitioned to a boot or Charcot restraint orthotic walker (CROW).
- Non-weight-bearing (NWB) was previously thought to decrease the risk of collapse and progression. However, there are recent data to support weight-bearing in a cast.[21,22] Authors of this chapter currently prefer NWB if feasible, particularly for more unstable patterns of Charcot.
- If the patient is clinically and radiographically plantigrade, weight bearing in a total contact cast may be entertained until the swelling stabilizes and the Charcot begins to consolidate.

18.5.3 Eichenholtz Stages II and III

- The goal of treatment remains the same, and the focus is on preventing any limb-threatening complications. Once the foot has reached the consolidation phase, the risk of deformity progression decreases, and attention is directed toward accommodating any residual deformity to prevent ulceration.
  - Accommodative custom-molded orthosis with rocker bottom sole modification can be fabricated to address residual midfoot deformity, assuming it is not severe.
  - For more severe midfoot deformity, or Charcot involving the ankle/hindfoot, an ankle–foot orthosis (AFO), double-upright brace, or (CROW) should be considered (► Fig. 18.4). This provides more offloading to the tibia and better coronal plane stability,[23,24] but it does require maintenance/frequent inspection and is cumbersome, making compliance more difficult.

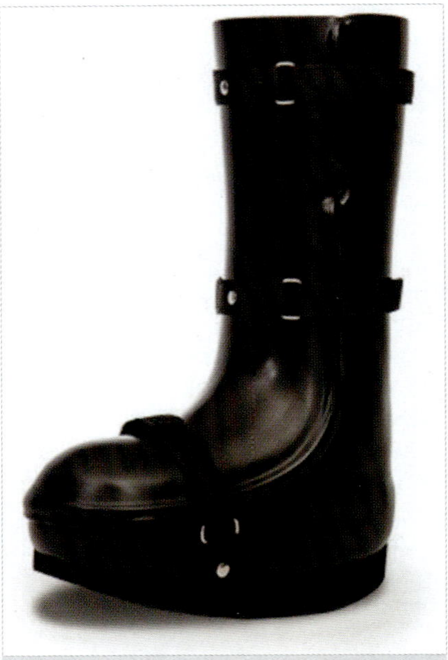

Fig. 18.4 Charcot restraint orthotic walker (CROW).

18.6 Surgical Intervention

18.6.1 General Principles

- Ideally, during the course of treatment, the foot/ankle is protected until the Charcot process reaches stage III, and deformity/ulceration is avoided.
- Ultimately the goal is to obtain and maintain a plantigrade (near normally aligned) foot/ankle.
- As you move from distal to proximal (foot to ankle), the Charcot disease is generally less stable and more likely to require surgery.

Absolute Indications for Surgical Intervention

- A progressive deformity despite appropriate immobilization.
- A deformity that has progressed to the point that it is not brace-able or cannot be accommodated with shoe wear/insert modification.
- A persistent or recurrent ulceration related to Charcot deformity despite offloading attempts.
- A Charcot foot with an established deep infection.

Relative Indications for Surgical Treatment

- A painful deformity related to mechanical instability—typically an unstable midfoot Charcot that fails to consolidate.
- A severe deformity with high risk of ulceration secondary to malalignment.

18.6.2 Surgical Principles

- Deformity correction, even if severe, can typically be achieved acutely during surgery.
- Correction is primarily achieved through bone resection and arthrodesis.
- Joint-preserving osteotomies have a limited role in Charcot reconstruction.
- Shortening the foot or extremity is acceptable for these limb salvage procedures.
- If a significant deep infection is present, a staged approach may be preferable (stage I: debridement/ spacer; stage II: formal realignment arthrodesis).
- Adjuvant biologics, particularly for clean cases, are highly recommended.

Preoperative Consideration

- Although usually *not* a problem in Charcot, always check the vascularity of the foot (i.e., pedal pulses, arterial Doppler, and arteriogram).
- If there is a concern for deep infection, obtain infection markers (ESR, CRP) and advanced imaging if necessary (i.e., MRI, three-phase tagged WBC scan).

- For suspected infected cases, hold antibiotics 1 to 2 weeks preoperatively if clinically feasible and obtain intraoperative cultures and biopsies to guide postoperative antibiotic treatment.
- Always check the HgbA1C; high levels correlate strongly with surgical complications and failures.[25]

Fixation Principles

- If a deep infection or large ulceration is present, a thin-wire frame is the preferred choice of fixation.
- For "clean" cases, internal fixation and/or external fixation may be utilized.
- Midfoot Charcot: Medial and lateral column "beaming" is evolving to be the gold standard for internal fixation.
- Hindfoot Charcot: Fixation is similar to the midfoot, often with the addition of an ST arthrodesis screw.
- Ankle Charcot: A hindfoot fusion nail is the most common construct utilized if the case is considered "clean."

Technique: Midfoot

- The midfoot is the most common location for Charcot—most often a "rocker-sole" deformity (abducted dorsiflexed midfoot, apex plantar).
- Achilles lengthening is routinely performed, usually percutaneously.
- A medial approach to the midfoot from the first metatarsal base to the talus is utilized.
- A biplanar closing wedge osteotomy at the apex of the deformity across the width of the foot is performed to restore plantigrade alignment (▶ Fig. 18.5).
- All joints not resected in the osteotomy along the medial column are individually prepared for arthrodesis (including the TN articulation).
- The lateral column is almost always involved in the Charcot process, and should be addressed by at least resecting and/or preparing the CC joint for fusion through a separate short lateral incision. If the lateral column is entirely uninvolved or near normal, and the

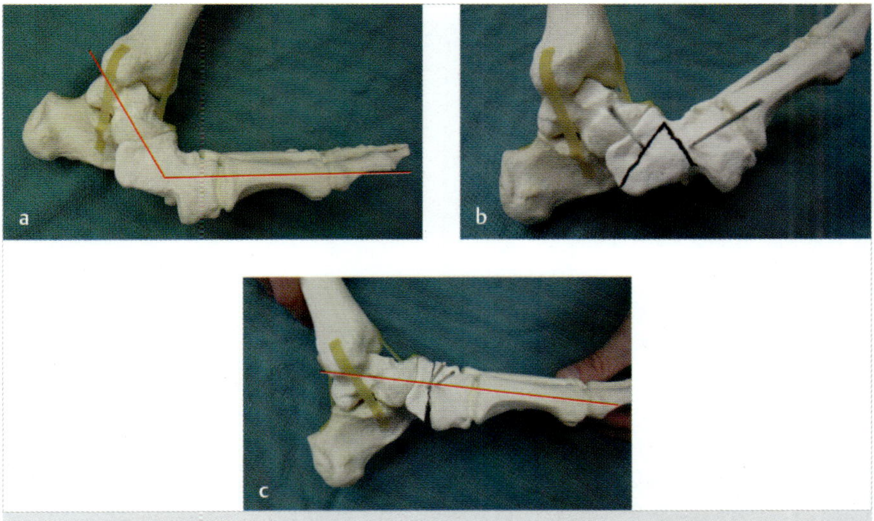

Fig. 18.5 (a) Saw bones model demonstrating rocker bottom deformity with disruption of Meary's lines. **(b)** Biplanar closing wedge osteotomy is drawn through the midfoot at the apex of the deformity. **(c)** Correction of the deformity can be seen following biplanar osteotomy, and Meary's lines are restored.

Charcot deformity is isolated to the medial column, it may be left alone.

- Fixation can be achieved with a plate and/or a combination of beams.
  - It is critical to incorporate the entire medial column (the first metatarsal to the talus) in most cases.
- A retrograde-placed medial column intramedullary rod provides excellent compression and stability, often in combination with central and lateral column beams (▶ Fig. 18.6).
- Alternatively, a thin-wire external fixator may be used if there is concern for deep infection (▶ Fig. 18.7).

Technique: Hindfoot

- Achilles lengthening is routinely performed.
- Assuming the talus is salvageable and the hindfoot is reducible, the goal is a triple arthrodesis with an extended medial column fusion.
- A similar medial approach is utilized, as outlined earlier for midfoot Charcot.
- A lateral incision is used to approach and reduce the ST and CC joints.
- Aggressive soft-tissue releases may be necessary to achieve adequate reduction (i.e., peroneal tendons).
- All joints are prepared for arthrodesis, by either resection or in situ preparation.
- Fixation for the medial and lateral columns is similar to that for midfoot Charcot (see above).
- Large-diameter screw fixation for ST arthrodesis is also employed.
- Irreducible hindfoot Charcot may require a complete talectomy and tibiocalcaneal (TC) arthrodesis.

Technique: Ankle

- Ankle Charcot is most likely to require surgery due to coronal plane instability (varus/valgus) and resultant associated soft-tissue pressures and difficulty bearing weight.
- The goal is to achieve a stable and plantigrade tibiotalocalcaneal (TTC) or TC arthrodesis.

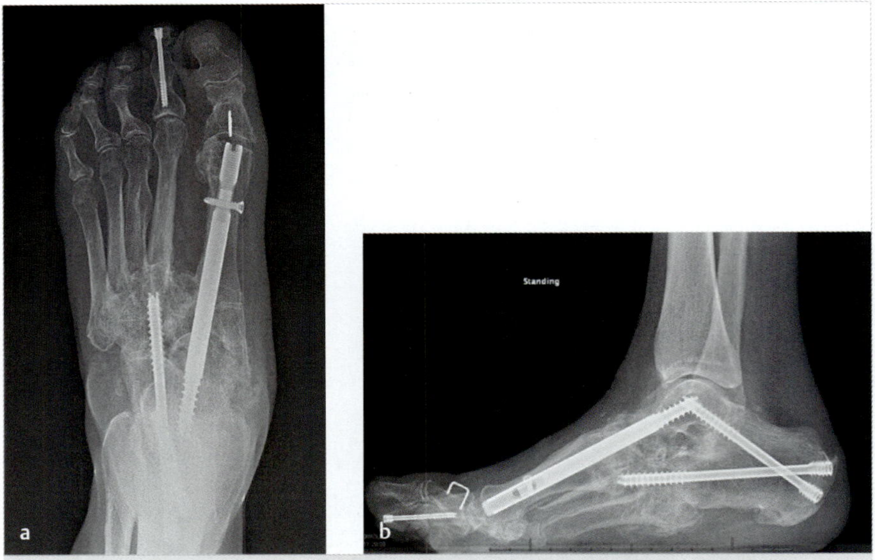

Fig. 18.6 (a) Anteroposterior (AP) and **(b)** lateral views of the foot demonstrating medial column fixation with a retrograde nail, lateral column fixation with an intramedullary beam, and (in this case) with the addition of a subtalar fusion.

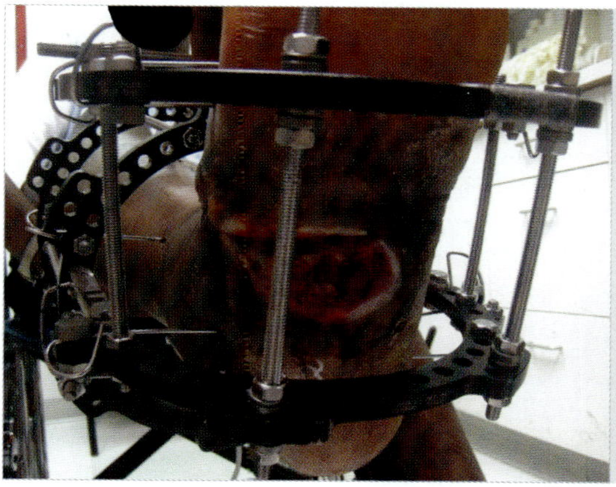

Fig. 18.7 Clinical photograph demonstrating a thin-wire external fixator used in the treatment of midfoot Charcot with ulceration and concern for deep infection.

- A transfibular approach is almost always utilized.
- The distal fibula is cut and resected to provide access to the lateral aspect of the ankle and ST joints.
- If the fibular bone is clean, it may be morselized for autograft.
- The surgeon may choose either an in situ preparation of the ankle joint or flat-cut resection of the distal tibia and dorsal talus (the latter may be necessary for more severe deformities with bone loss).
- Additionally, the ST joint is typically prepared for arthrodesis.
- If the talus is not viable or salvageable, it may be resected and a TC arthrodesis is performed.
- For clean cases, a hindfoot fusion nail is typically utilized for fixation (a plate is a reasonable option as well).
- Cases with suspected infection are treated with a thin-wire circular fixator.

18.6.3 Postoperative Care

- Cases treated with internal fixation are placed in a splint for 1 to 2 weeks followed by a short-leg cast until 10 to 12 weeks post-op.
- External fixators are generally left on for 3 months.
- Patients are kept NWB for 10 to 12 weeks, although earlier weight bearing may be permitted for patients in thin-wire fixators.

Postoperative Considerations

- Vitamin D and calcium supplementation is strongly recommended.
- The use of an external bone stimulator should be considered as well.

18.7 Rehabilitation

- Rehabilitation has a limited role for the affected Charcot foot/ankle.
- Once the patient has recovered, whether operative or nonoperative, rehabilitation is recommended for generalized strengthening and gait training.
- Blood sugar control, appropriate nutrition, and weight loss are very important for short- and long-term Charcot outcomes and the general health of the patient.

18.8 Key Testing Facts

Charcot's arthropathy	• Osteolytic/destructive process primarily seen in patients with diabetes and neuropathy that may lead to deformity, ulceration, and infection. • Morbid condition placing patients at risk of amputation. • Neurotraumatic, neurovascular, and inflammatory-mediated process.
Diagnosis	• Patients may complain of warmth, swelling, and erythema, which is often nontraumatic, and at later stages may present with complaints of deformity. • Erythema is dependent on gravity on examination, which may help distinguish from infection. • Plain radiographs are typically all that is necessary to make a diagnosis. • Advanced imaging such as MRI and three-phase tagged WBC scan along with laboratory studies and detailed physical examination may be used to help distinguish from infection. • Eichenholtz's and Brodsky's classification schemes are most commonly used.
Nonoperative treatment	• The primary goal of all treatment is to obtain a plantigrade and ulcer-free foot. • Total contact casting is the gold standard in the early stages of Charcot. • Transition to an accommodative custom orthosis with rocker bottom sole in Eichenholtz stages II and III with minimal residual deformity. • AFO or CROW boot may be used in later stages for more significant residual deformity.
Surgical treatment	• Performed in patients with progressive or nonbraceable deformity, or with recurrent or recalcitrant ulceration, or in those with established deep bone infection. • Mainstay of surgical treatment is bone resection and arthrodesis to correct alignment and reduce pressure on the skin. • Plates and screws, intramedullary beaming, and thin-wire frames may all be utilized when ulceration/infection is not present. Generally, thin-wire frames are used when there is ulceration or infection. • For ankle and hindfoot Charcot, tibiotalocalcaneal or tibiocalcaneal arthrodesis may be performed and may use intramedullary nail fixation when appropriate.
Aftercare	• Rehabilitation including strengthening and gait training are generally recommended. • Blood sugar control, appropriate nutrition, and weight loss are key to a successful outcome.

References

[1] Charcot J. Lecons sur les maladies du systeme nerveux. Archives de Physiologie. 1868

[2] Pinzur MS. Current concepts review: Charcot arthropathy of the foot and ankle. Foot Ankle Int. 2007; 28(8):952–959

[3] Saltzman CL, Hagy ML, Zimmerman B, Estin M, Cooper R. How effective is intensive nonoperative initial treatment of patients with diabetes and Charcot arthropathy of the feet? Clin Orthop Relat Res. 2005(435):185–190

[4] Jones CP. Beaming for Charcot foot reconstruction. Foot Ankle Int. 2015; 36(7):853–859

[5] Jones C, McCormick JJ, Pinzur MS. Surgical management of Charcot arthropathy. Instr Course Lect. 2018; 67:255–267

[6] Pinzur M. Surgical stabilization of nonplantigrade Charcot arthropathy of the midfoot. In: Easley M, Weisel SW, eds. Operative Techniques in Foot and Ankle Surgery. 2nd ed. Philadelphia, PA: Wolters Kluwer; 2017:400–409

[7] Pinzur MS, Schiff AP. Deformity and clinical outcomes following operative correction of Charcot

foot: a new classification with implications for treatment. Foot Ankle Int. 2018; 39(3):265–270

[8] Ford SE, Cohen BE, Davis WH, Jones CP. Clinical outcomes and complications of midfoot Charcot reconstruction with intramedullary beaming. Foot Ankle Int. 2019; 40(1):18–23

[9] Fabrin J, Larsen K, Holstein PE. Long-term follow-up in diabetic Charcot feet with spontaneous onset. Diabetes Care. 2000; 23(6):796–800

[10] Smith DG, Barnes BC, Sands AK, Boyko EJ, Ahroni JH. Prevalence of radiographic foot abnormalities in patients with diabetes. Foot Ankle Int. 1997; 18 (6):342–346

[11] Cofield RH, Morrison MJ, Beabout JW. Diabetic neuroarthropathy in the foot: patient characteristics and patterns of radiographic change. Foot Ankle. 1983; 4(1):15–22

[12] Herbst SA, Jones KB, Saltzman CL. Pattern of diabetic neuropathic arthropathy associated with the peripheral bone mineral density. J Bone Joint Surg Br. 2004; 86(3):378–383

[13] Baumhauer JF, O'Keefe RJ, Schon LC, Pinzur MS. Cytokine-induced osteoclastic bone resorption in Charcot arthropathy: an immunohistochemical study. Foot Ankle Int. 2006; 27(10):797–800

[14] Jeffcoate WJ, Game F, Cavanagh PR. The role of proinflammatory cytokines in the cause of neuropathic osteoarthropathy (acute Charcot foot) in diabetes. Lancet. 2005; 366(9502):2058–2061

[15] Ndip A, Williams A, Jude EB, et al. The RANKL/RANK/OPG signaling pathway mediates medial arterial calcification in diabetic Charcot neuroarthropathy. Diabetes. 2011; 60(8):2187–2196

[16] Labovitz JM, Shapiro JM, Satterfield VK, Smith NT. excess cost and healthcare resources associated with delayed diagnosis of Charcot foot. J Foot Ankle Surg. 2018; 57(5):952–956

[17] Eichenholtz S. Charcot Joints. Springfield, IL: Charles C. Thomas; 1966

[18] Shibata T, Tada K, Hashizume C. The results of arthrodesis of the ankle for leprotic neuroarthropathy. J Bone Joint Surg Am. 1990; 72(5):749–756

[19] Rosenbaum AJ, DiPreta JA. Classifications in brief: Eichenholtz classification of Charcot arthropathy. Clin Orthop Relat Res. 2015; 473(3):1168–1171

[20] Brodsky J. The diabetic foot. In: Coughlin MJ, Mann RA, Saltzmann CL, ed. Surgery of the Foot and Ankle. Philadelphia, PA: Mosby Elsevier; 2007:1341

[21] Pinzur MS, Lio T, Posner M. Treatment of Eichenholtz stage I Charcot foot arthropathy with a weightbearing total contact cast. Foot Ankle Int. 2006; 27(5):324–329

[22] de Souza LJ. Charcot arthropathy and immobilization in a weight-bearing total contact cast. J Bone Joint Surg Am. 2008; 90(4):754–759

[23] Mehta JA, Brown C, Sargeant N. Charcot restraint orthotic walker. Foot Ankle Int. 1998; 19(9): 619–623

[24] Pinzur M. Surgical versus accommodative treatment for Charcot arthropathy of the midfoot. Foot Ankle Int. 2004; 25(8):545–549

[25] Wukich DK, Crim BE, Frykberg RG, Rosario BL. Neuropathy and poorly controlled diabetes increase the rate of surgical site infection after foot and ankle surgery. J Bone Joint Surg Am. 2014; 96 (10):832–839

19 Foot and Ankle Amputations

Michael S. Pinzur and Adam P. Schiff

Abstract

Foot and ankle amputations are among the most common amputations performed. A well-done and appropriately indicated amputation can help restore function and quality of life. Foot and ankle amputations are performed for gangrene, infection, trauma, tumor, and congenital anomaly. Whatever the etiology, the goals of modern amputation surgery are to remove all nonviable and infected tissue, followed by creation of a functional terminal organ of weight bearing.

Keywords: foot amputation, ankle amputation, transtibial amputation, diabetes

19.1 Terminal Organ of Weight Bearing

- The foot is composed of 28 bones and a durable soft-tissue envelope that, combined, function as a terminal organ of weight bearing.
- The foot serves as a "shock absorber" at heel strike, that is, initial loading. This is accomplished by positioning the ankle in dorsiflexion and the hindfoot in the unlocked position of supination to allow dampening of the impact associated with loading.
- Transition of the hindfoot from supination to pronation during terminal stance phase "locks" the hindfoot in a stable position to become a stable platform to facilitate knee extension against a stable foot to achieve forward propulsion.
- One must take into account the functional loss that occurs with each prospective amputation level, in order to determine the most functional amputation level for an individual patient.[1]

19.2 Initial Wound Management

- Traumatic amputation is generally associated with some element of crushing injury. Following the principles of "damage control" orthopaedics, the first step of treatment is debridement of all nonviable tissue.
- Determination of the extent of tissue damage at the time of injury is virtually impossible within the "zone of injury," so most traumatic wounds are initially managed with open wound treatment or negative pressure wound care.
- The extent of tissue viability within the zone of injury generally becomes apparent within 7 to 10 days, when staged wound closure and definitive amputation can be accomplished.
- A similar staged approach is often the best option in diabetic foot infection or infected gangrene. Akin to "damage control," the first step is the removal of all infected and nonviable tissue. Tissue cultures obtained at the initial debridement direct antibiotic therapy.
- Open wounds are best managed with negative pressure wound therapy. Immobilization can be accomplished with a splint or external fixator.
- Determination of the ultimate level of amputation is deferred until the zone of tissue injury is clearly defined. This often requires 7 to 10 days, even in healthy individuals.
- The clinical characteristics of a viable soft-tissue flap are normal tissue turgor, warm skin, and hair growth.

19.3 Determination of Amputation Levels

- The decision-making process to determine amputation and amputation level will be based on the inciting etiology and an assessment of key wound healing parameters.

- The first wound healing consideration is the availability of a bony platform for weight bearing and a functional soft-tissue envelope.
- The key wound healing parameters to be considered next are vascular inflow, tissue nutrition, and immunocompetence.
- The ultrasound Doppler ankle brachial index (ABI) is the most reliable measure of vascular inflow for amputation levels within the foot. The ABI is determined by a ratio of the ultrasound Doppler pressure of either the dorsalis pedis artery at the ankle or the posterior tibialis artery behind the medial malleolus to the brachial arterial pressure.
  - Greater than 0.5 suggests adequate vascular inflow to support wound healing.
  - Calcification of the dorsalis pedis and posterior tibial arterials makes the ABI unmeasurable in approximately 15% of diabetic patients.[2]
  - The best alternative measure in such patients is the ultrasound Doppler toe pressure, where the key threshold value is 30 mm Hg.
  - Other methods, including transcutaneous oximetry, have shown promise, but are either not readily available, too expensive, or too resource intensive.[3,4]
- A serum albumin level of 3.0 g/dL suggests adequate tissue nutrition to support wound healing.[5,6,7]
  - Infection or trauma may deplete protein stores.
  - In such patients, infection should be resolved by debridement of infected or nonviable tissue, followed by culture-specific antibiotic therapy and open wound care should be used to allow the zone of injury to become defined.
  - Oral nutritional support can then be initiated to achieve threshold wound healing parameters.[6,8]
  - Renal failure patients with low serum albumin levels are unlikely to improve serum albumin levels and are unlikely to achieve successful partial foot amputations.
- Total lymphocyte count was initially felt to be a predictive measure of immunocompetence, but its reliability has not been supported over time.[5,6,7]
- The next step is a determination of the functional ambulatory potential of the patient.
- The specific surgical amputation level can be determined by the availability of a bony platform and viable soft-tissue envelope.

19.4 Successful Amputation Levels

19.4.1 Hallux Amputation

- A functional hallux (great toe) is essential for normal walking. In the normal foot, the flexor hallucis longus creates stability along the medial column of the foot during terminal stance phase. It is the stability of the medial column of the foot that allows the quadriceps to extend the knee against a stable foot platform during the push-off phase of gait.[6]
- Loss of flexor hallucis longus or brevis function leads to medial column instability and a relatively apropulsive gait. These tendons can be transferred to the distal aspect of the metatarsal to preserve some strength, but will still lead to weakness in ambulation.
- Adequate functional stability can be achieved by retention of the proximal metaphysis of the proximal phalanx and the insertion of the flexor hallucis brevis.
- The optimal soft-tissue envelope in hallux amputation is accomplished with the so-called terminal Syme's

amputation. The nail and involved bone of the distal phalanx are removed through a dorsal approach.

- If infection or trauma dictates removal of the terminal proximal phalanx, care should be taken to preserve the proximal metaphysis with the attachment of the flexor halluces brevis. The plantar flap can then be loosely reattached to create a stable hallux (▶ Fig. 19.1).[9] Rotational or "fish-mouth" types of flaps are reasonable second choices.
- There is no necessity for orthotic modification to footwear following hallux amputation. Patients with perceived weakness or instability at terminal stance phase of gait can use a carbon graphite "Morton's extension" to substitute for absent flexor hallucis longus.

19.4.2 Lesser Toe Amputation

- There is little functional loss from lesser toe amputations.
- The exception is the second toe, where disarticulation may lead to a severe

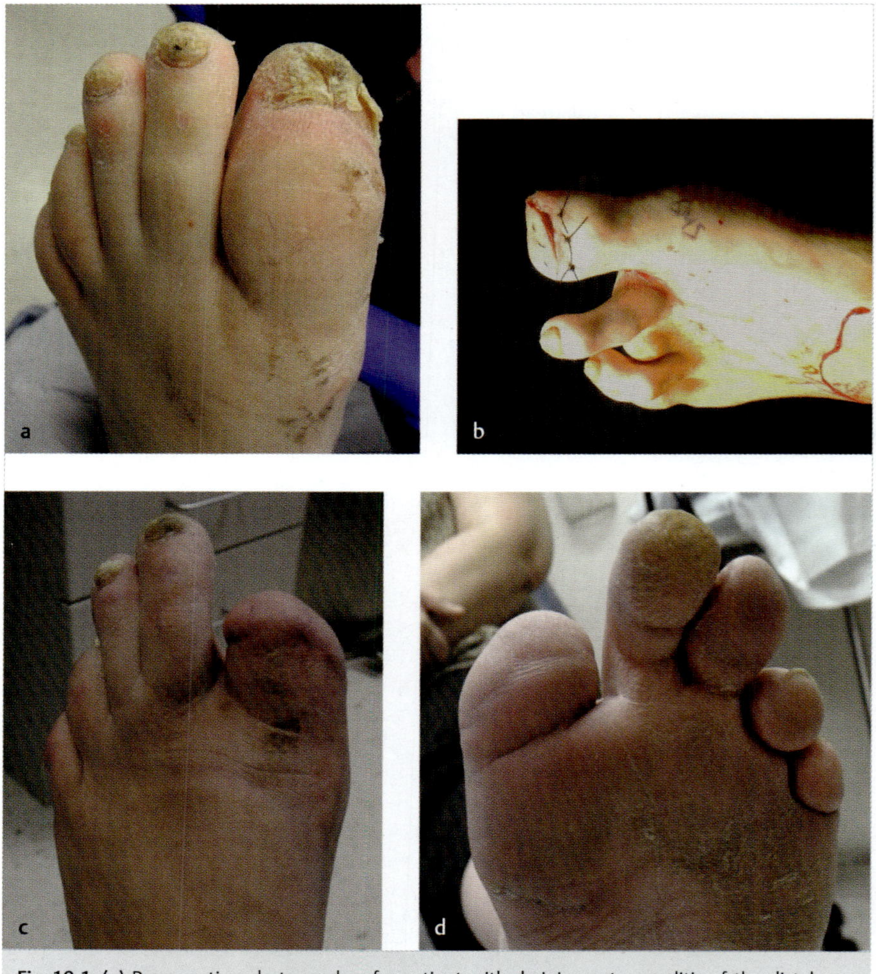

Fig. 19.1 **(a)** Preoperative photographs of a patient with draining osteomyelitis of the distal phalanx. **(b)** Typical long posterior flap for hallux amputation. **(c,d)** Photograph 2 years later.

hallux valgus with prominence of the medial border of the first metatarsal. For this reason, an attempt should be made to retain the proximal metaphysis of the second toe (▶ Fig. 19.2). The second important consideration in lesser toe amputation is maintenance of a nonprominent parabola of the forefoot (▶ Fig. 19.3).

- The local pressure on a retained single prominent toe makes accommodation difficult within a depth-inlay shoe.

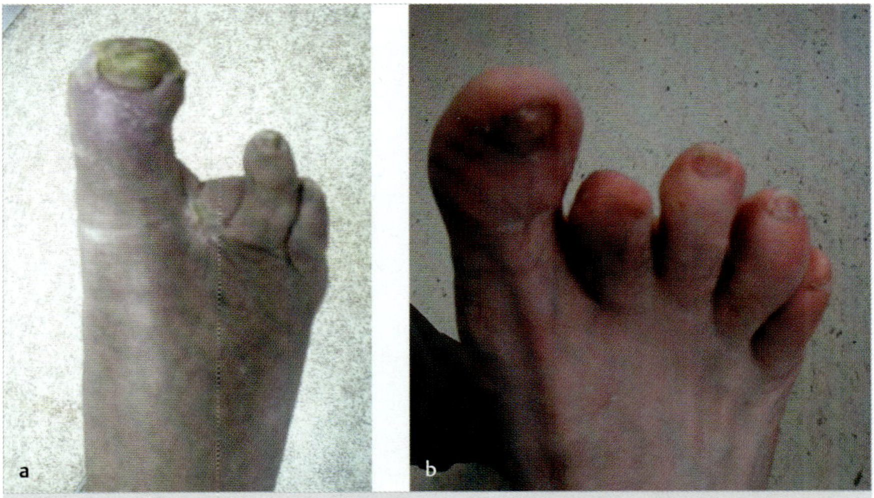

Fig. 19.2 **(a)** This patient underwent second toe amputation for osteomyelitis. He is at increased risk of developing a severe hallux valgus leading to a pressure ulcer when he resumes wearing shoes. **(b)** Late hallux valgus can be avoided by retaining even half of the proximal phalanx of the second toe.

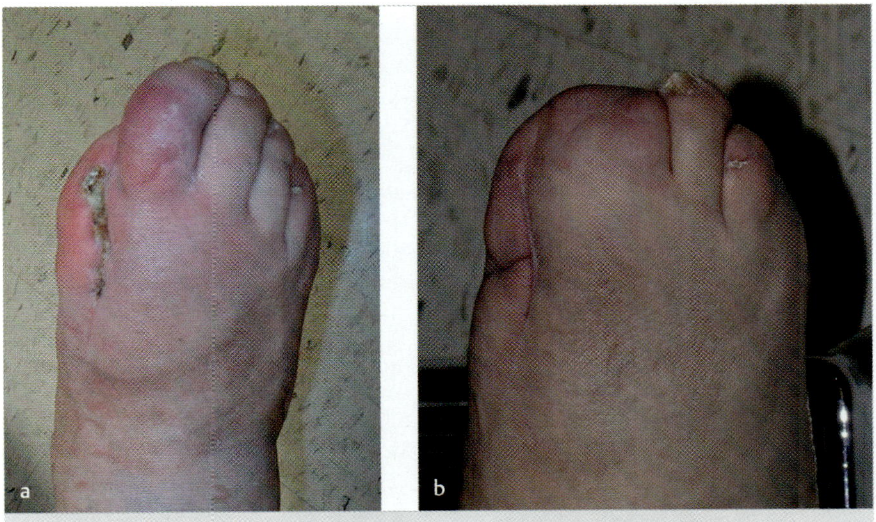

Fig. 19.3 **(a)** The patient on the left recently underwent a first ray resection. The second toe became relatively long and developed a pressure-induced infection. **(b)** A more reasonable parabola allowing easy shoe fit was accomplished following removal of the prominent second toe.

- These patients often benefit from some type of orthotic insole with a "toe filler" to prevent the residual foot from sliding within the shoe.

19.4.3 Ray Resection

- Single outer (first or fifth) ray resection is generally used for osteomyelitis of an involved outer metatarsal. It is rarely indicated in dysvascular disease due to the geographic nature of the disease process.
- The downside deformity associated with first ray resection is instability of the medial column with a resultant apropulsive gait pattern.
- The downside deformity associated with fifth ray resection is the late development of a severe varus deformity secondary to muscle imbalance following disengagement of the peroneus brevis. Care should be taken to retain the base of the fifth metatarsal with the attachment of the peroneus brevis during fifth ray resection. Oblique osteotomy of the metatarsal will allow maintenance of a smooth lateral border of the residual foot. If the base of the 5th metatarsal needs to be resected, one should transfer the brevis to the cuboid.
- Surgery is performed with the so-called tennis racquet incision. Wound management can be accomplished with primary or delayed primary closure, open wound management, or loose approximation of wound edges to allow sufficient drainage during the perioperative period (▶ Fig. 19.4).
- Central ray resections can be accomplished as a primary method of debridement of infection. When used as a definitive treatment, the management of the resultant wound can be complex and may not justify the prolonged time to healing. These patients often benefit with a custom foot orthosis that fills the geographic deficit.[10]

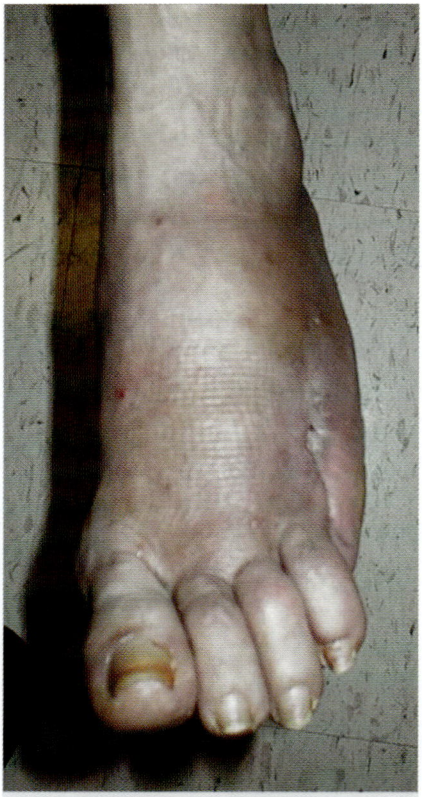

Fig. 19.4 Lateral ray resection leaves minimal deformity if the base of the metatarsal and the attachment of the peroneus brevis are retained.

19.4.4 Midfoot Amputation

- Midfoot amputation can be performed at the transmetatarsal or tarsometatarsal levels.
- Both levels leave the patient with limited propulsion during terminal stance phase of gait due to the very short lever arm of the residual foot.
- The most durable soft-tissue envelope is accomplished with a plantar-based flap. This flap will generally require performing the bony transection at the level of the proximal metaphysis of each of the metatarsals (▶ Fig. 19.5).
- A longer lever arm can be accomplished by performing the bony transection

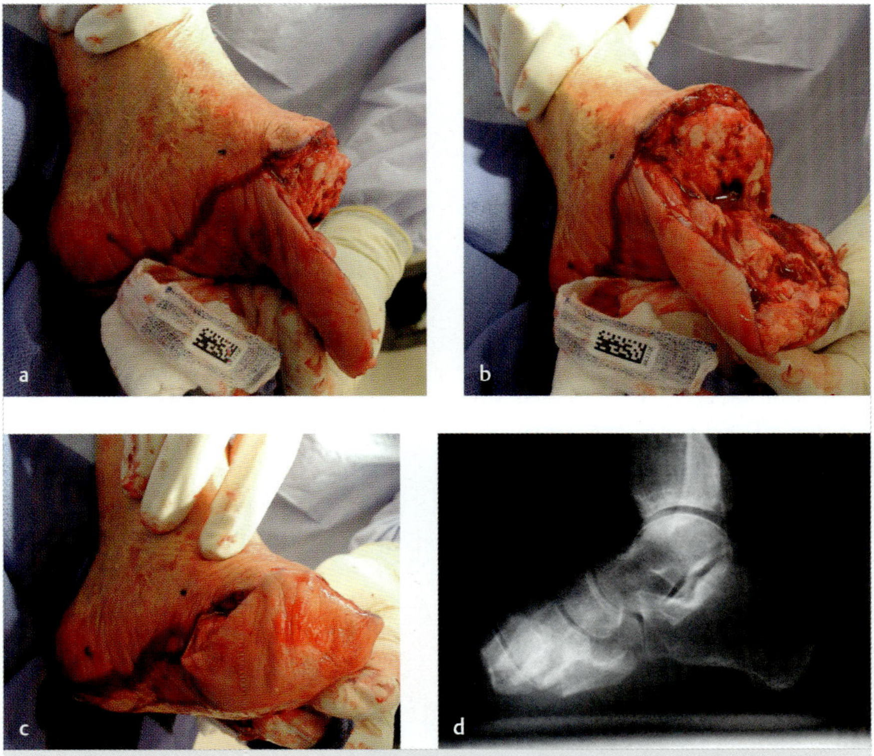

Fig. 19.5 (a,b) Long plantar flap used in transmetatarsal amputation. **(c)** Flap prior to closure. **(d)** Radiograph representing platform for weight bearing.

through the distal metatarsal shafts. The down side tradeoffs to achieve this improved lever arm for push-off is the necessity to use less durable "fish-mouth" dorsoplantar flaps and the risk of late plantar pressure ulcers under the residual metatarsal shafts.

- Surgery should almost always include either a percutaneous Achilles tendon lengthening or gastrocnemius muscle lengthening to balance the loss the foot and ankle dorsiflexors.[6,11,12]
- Orthotists argue that a "prosthetic" combining a toe filler with ankle foot orthosis makes this a very functional level. While this is functionally correct, most patients reject using the complex "prosthesis." Postoperative management should include a short-leg cast to avoid heal ulcers secondary to overlengthening of the Achilles tendon with either tendon Achilles lengthening or gastrocnemius muscle lengthening.

19.4.5 Hindfoot Amputation

- Hindfoot amputation is generally performed as a method of accomplishing debridement of infected gangrene of the forefoot.
- Amputation through the transverse tarsal joint, that is, "Chopart's joint," should be avoided due to the high risk of the development of a late equinus deformity even when a section of the Achilles tendon is removed (▸ Fig. 19.6).

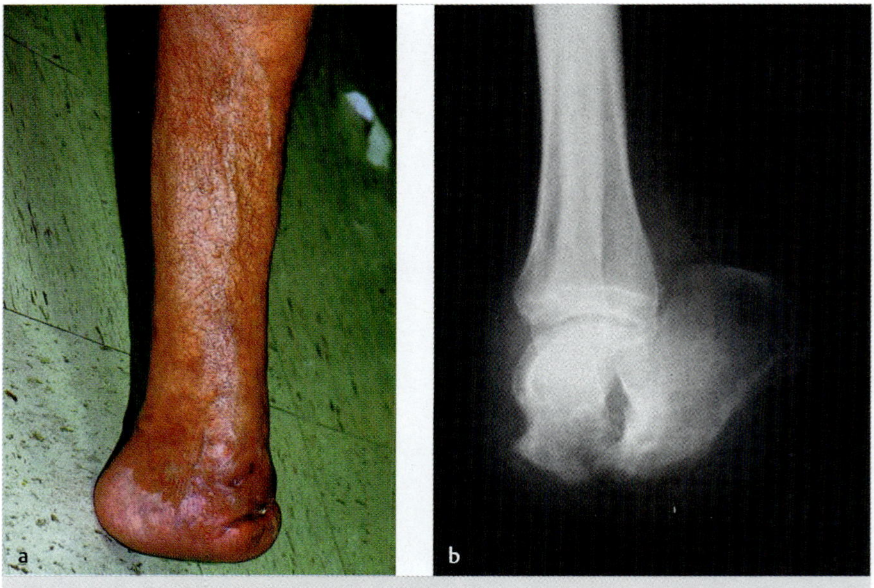

Fig. 19.6 **(a)** Successful hindfoot amputation. Even when a plantigrade residual foot can be achieved, the patient has an inadequate lever arm for propulsion. **(b)** This X-ray was taken 6 weeks after hindfoot amputation combined with resection of 1 cm of the Achilles tendon and cast immobilization for 1 month. Late equinus deformity is too often the end result of hindfoot amputation.

- Even when successful, the patient is left without a forefoot to act as a lever arm during terminal stance, leaving the patient with an apropulsive gait pattern.
- These patients are functionally far better served with Syme's ankle disarticulation, which allows end bearing and space for a dynamic elastic response prosthetic foot.

19.4.6 Syme's Ankle Disarticulation

- Syme's ankle disarticulation is an end-bearing amputation that retains the weight-bearing surface of the distal tibia and the normal soft-tissue envelope of the retained heel pad.
- The metabolic cost of walking is close to age-matched controls, and far less than transtibial amputees. Patients require minimal gait training and rarely require hospitalization in a rehabilitation unit.[7,11,12,13,14]

Technique

- The apices of the fish-mouth incision are placed at the anterior midpoints of the medial and lateral malleoli.
- The incision is taken down to the bone, followed by removal of the talus and calcaneus via sharp dissection.
- Care is taken to protect the posterior tibial artery, which is the primary blood supply of the flap.
- The malleoli are removed flush with the articular surface of the retained tibia and the metaphysical flares of the distal tibia and fibula are removed with a small power saw.
- The heel pad is then secured to the retained tibia with a nonabsorbable suture placed through a drill hole in the anterior corner of the residual tibia (▶ Fig. 19.7).
- Weight bearing with a walking cast with rubber heel can be initiated as early as 2 weeks if the surgical wound appears

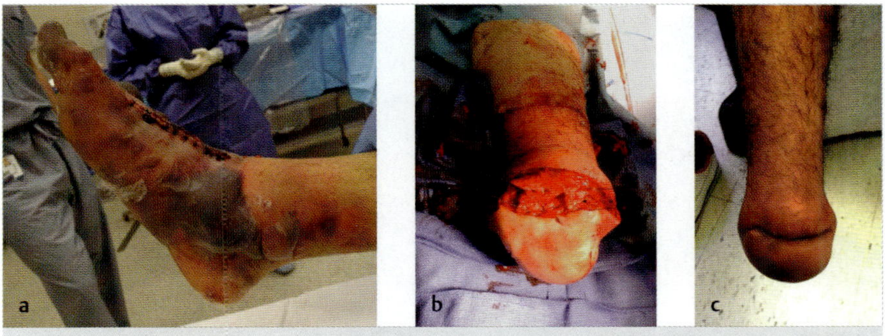

Fig. 19.7 (a) Crush injury with avascular foot. (b) Intraoperative photograph following single-stage Syme's amputation. (c) 1 year later.

secure. Early prosthetic fitting can be accomplished with a preparatory prosthesis as early as 2 weeks following surgery.

19.4.7 Transtibial (Below-Knee) Amputation

- Transtibial amputation is the default amputation level performed when partial foot amputation is not indicated.
- The tibial length is best performed at a level of 10 to 12 cm below the joint line. This level allows creation of the most durable gastrocnemius soft-tissue envelope.
- Historical fibular transection is performed 1 cm proximal to the tibia. Fibular transection at essentially the same level creates an excellent bony platform for load transmission when walking with a prosthesis.[15]
- The long posterior flap should be equal to the length of the diameter of the limb at the level of amputation, + 1 cm.
- The anterior flap should be 2 cm distal to the planned tibial resection to allow creation of the extended posterior flap, which will lessen the shearing forces applied to the limb and surgical scar during early weight bearing.[16]
- The anterior surface of the tibia should be beveled to accommodate shearing during weight bearing.
- The posterior gastrocnemius muscle fascia is attached to the anterior compartment fascia of the leg and the periosteum of the tibia 1 to 2 cm proximal to the tibial transection. This allows creation of a bulky extended posterior flap that will facilitate early prosthetic fitting. This bulky tissue is valuable during early prosthetic fitting as it dampens the shearing forces applied to the region of the surgical wound during early prosthetic fitting (▶ Fig. 19.8).
- A rigid plaster dressing protects the wound during the preoperative period and facilitates shaping the stump for prosthetic fitting.[2]
- Preparatory prosthetic fitting can be initiated as early as 2 weeks, dictated by the early healing of the surgical wound.

19.5 Conclusions

- When performed properly, partial or whole foot amputation allows retention of a reasonable platform for weight bearing and the normal soft-tissue envelope of the durable plantar skin.
- The energy cost of walking, that is, disability, can be minimized by good surgical planning.
- Early weight bearing can be achieved with a well-contoured short-leg walking cast.
- Custom insoles and mild shoe modification can preserve a high level of functional independence.

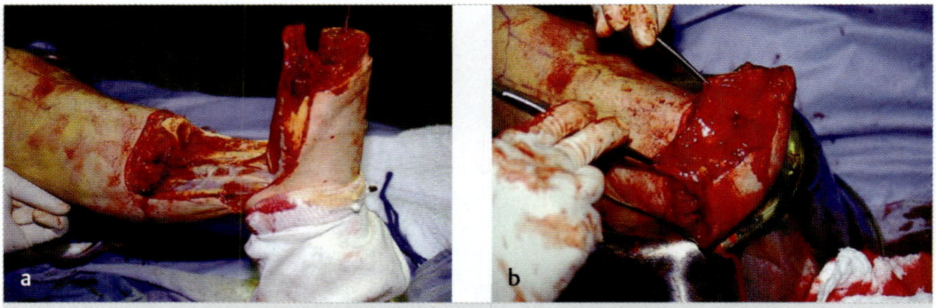

Fig. 19.8 **(a)** Long posterior flap for transtibial amputation. **(b)** The posterior gastrocnemius fascia is repaired to the anterior compartment fascia and the periosteum of the tibia 1 to 2 cm proximal to the tibial transection, to create additional stump padding to allow early weight bearing.

19.6 Key Testing Facts

Indications for Foot and Ankle Amputations:

- Common causes include gangrene, infection, trauma, tumors, and congenital anomalies. The primary goal is to remove nonviable tissue and create a functional weight-bearing terminal organ to enhance quality of life.

Initial Wound Management:

- Open wounds resulting from traumatic amputations or infections should be managed with debridement and negative pressure wound therapy. It is essential to wait for the zone of injury to become defined (7-10 days) before determining the final amputation level.

Determination of Amputation Levels:

- Amputation level depends on wound healing parameters, availability of a bony platform for weight-bearing, and a viable soft-tissue envelope.
- Reliable assessments include the ankle-brachial index (ABI), with a value of greater than 0.5 being a key indicator for vascular inflow.

Hallux Amputation:

- The hallux is crucial for stability and propulsion during gait.
- Preserving the proximal phalanx and flexor hallucis brevis attachment ensures medial column stability. Hallux amputation requires minimal to no orthotic modification.

Lesser Toe Amputation:

- There is minimal functional loss with lesser toe amputations, except for the second toe. Amputation of the second toe may cause severe hallux valgus, so preserving part of the proximal phalanx can help prevent deformities.

Ray Resection:

- First or fifth ray resection is often performed for osteomyelitis.
- First ray resection may cause medial column instability, while fifth ray resection can result in varus deformity. Proper surgical technique can mitigate complications.

Midfoot Amputation:

- Midfoot amputations (transmetatarsal or tarsometatarsal) result in a short residual foot and reduced propulsion. A durable plantar-based flap is preferred, and tendon lengthening procedures are often required for balance.

Syme's Ankle Disarticulation:

- This end-bearing amputation retains the heel pad for weight bearing and offers metabolic benefits similar to normal walking. It is preferred over hindfoot amputation due to better functional outcomes and fewer complications.

References

[1] Queen RM, Orendurff M. Amputee gait. Normal and abnormal. In: Krajbich I, Pinzur MS, Potter BK, Stevens PM, eds. Atlas of Amputations and Limb Deficiencies. 4th ed. Rosemont, IL: American Academy of Orthopaedic Surgeons; 2016:69–80

[2] AbuRahma AF, Adams E, AbuRahma J, et al. Critical analysis and limitations of resting ankle-brachial index in the diagnosis of symptomatic peripheral arterial disease patients and the role of diabetes mellitus and chronic kidney disease. Vasc Surg. 2020; 71(3):937–945

[3] Pinzur MS. New concepts in lower-limb amputation and prosthetic management. Instr Course Lect. 1990; 39:361–366

[4] Pinzur MS, Bowker JH, Smith DG, Gottschalk F. Amputation surgery in peripheral vascular disease. Instr Course Lect. 1999; 48:687–691

[5] Dickhaut SC, DeLee JC, Page CP. Nutritional status: importance in predicting wound-healing after amputation. J Bone Joint Surg Am. 1984; 66 (1):71–75

[6] Pinzur M, Kaminsky M, Sage R, Cronin R, Osterman H. Amputations at the middle level of the foot. A retrospective and prospective review. J Bone Joint Surg Am. 1986; 68(7):1061–1064

[7] Pinzur MS, Stuck RM, Sage R, Hunt N, Rabinovich Z. Syme ankle disarticulation in patients with diabetes. J Bone Joint Surg Am. 2003; 85(9): 1667–1672

[8] Pinzur MS, Stuck R, Sage R, Osterman H. Transcutaneous oxygen tension in the dysvascular foot with infection. Foot Ankle. 1993; 14(5):254–256

[9] Pinzur MS. Amputations in the foot and ankle. In: Kelikian A, ed. The Surgical Treatment of the Foot and Ankle. Stamford, CT: Appleton & Lange; 1999:607–620

[10] Pinzur MS, Sage R, Schwaegler P. Ray resection in the dysvascular foot. A retrospective review. Clin Orthop Relat Res. 1984(191):232–234

[11] Pinzur MS, Wolf B, Havey RM. Walking pattern of midfoot and ankle disarticulation amputees. Foot Ankle Int. 1997; 18(10):635–638

[12] Pinzur MS, Gold J, Schwartz D, Gross N. Energy demands for walking in dysvascular amputees as related to the level of amputation. Orthopedics. 1992; 15(9):1033–1036, discussion 1036–1037

[13] Wagner FW, Jr. Amputations of the foot and ankle. Current status. Clin Orthop Relat Res. 1977(122): 62–69

[14] Finkler ES, Marchwiany DA, Schiff AP, Pinzur MS. Long term outcomes following Syme's amputation. Foot Ankle Int. 2017; 38(7):732–735

[15] Keeling JJ, Shawen SB, Forsberg JA, et al. Comparison of functional outcomes following bridge synostosis with non-bone-bridging transtibial combat-related amputations. J Bone Joint Surg Am. 2013; 95(10): 888–893

[16] Assal M, Blanck R, Smith DG. Extended posterior flap for transtibial amputation. Orthopedics. 2005; 28(6):542–546

20 Foot and Ankle Trauma

Tobin Eckel, Thomas M. Hearty, and Scott B. Shawen

Abstract

In this chapter, we explore the etiology, diagnosis, management, and rehabilitation of lower extremity trauma. We examine both high- and low-energy traumas, with a regional approach. Specific areas covered include the ankle, hindfoot, midfoot, and forefoot.

Keywords: pilon fracture, ankle fracture, calcaneus fracture, peritalar and Chopart dislocations, talus fracture, Lisfranc injury, metatarsal fracture, phalanx fracture

20.1 Pilon Fractures

20.1.1 Etiology and Pathophysiology

- Tibial plafond or pilon fractures generally occur by one of two mechanisms: rotational forces or axial load.
  - *Rotational*: Lower-energy injuries that typically have large intra-articular fracture fragments with minimal comminution and joint impaction, and less soft-tissue injury.
  - *Axial*: Result from falls from height or motor vehicle accidents.
    - The term "pilon fracture" describes the talus acting as a hammer impacting the tibial plafond.
    - Axial load injuries differ from rotational injuries in that there is often marked articular and metaphyseal comminution, joint impaction, and severe soft-tissue trauma, all of which result in a much less favorable prognosis[1] (▶ Fig. 20.1a, b).

20.1.2 Symptoms

- Often seen in polytraumatized patients.
- May be visible bony deformity, but soft-tissue damage will be most evident to include swelling, ecchymosis, fracture blisters, skin tenting from underlying bony fragments, open wounds, and/or fractures.
- Patients should be monitored for the development of compartment syndrome.[1,2]

20.1.3 Diagnostics/ Classification

- Vascular examination to confirm adequate perfusion.
- Plain radiographs.
- Computed tomography (CT) scan is vital in characterizing the fracture and in developing the surgical plan; however, this is best done after initial reduction of the fracture.
  - In fact, the CT scan has been shown to add information in 82% of patients and change the initial surgical plan in 64% of patients.[1,3]

20.1.4 Conservative Management

- All managed surgically.
  - Initial conservative measures may assist in improving outcomes.
- In the event of open wounds, intravenous antibiotics can be started initially, and gross contamination can be removed and saline irrigation performed to decrease foreign material and infectious burden.
- Any skin tenting or extruded bony fragments may be reduced to prevent further tension or compromise on the soft tissues.
- Medical optimization can also improve long-term results.
- Nicotine use and poorly controlled diabetes have both been shown to increase wound healing complications

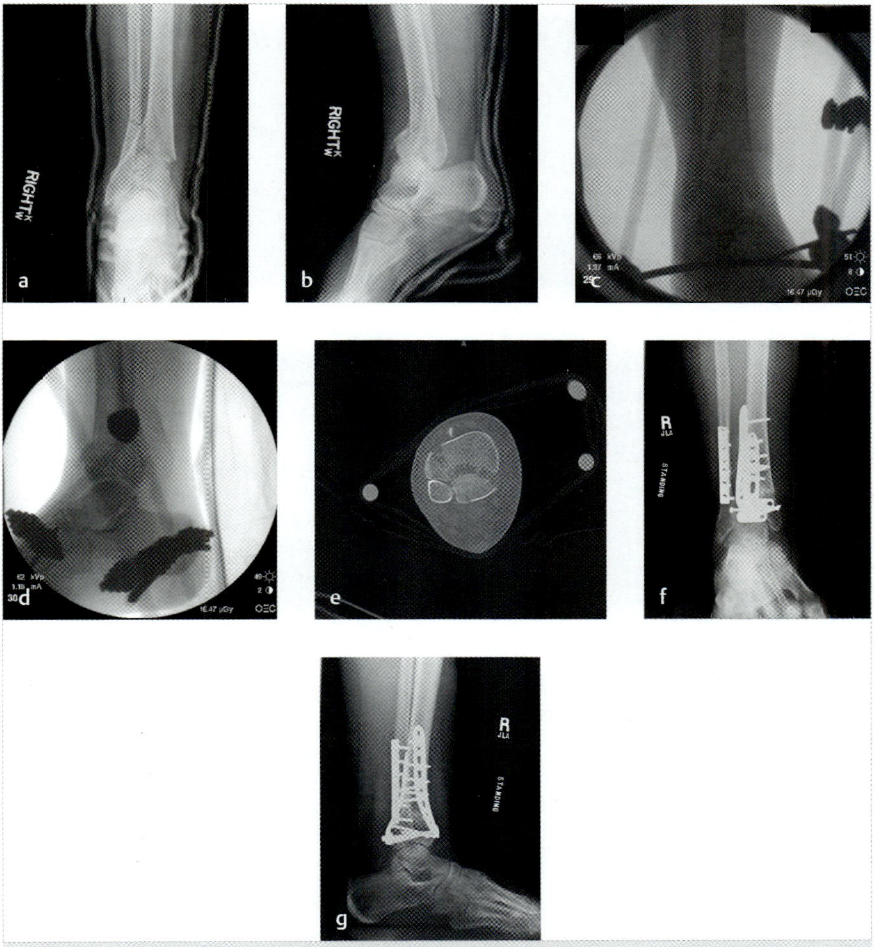

Fig. 20.1 (a,b) Displaced intra-articular pilon fracture from motor vehicle collision with extension and fibular involvement. **(c,d)** Fracture as seen above after external fixation and reduction. Note the reduction of the joint and realignment of the ankle held with the external pins and rods. **(e)** Computed tomography (CT) scan after reduction with external fixation. Note the starlike pattern of the fracture typically seen with higher-energy pilon fractures. **(f,g)** After open reduction with plates and screws using a combined posterolateral, posteromedial, and anterolateral approaches.

and the need for revision surgery, so initial management should include improved glycemic control and smoking cessation counseling.[2]

20.1.5 Surgical Intervention

- Soft-tissue impairment secondary to inflammation is greatest from 6 hours to 6 days postinjury, and this time frame should be avoided for definitive fixation of these injuries.
- Historically, when these injuries underwent immediate open reduction and internal fixation (ORIF), wound complications approached 100%.[2,3]
- While some experienced trauma surgeons still advocate for immediate

ORIF, the vast majority favor a staged protocol.

- Goals of surgery:
  - Restoration of alignment and joint congruity.
  - Stable fixation to allow for early motion.[4]
- The first stage focuses on adequate debridement, soft-tissue stabilization, and temporary external fixation to maintain a provisional reduction (▶ Fig. 20.1c, d).
  - This allows for soft-tissue rest and CT scan to plan for definitive ORIF when the soft tissue allows, which can be anywhere from 10 to 21 days postinjury (▶ Fig. 20.1e).
- There is no consensus on when to fix the fibula fracture.
  - Potential advantages for fixing the fibula fracture in the initial stage is that it can assist in maintaining length and alignment of the tibia.
    - It may only require monoplanar external fixation.
  - Increased risk of fibular wound complications with initial plate fixation.
  - With significant fibular comminution, anatomic reduction may be difficult.
  - Malreduced fibula will impede tibial reduction at the time of definitive fixation.
- The "work horse" incision is usually determined after the CT scan is obtained.
  - Delay fibular fixation until the surgical approach/es have been determined.
- If unsure where definitive incisions will be, or you will not be the definitive treating surgeon, then the fibula should not be fixed at the initial stage of treatment.
  - Tornetta et al questioned whether the fibula needs fixed at all in pilon fractures.
  - No difference in reduction or maintenance of alignment between those with or without fibula fixation.
  - Higher number of complications in the group treated with fibular fixation.[4]
- Surgical approaches are based on the fracture pattern and existing soft-tissue envelope.
- Posterolateral approach:
  - It can be used for the fibula as well as the posterior tibia, and the anterior fragments can be approached through an anteromedial or anterolateral approach.
- A straight anterior approach has the advantage of the most visualization of the anterior approaches and can also be used for revision to arthrodesis in the future[2] (▶ Fig. 20.1f, g).

20.1.6 Rehabilitation

- Prolonged period of non-weight-bearing, typically between 8 and 12 weeks.
- Early range of motion (ROM), but there is no clear consensus on what period of time defines early motion.
- We recommend 6 weeks of cast immobilization, followed by initiation of motion and weight bearing at 12 weeks.
- Functional outcomes after pilon fracture tend to be poor, regardless of the rehabilitation protocol.[3]

20.2 Ankle Fractures

20.2.1 Etiology and Pathophysiology

- Rotational injuries that occur in younger, more active people as well as an older, more sedentary population.
- The ankle accounts for 10% of all fractures, is the most commonly fractured weight-bearing joint, and is the most frequent surgically treated orthopaedic injury.
- They are responsible for nearly 25% of all sports-related injuries.
- Likewise, the incidence is increasing in the geriatric population, and expected to continue to climb with increases in mobility and life expectancy.[5,6,7]

20.2.2 Symptoms

- Patients present after an inciting traumatic event with pain, swelling, and inability or difficulty bearing weight.
- Bony tenderness is used to distinguish from soft-tissue tenderness, and is more indicative of fracture rather than a ligamentous sprain.
- With increasing fracture displacement and/or dislocation, visible deformity may be present.

20.2.3 Diagnostics/ Classification

- Plain radiographs are sufficient to characterize ankle fractures.
- CT scan is rarely needed.
- Full-length tibia films may be necessary to rule out proximal fibula fracture, consistent with a Maisonneuve injury, and should be considered whenever a patient presents with ankle pain and swelling and a mechanism of injury, with or without a medial malleolar fracture, but no fibula fracture on ankle radiographs (▶ Fig. 20.2).
- The Lauge-Hansen classification was developed in the 1950s after experimentally produced fracture patterns were created with cadaver specimens.
  - Supination-external rotation, supination-adduction, pronation-external rotation, and pronation-abduction.
  - Still remains widely in use today, likely because of its descriptive familiarity among surgeons, as well as the relative utility in guiding management of the various fracture patterns.[5,8]
- The Danis–Weber classification is also frequently used, and describes the level of the fibula fracture relative to the ankle joint, and can also help guide treatment strategies.[9]
  - We feel it is most useful to think of ankle fractures in terms of stability, and whether or not operative intervention is warranted.
- Fracture-dislocations, widely displaced factures, and bi- and trimalleolar fractures are regarded as unstable and necessitate surgical fixation.
- Isolated malleolar fractures with minimal displacement and ankle mortise congruity, on the other hand, can be treated nonoperatively.[10]

20.2.4 Conservative Management

- All ankle fractures can initially undergo reduction and splint immobilization, and in the absence of an open wound, an

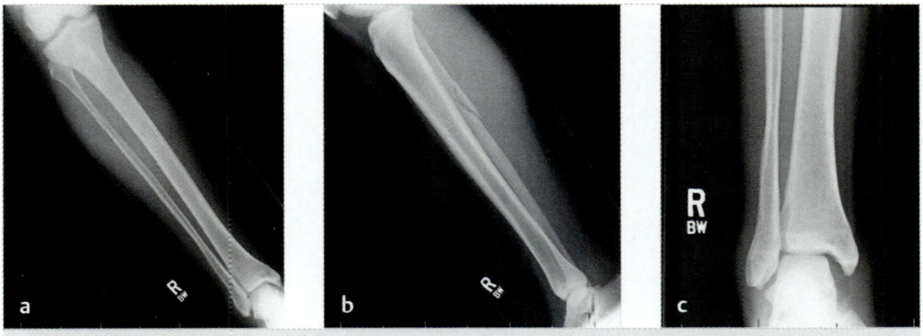

Fig. 20.2 (a) Ankle injury demonstrating what initially appears to be a normal ankle without fracture on radiographs **(b,c)**, but with a high fibular fracture and medial clear space and syndesmosis widening seen on closer examination.

impending open wound, neurovascular compromise, or irreducible dislocation, surgery can be scheduled on an elective basis if needed.
- A period of soft-tissue elevation to decrease edema is beneficial to wound healing.
- Isolated malleolar fractures with concomitant ligamentous injury, are more appropriately managed with operative fixation:
  - The key ligaments regarding ankle stability are the deltoid and the syndesmosis.
- Measuring the tibiofibular overlap and clear space can be cumbersome when trying to assess for syndesmotic injury, plus, the majority of injury films are non-weight-bearing.
- Much easier to assess the medial clear space looking for deltoid incompetence.
- Widening on injury films indicates a deltoid injury:
  - *Stress test:* External rotation stress test, or a gravity stress test, the latter of which does not require a physician to administer the stress, and is better tolerated by the patient.[5]
  - Some have advocated against the stress radiograph, in support of weight-bearing radiographs at initial follow-up or even magnetic resonance imaging (MRI) to assess deltoid competence.[11,12]
- The initial stress test performed is looking at deltoid competence and fracture instability, while the intraoperative stress test, the Cotton test, is performed after fibula fixation and is looking for syndesmotic instability.

20.2.5 Surgical Intervention

- Treatment is based on the fracture pattern.
- Oblique fibula fractures are typically treated with lag screw stabilization, followed by a neutralization plate.
- Very distal fractures or osteoporotic bone may require an anatomic locking plate.
- Severely comminuted fractures are not amenable to lag compression, and instead require bridge plating to maintain length (► Fig. 20.3).
- There is some biomechanical evidence that suggests posterior fibula plating is superior to lateral plating in osteoporotic bone, although it comes with an increased incidence of peroneal tendon irritation.[13]
- Oblique medial malleolus fractures are often treated with traversing screw fixation, whereas more vertical fracture patterns may require an antiglide plate or screw trajectory paralleling the ankle joint, to prevent fracture displacement.

20.2.6 Posterior Malleolar Fractures

- There is considerable debate regarding the treatment of posterior malleolus fractures and the syndesmosis:
  - Historically, if the posterior malleolus involved more than 25% of the articular surface, then this would lead to posterior instability if not surgically stabilized.
  - Posttraumatic arthritis has been shown to develop in the cases where the posterior malleolar fragment represented as little as 5% of the articular surface.[14]
  - Others argue that there is minimal reduction in tibiotalar contact area with fragments less than 25%, particularly if the medial and lateral columns have been stabilized, and perhaps articular congruity is more predictive of outcome, rather than fragment size.
  - For this reason, some advocate posterior plating over anteroposterior

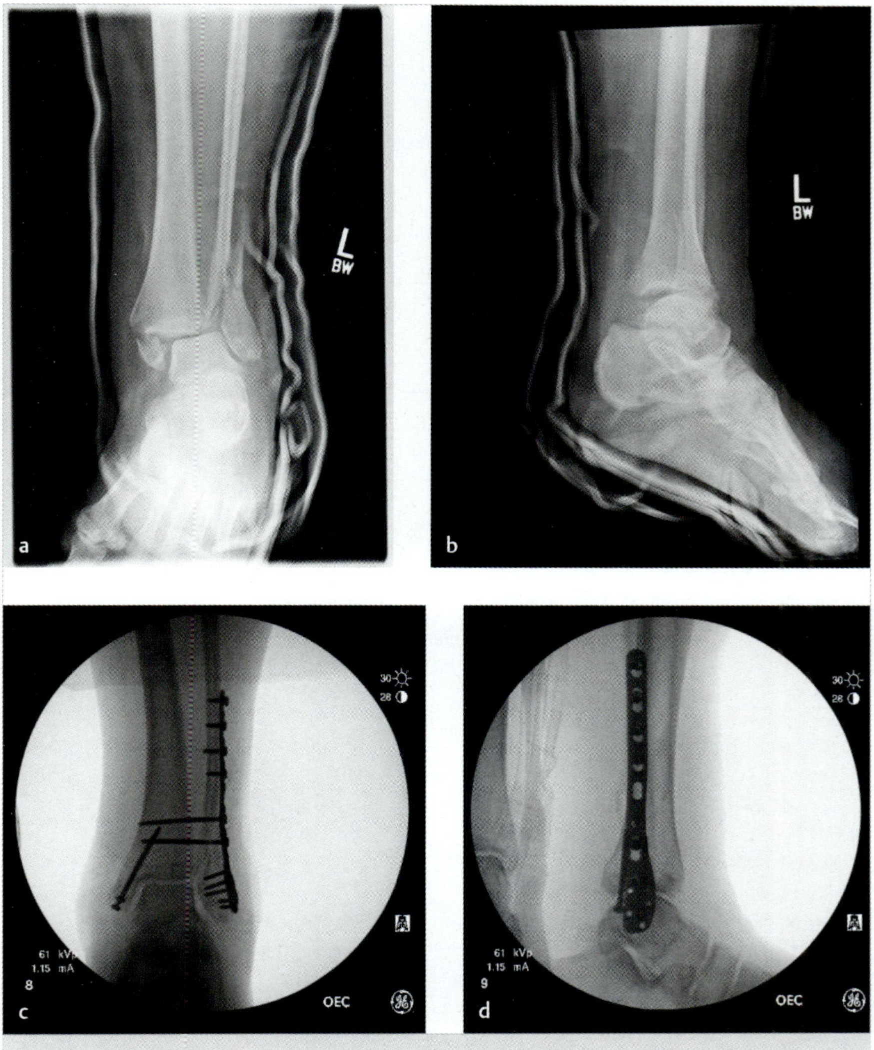

Fig. 20.3 (a) Trimalleolar ankle fracture with comminution of the fibula **(b)** minimally displaced posterior malleolar fracture on lateral radiograph. **(c,d)** Bridge plating of the fibula performed with syndesmotic fixation to help maintain the length and reduction of the fibula.

(AP) screw fixation, as plating is a biomechanically more stable construct and affords better articular reduction than AP screws.[15,16,17]

20.2.7 Syndesmosis

- Incidence of syndesmosis injury: 23%.
  - Operative ankle fractures are inherently more unstable and have a higher incidence of syndesmotic injury, with reports as high as 45%.[18]
- Surgical options to treat syndesmosis instability:
  - One or two screws spanning three or four cortices.

- Suture button devices.
- Anatomic reduction and fixation of the posterior malleolus to restore the posteroinferior tibiofibular ligament.
- Deltoid ligament repair.
- No one technique has demonstrated superior results when compared.
- Further complicating the issue of syndesmosis stabilization is that malreduction rates have been reported to be between 16 and 52% with screw fixation, of which 89% spontaneously reduces after screw removal.[9,19,20,21]

- Growing number of geriatric ankle fractures:
  - Complication rates are 20 to 40%, with the only modifiable risk factor being operative time.
  - These patients need to be optimized with regard to medical comorbidities, and strategies employed to reduce operative time.[6]

20.2.8 Rehabilitation

- Great variability within rehabilitation protocols.
- Non-weight-bearing for 6 weeks.
- ROM beginning between 2 and 4 weeks.
- If syndesmotic fixation was performed, then the non-weight-bearing period is extended between 8 and 12 weeks:
  - We prefer suture button devices for syndesmotic fixation and allow weight bearing after 8 weeks when the syndesmosis is involved.
- We prefer cast immobilization for 4 weeks, followed by ROM in a controlled ankle motion (CAM) boot, but no weight bearing until 6 weeks postoperatively.

20.3 Calcaneal Fractures

20.3.1 Etiology and Pathophysiology

- The calcaneus is the most commonly fractured tarsal bone:
  - Seventy percent of all tarsal fractures.
- Typically the result of high-energy loading, commonly seen in falls from height or motor vehicle accidents.
- As the talus is driven down into the calcaneus, the primary fracture line occurs, separating the medial sustentaculum from the calcaneal tuberosity.
- Secondary fracture lines occur in the sagittal plane and are responsible for posterior facet comminution:
  - This axial force results in the characteristic deformity of a shortened calcaneus and lateral displacement or blowout of the lateral wall.
- Calcaneal shortening leads to anterior ankle impingement and decreased push-off strength secondary to a shorter Achilles lever arm:
  - This, in addition to lateral displacement, can lead to subfibular impingement, sural neuritis, and difficulty with shoe wear.
- Long-term sequelae include posttraumatic arthritis, pain, and stiffness.
- These injuries have major socioeconomic implications as the vast majority occur in young people and laborers.[22]

20.3.2 Symptoms

- Patients present after high-energy trauma, with pain, swelling, and inability to bear weight.
- Fracture blisters are also common.
- Open fractures can occur in 1 to 10% of calcaneal fractures.
- Posterior displaced tongue-type fractures are rare, but need to be recognized immediately, as the posterior skin tenting can lead to full-thickness skin breakdown if not reduced urgently[23] (► Fig. 20.4a, b).

20.3.3 Diagnostics/ Classification

- Plain radiographs of the foot are obtained, with the lateral view

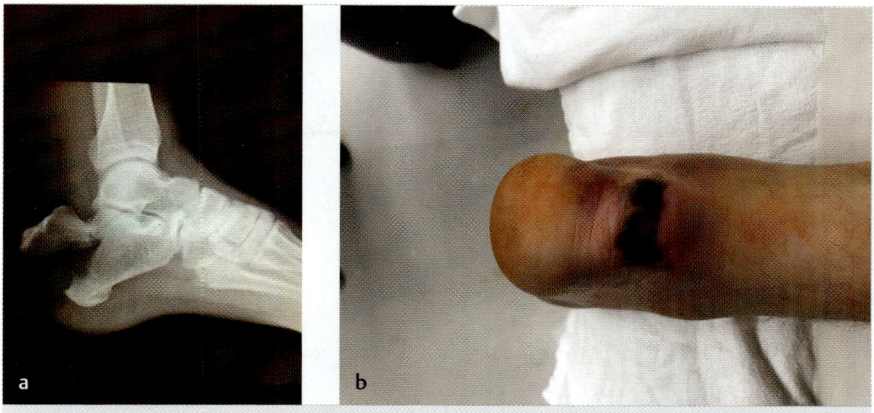

Fig. 20.4 (a,b) Tongue-type fracture with skin breakdown in a patient who presented 48 hours after injury.

demonstrating loss of height of the posterior facet (► Fig. 20.5a).

- CT scan is also routinely obtained to further delineate these injuries (► Fig. 20.5b).
- Sanders' classification:
    - Utilizes semi-coronal images through the posterior facet.
    - Characterizes these fractures based on the number of posterior facet fracture fragments.
- Essex-Lopresti classification scheme is based on plain films:
    - Defines fractures as joint depression or tongue type, with the latter having a secondary fracture line that exits posteriorly, often with the Achilles attached to this tuberosity fragment, which leads to superior displacement and often tenting of the posterior skin.[24]

20.3.4 Conservative Management

- Given the extensive soft-tissue swelling and trauma, these fractures are typically placed in a well-padded splint with definitive treatment delayed until soft-tissue swelling resolves.
    - Exceptions include open fractures or those with skin tenting that are impending open fractures, that require urgent reduction to prevent open wound formation, or that require surgical debridement for existing open wounds.
- Foot compartment syndrome is also a concern with these injuries, although fasciotomies are rarely performed, as the main sequela of compartment syndrome is claw-toe deformity.
- Others may advocate for early fixation for patients who are already admitted to the hospital for polytrauma.
    - Assessment for lumbar issues is paramount given the high incidence of concomitant injury
- Nonoperative management is generally avoided, as it leads to malunion and higher incidence of subtalar arthritis.
- Malunion leads to anterior ankle impingement, subfibular impingement, pain, and difficulty with shoe wear.[23,25]

20.3.5 Surgical Intervention

- Can be delayed up to 3 weeks to allow the resolution of soft swelling.
- *Lateral extensile approach:* Postsurgical wound breakdown can still occur in 25%

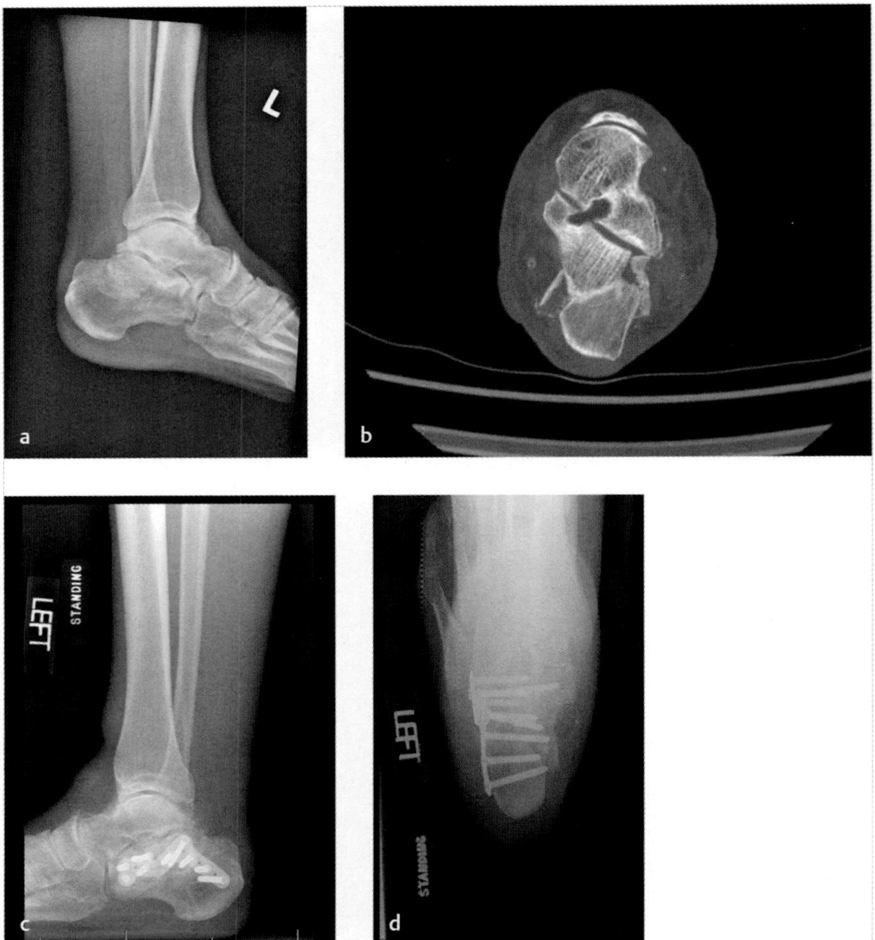

Fig. 20.5 **(a)** Subtle intra-articular calcaneus fracture seen on lateral radiograph. **(b)** The same patient with calcaneus fracture seen on computed tomography (CT) scan with involvement of the posterior facet and the major fracture line between the sustentaculum and the posterior portion of the calcaneus. **(c,d)** Combined sinus tarsi and percutaneous techniques to perform open reduction and fixation of the calcaneal fracture presented in **(a)** and **(b)**.

of patients, with osteomyelitis occurring in 1 to 4% of closed and up to 19% of open fractures.[26]

- Percutaneous techniques and limited sinus tarsi approaches have been utilized with less wound healing complications:
  - These are often limited to simpler fracture patterns with less articular comminution (► Fig. 20.5c, d).
- Goals:
  - Restoring hindfoot alignment to prevent varus malunion.
  - Restoring posterior facet height and articular congruity, to prevent anterior impingement, and minimize secondary arthrosis
  - Restore calcaneal width to prevent chronic subfibular impingement, sural neuritis, and difficulty with shoe wear.

- More anatomic restoration with surgery includes fewer complications and better outcomes with delayed subtalar arthrodesis when compared to arthrodesis after nonoperative management.[25,27]

20.3.6 Rehabilitation

- Depending on the severity of injury, patients can expect to be non-weight-bearing for 8 to 12 weeks.
- Early ROM after the wound is important to help minimize stiffness.
- Typically, these are polytrauma patients and therefore they have other injuries that may dictate their rehabilitation.

20.4 Peritalar Dislocations—Subtalar

20.4.1 Etiology and Pathophysiology

- Usually dislocation of the subtalar joint occurs with a talonavicular joint dislocation.
- Comprises of 1 to 2% of all dislocations.
- Frequently associated with bony injuries, although these can be purely ligamentous.
- High-energy injuries typically cause this injury but can occur with sports and other low-energy injuries.
- Medial (75%) and lateral (17–26%) are the most common dislocations and the injury usually occurs by forced inversion of the plantarflexed foot (medial) or forced eversion of the dorsiflexed foot (lateral).[28,29]

20.4.2 Symptoms

- Patients will present with a locked foot and ankle, severe pain, and obvious deformity of their hindfoot and midfoot.

20.4.3 Diagnostics/ Classification

- Medial dislocations will have medially displaced hindfoot, and an inverted/ plantarflexed foot.
- Lateral dislocations will present with a laterally displaced hindfoot and an everted/abducted/dorsiflexed foot.
- Anterior and posterior dislocations are rare.
- Examine carefully for open injuries, particularly with lateral dislocations and assess neurovascular status carefully.
- Attain anterior/posterior and lateral radiographs of the ankle and foot to diagnose and evaluate for bony injuries and accuracy of reduction with a postreduction CT scan.[28,29]

20.4.4 Conservative Management

- An urgent closed reduction is vital.
- Sedate the patient and flex the hip and knee to 90 degrees.
- Medial dislocations:
  - Accentuate the deformity bringing the foot into plantarflexion/inversion, pull traction, and dorsiflex/evert the foot and push medially on the prominent lateral talar head.
  - Blocks to reduction:
    - Incarcerated superior extensor retinaculum.
    - And/or the extensor digitorum brevis muscle (possible talonavicular joint capsule, neurovascular bundle, or peroneal tendons) 10% of the time.
- Lateral dislocations:
  - Accentuate the deformity by dorsiflexing/everting the foot, pull traction, and then bring the foot into plantarflexion/inversion while providing lateral directed pressure on the prominent medial talar head.
  - Audible click is typically heard in both reductions.
  - Blocks to reduction:
    - Posterior tibialis tendon.
    - Flexor digitorum longus tendon in 40% of cases.

- After reduction, if there are no other injuries, the foot can be managed in a non-weight-bearing short-leg cast for 6 weeks.[28,29]

20.4.5 Surgical Intervention

- Surgical management is necessary for open injuries, unstable or irreducible closed injuries, vascular injuries, and for displaced fractures.
- Open injuries are treated with irrigation and debridement and irreducible dislocations require open reduction and possible repair of injured soft-tissue structures (posterior tibialis tendon may be lacerated in lateral dislocations).
- K-wire fixation and/or external fixation may be required in unstable injuries and/ or severe soft-tissue injuries[28,29] (▶ Fig. 20.6a–d).

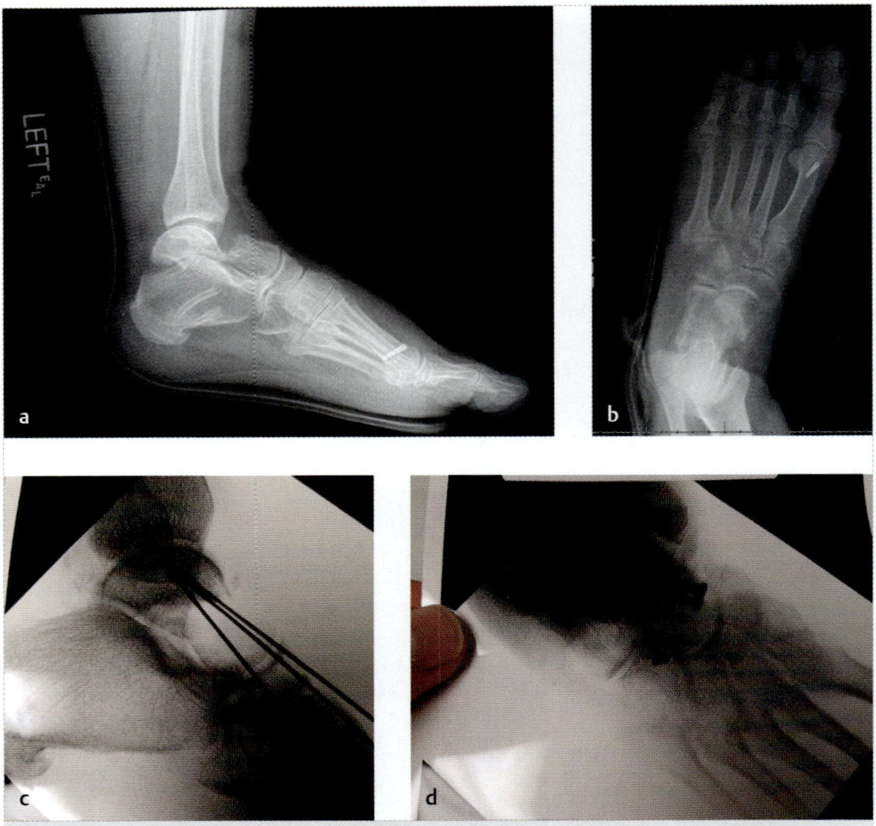

Fig. 20.6 (a–d) Fracture and dislocation of the talus with involvement of the talar neck and subtalar dislocation treated with closed reduction of the subtalar dislocation and open reduction and internal fixation of the talar neck fracture.

20.4.6 Rehabilitation

- Unstable injuries and/or fracture dislocation injuries that involve the articular surface should be kept non-weight-bearing for 8 to 12 weeks with ROM exercises once the soft tissue is healed.
- Physical therapy should be considered after cast is removed for gait training, ROM/stretching, strengthening, as well as balance and proprioception training.
- Orthotics and bracing may be required for instability and/or posttraumatic arthritis symptoms.

20.5 Chopart Dislocations

20.5.1 Etiology and Pathophysiology

- *Chopart joint:* Combined talonavicular and calcaneocuboid joints.
- These injuries are rare but commonly overlooked.
- Caused by axial load and is dependent on if the foot is plantarflexed or dorsiflexed.
- Typically a compression injury on one side and corresponding traction injury on the other side with fracture at either two or more areas in addition to ligamentous injury.[30]

20.5.2 Symptoms

- Present with midfoot pain with weight bearing, swelling and hematoma, or severe pain with deformity and inability to bear weight with dislocations.
- Plantar ecchymosis may be present along the midfoot.
- Open wounds are possible given that many of these injuries are high energy.
- But consider Charcot's arthropathy in the setting of neuropathy with a low-energy injury or idiopathic presentation.[30]

20.5.3 Diagnostics/ Classification

- Standard lateral, AP, and oblique foot radiographs should be taken.
- Low threshold to evaluate with a CT scan to evaluate complex fractures or occult fractures and to assess for articular displacement.

Injuries are classified according to the Zwipp classification[30]:

1. Transligamentous.
2. Transtalar.
3. Transcalcaneal.
4. Transnavicular.
5. Transcubiod.
6. Combinations 2 to 5.

20.5.4 Conservative Management

- If the injury is stable, mostly ligamentous with bony avulsions, treatment consists of weight bearing as tolerated in an orthosis.
- Nondisplaced tarsal fractures need to be treated in a below-knee cast with either non-weight-bearing or partial weight bearing for 6 to 8 weeks, then progression to orthosis with weight bearing as tolerated.[30]

20.5.5 Surgical Intervention

- Simple dislocations and fracture dislocations need emergent reduction but often need open reduction as closed reductions are often unsuccessful.
- All displaced fractures need ORIF with consideration of transarticular pinning of the joints if unstable after fixation.
- Restore the medial column length (talar head, navicular, cuneiforms) and the lateral column length (anterior calcaneus process, cuboid).[31]
- External fixation should be considered in cases with severe soft-tissue swelling

and defects as well as with unstable injuries.
  - Hybrid internal/external fixation constructs can be used as well.
- Open fracture/dislocations need emergent reduction, irrigation, and debridement with internal and/or external fixation.
- Primary fusion can be considered for severe articular destruction.[30]

20.5.6 Rehabilitation

- Unstable injuries and/or fracture dislocation injuries that involve the articular surface should be kept non-weight-bearing for 8 to 12 weeks with ROM exercises once the soft tissue is healed.
- Physical therapy should be considered after cast removal.
- Orthotics and bracing may be required for instability and/or posttraumatic arthritis symptoms.

20.6 Talus Fractures

20.6.1 Etiology and Pathophysiology

- Second most common tarsal fracture.
- Account for 0.15% of all fractures.[32]
- High-energy trauma but can occur from sports injuries as well.
- Medial-sided forefoot compression causes talar head fractures.
- Forced dorsiflexion of the foot is the primary cause of talar neck fractures.
- Axial compression between the tibia and calcaneus is the primary cause of talar body fractures.[32,33]

20.6.2 Symptoms

- After high-energy trauma, there will be significant deformity and/or swelling in the ankle and hindfoot, particularly with displaced talar neck fractures, which are often associated with dislocation.
- Be highly suspicious for open injuries or pending open injuries with associated dislocations.
- With lower-energy trauma (sports, snowboarding), be suspicious of occult talus fracture with negative radiographs but swelling and inability to bear weight.

20.6.3 Diagnostics/ Classification

- Ankle and foot radiographs should be taken for all patients with suspected foot or ankle fractures.
- Any irregularities of the talus seen on radiographs should be further evaluated with a CT scan.[32,33]
- Consider getting contralateral radiographs for comparison as well a Canale view radiograph to evaluate talar neck fractures.
- Classified by anatomic location:
  - Head (10%).
  - Neck (50%):
    - Nondisplaced (OTA 81-B1; Hawkins 1).
    - Subtalar joint incongruity (81-B2; Hawkins 2).
    - Subtalar and tibiotalar joint incongruity (81-B3; Hawkins 3).
    - Complete peritalar dislocation (Hawkins 4).
  - Body (posterior to lateral tubercle, 38%):
    - Talar dome (OTA 81-C1).
    - With subtalar involvement (B1-C2).
    - Subtalar and tibiotalar joint involvement (81-C3).[33]

20.6.4 Conservative Management

- Tenuous extraosseous blood supply of the talus creates significant areas of anastomosis:
  - High rates of osteonecrosis after fracture displacement.
  - Higher rates occur with more displacement, particularly seen with neck fractures.

- Nonoperative management is reserved for nondisplaced fractures only.
- Immobilization with protected weight bearing for 6 to 8 weeks is typical for nondisplaced fractures.
- Small avulsion injuries are treated symptomatically and usually do not require immobilization.[32,33]

20.6.5 Surgical Intervention

- Displaced fractures are best treated with ORIF.
- External fixation may be needed for temporary fixation in the setting of poor soft-tissue envelope and instability.
- Fracture dislocations and open injuries are treated emergently and require open reduction:
  - Internal and/or external fixation is used at the time of open reduction.
- For closed injuries, accuracy of reduction is more important than timing of fixation.
- Emergent reduction of talar neck fractures is no longer considered important in decreasing rates of osteonecrosis.
- *Neck fractures* are treated with a dual approach, medial and lateral, and often require medial and lateral fixation.
  - Care must be taken not to compress comminution of the medial side, as this can lead to varus malunion.
- *Talar head fractures* are approached medially and treated with extra-articular screws and/or intra-articular countersunk or headless screws:
  - Medial column length preservation is needed and may require bridge plating or external fixation.
- *Body fractures* are treated primarily with screws, countersunk or headless if overlying the articular cartilage (60% of talus is intra-articular):
  - Screws may be inserted from anteromedial, anterolateral, posterolateral, posteromedial, or through a medial malleolus osteotomy.
  - Small lateral process fractures are excised if small or fixed with a screw and osteochondral fragments are fixed with headless screws or bioabsorbable pins.[32,33,34]

20.6.6 Rehabilitation

- For associated dislocations that are deemed unstable after surgery, cast immobilization may be required for several weeks; otherwise, ROM exercises should commence once skin incisions are healed.
- ROM exercises can be delayed for severely comminuted fractures or joint instability.[34]
- Protected weight bearing should be ordered until there are radiographic signs of healing, typically 8 weeks postoperatively but possibly longer.
- The Hawkins sign (radiographic subchondral lucency) seen at 6 to 8 weeks postoperatively after talar neck internal fixation is a sign of viability of the talus.

20.7 Lisfranc Injuries

20.7.1 Etiology and Pathophysiology

- Lisfranc injuries are ligamentous ruptures and/or fractures across the tarsometatarsal (TMT) joints.
- The primary ligament involved is the Lisfranc ligament that connects the medial cuneiform to the base of the second metatarsal.
- Injuries can occur across all five TMT joints and the strong plantar ligaments connecting metatarsals 2 to 5.
- Over 20% of Lisfranc injuries are missed.
- It is important to distinguish lower-energy injuries (sports, twisting/falls) from true fracture/dislocations that typically occur with high-energy injuries (motor vehicle accidents, falls from height, crush injuries).[35,36]

- The true Lisfranc fracture dislocation is a rare injury that occurs 1 in 50,000 people in the United States or 0.2% of all fractures.[35,37]
  - These injuries occur from forceful torsion of the foot, axial loads in equinus, or direct crush injuries onto the midfoot.
- Midfoot sprains (lower energy) are the second most common sports foot injury, which make up 16% of all sports injuries:[37]
  - These occur from indirect mechanisms including axial load to a plantarflexed foot, or a twisting force through the midfoot particularly seen with cleated athletes.[35]

20.7.2 Symptoms

- High-energy injuries will have significant midfoot swelling and ecchymosis (plantar and dorsal) at the midfoot, possible deformity, soft-tissue injury, as well as possible foot compartment syndrome.
- Lower-energy injuries may or may not have swelling in the midfoot, inability to bear weight, tenderness over the midfoot, as well as plantar ecchymosis.
- The missed Lisfranc injury often presents with continued pain with weight bearing after several months with or without previous immobilization.[35,37]

20.7.3 Diagnostics/ Classification

- For high-energy injuries, AP, lateral, and oblique radiographs of the foot along with CT scan to evaluate the fracture pattern is needed (▶ Fig. 20.7a–d).
- For lower-energy injuries, in addition to radiographs of the foot, bilateral weight-bearing AP radiographs are needed to compare to the contralateral side and evaluate for gapping at the first intermetatarsal space at the base as well as subluxation of the second and third TMT joints (▶ Fig. 20.7e, f).
  - A CT scan can help evaluate fractures and joint incongruity and MRI can evaluate the continuity of the Lisfranc ligament in equivocal cases or for patients who cannot bear weight.[35,36,37]
  - Abduction stress radiographs or fluoroscopy can demonstrate instability as well.[38]
  - This should be done after anesthetizing the patient or in the operation room under anesthesia for surgical planning.
- High-energy injuries are often described using the Myerson classification:
  - *Type A*: Total incongruity (lateral or medial) of all five TMT joints.
  - *Type B*: Partial incongruity (B1: medial, B2: partial lateral, and B3: total lateral).
  - *Type C:* Divergent (C1: partial and C2: total).[37]
- Low-energy injuries are best described by Nunley and Vertullo:
  - *Stage 1*: No diastasis at the Lisfranc space with weight-bearing X-rays.
  - *Stage 2*: 2 to 5 mm of diastasis of AP weight-bearing X-rays.
  - Stage 3: > 5 mm diastasis and loss of longitudinal arch seen on lateral foot weight-bearing X-rays.[35,36]

20.7.4 Conservative Management

- Only stage 1 injuries should be treated without surgery.
- Protected weight bearing in an orthosis or a short=leg cast is an option for 4 to 6 weeks:
  - Many patients do fine with orthosis and weight bearing as tolerated with avoidance of prolonged standing or walking for several weeks.

20.7.5 Surgical Intervention

- Most other injuries do better in the long term with surgery.
- The goal is anatomic reduction.

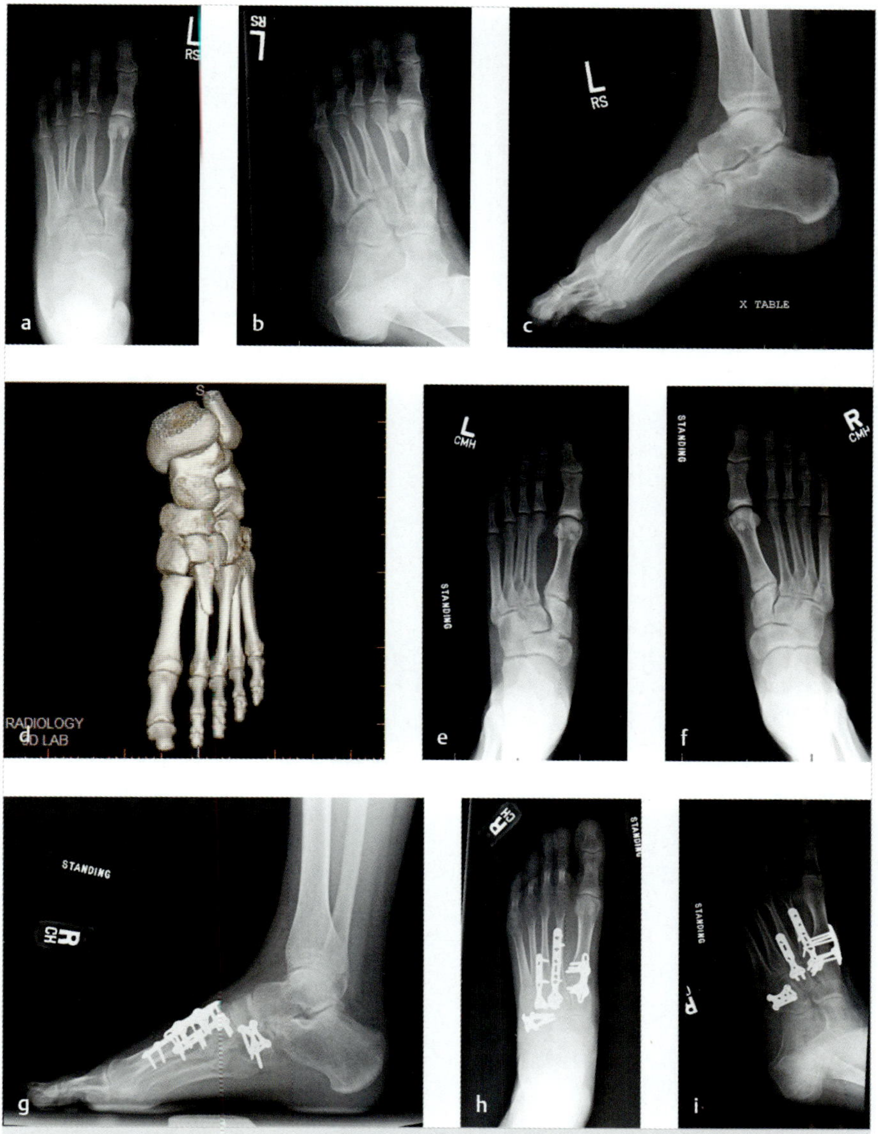

Fig. 20.7 (a–d) Lisfranc injury with radiographs demonstrating malalignment at the first tarsometatarsal joint, fracture of the base of the second metatarsal, malalignment of the base of the third metatarsal, and fracture of the cuboid. **(e)** Computed tomography (CT) scan reconstruction demonstrates the involvement of the Lisfranc articulation and a subtle lateral shift of the metatarsal on the cuneiforms. **(e,f)** Weight bearing films with a Lisfranc injury of the left foot **(e)** compared to a normal right foot radiograph **(f)**. **(g,i)** Bridge plating technique performed in the patient presented in Figures a-d because of relatively young age, 17, and joint sparing of the injury pattern.

- Options consist of primary arthrodesis or ORIF:
  - Controversy exists on choosing arthrodesis versus internal fixation (▶ Fig. 20.7g–i).

20.7.6 Rehabilitation

- Immobilized in a splint and with no weight bearing until incisions are healed.
- Some surgeons start ROM exercises at this point and others choose prolonged immobilization in a short-leg cast, but all agree on protected weight bearing for a total of about 8 weeks.
- Some surgeons will allow patients to return to all physical activity and take out the hardware at 6 months postoperatively, while others prefer to limit the physical activity and take the hardware out earlier.
- For primary arthrodesis, the hardware does not have to be removed and activity should be limited until radiographic signs of healing occur.[35,36,37]
- Most patients will return to physical activities although with possible limitations.

20.8 Metatarsal Fractures

20.8.1 Etiology and Pathophysiology

- Relatively common, accounting for 6% of all fractures seen in the primary care setting.
- Fractures occur through direct or indirect forces:
  - Direct force can happen acutely, such as a crushing-type injury from heavy objects landing on the foot, or it can be more chronic in nature, for instance, repetitive microtrauma leading to stress fractures.
  - A twisting injury in sports is an example of an indirect force that can lead to metatarsal fracture.
- The fifth metatarsal is the most commonly fractured metatarsal, and can be the result of an acute, twisting injury, or a chronic stress fracture.[39,41]

20.8.2 Symptoms

- Patients often present with pain overlying the metatarsal, swelling and ecchymosis, and difficulty or inability to bear weight.
- For stress fractures, they often report an insidious onset of pain that gradually worsens and is often exacerbated by increased impact activity.
  - These may often coincide with a recent increase in baseline level of activity, such as training for a marathon, or may be more subtle, like wearing a less supportive pair of shoes.

20.8.3 Diagnostics/Classification

- Plain radiographs are sufficient in the evaluation of metatarsal fractures, with the one exception being metatarsal base fractures, where CT or MRI may be warranted if there is an expected midfoot fracture/dislocation or associated midfoot ligamentous injury.
- Metatarsal fractures are often classified anatomically as neck, shaft, or base fractures.[39]
- Fifth metatarsal fractures are often classified by anatomic zones.
  - *Zone 1*: Proximal tuberosity fracture, the result of an avulsion force by either the lateral band of the plantar fascia or the insertion of the peroneus brevis and occurs with an acute inversion injury (▶ Fig. 20.8a, b).
  - *Zone 2 (Jones fractures)*: These occur in a watershed area of the bone 1.5 to 2 cm distal to the tuberosity with the fracture exiting into the four to five metadiaphyseal junctions (▶ Fig. 20.8c, d).
  - *Zone 3:* These occur in the metatarsal shaft, and are much less common.

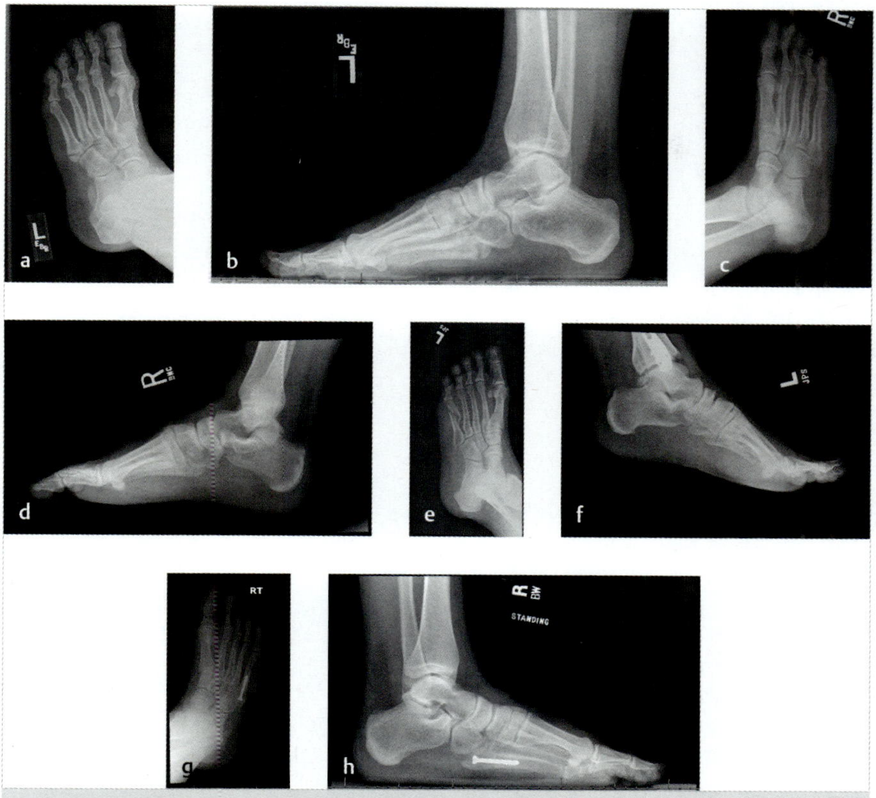

Fig. 20.8 **(a,b)** Zone I 5th metatarsal base fracture. **(c,d)** Zone II-III 5th metatarsal base fracture consistent with a Jones fracture. **(e,f)** Displaced spiral fracture of the 5th metatarsal shaft consistent with a Dancer's fracture. **(g,h)** Percutaneous screw fixation of the fracture presented in **(c,d)** performed for a rapid return to activity and work.

- Torg et al also classified these fractures based on acuity and thus healing potential:[40]
    - *Type I:* Acute injury.
    - *Type II*: Delayed union, where there was a history of previous injury, but incomplete radiographic healing and persistent pain.
    - *Type III*: Nonunion, with chronic pain and no radiographic healing.
- There is also a characteristic spiral oblique fracture of the mid to distal shaft of the fifth metatarsal fracture, commonly referred to as the "dancer's" fracture, as it was historically reported in ballet dancers[41,42,43] (▶ Fig. 20.8e, f).

20.8.4 Conservative Management

- No clear guidelines for when to operate on metatarsal fractures.
- Often managed nonoperatively with protected weight bearing in a CAM boot or post-op shoe.
- Fifth metatarsal fractures, on the other hand, typically require 6 to 8 weeks of non-weight-bearing when managed nonoperatively.
- Generally, up to 4 mm of translation and shortening and up to 10 degrees of angulation is well tolerated in metatarsal shaft fractures.
- The remaining intact metatarsals serve as internal splints and the

ligamentous connections confer stability and help minimize fracture displacement.
- Neck fractures are usually treated nonoperatively as well, unless there is significant rotational deformity or plantar angulation that could lead to metatarsalgia.[39]

20.8.5 Surgical Intervention

- Surgical options for metatarsal neck and shaft fractures:
  - Closed reduction and percutaneous pinning.
  - Open reduction and percutaneous pinning.
  - ORIF.
- Metatarsal base fractures in the absence of any midfoot dislocation or ligamentous injury are managed nonoperatively.[39]
- Treatment of fifth metatarsal fractures is based on location and chronicity.
  - *Zone 1 fractures* are almost universally managed nonoperatively.
  - *Acute Zone 2 and 3 fractures* can also be managed nonoperatively, although there is a trend toward surgery for zone 2 fractures to promote earlier fracture healing and return to sports (▶ Fig. 20.8g, h).
  - Stress fractures and delayed unions and nonunions should undergo surgery, and typically augmented with bone graft.[41,44,45]
  - Intramedullary screw fixation has shown to have superior bending stiffness and resistance to torsional loading when compared to plate fixation. Thus, we routinely use a solid intramedullary screw for fixation.
  - It is also important to assess for any cavovarus deformity, which can lead to stress fractures of the fifth metatarsal, and increased nonunion if not addressed at the time of surgery.[41,46]

20.8.6 Rehabilitation

- The vast majority of metatarsal fractures can be managed with protected weight bearing in a stiff postoperative shoe or CAM boot, with the exception being fifth metatarsal fractures.
- When managed nonoperatively, zone 2 and 3 fractures are placed in a non-weight-bearing cast for 6 to 8 weeks:
  - Conversely, when treated with screw fixation, patients are non-weight bearing for 2 weeks, then in a walking boot for 4 to 6 weeks.
- Return to sports is not allowed prior to radiographic healing.[41]

20.9 Phalanx Fractures

20.9.1 Etiology and Pathophysiology

- Most common lower extremity fractures, accounting for 3 to 8% of all injuries.
- Mechanism of injury is typically direct impact or axial load from a falling object.
- An estimated 9% of all referrals to fracture clinics are for phalangeal fractures, despite these injuries requiring operative intervention in less than 2% of cases.[47]

20.9.2 Symptoms

- Swelling, ecchymosis, and occasional deformity.
- The involved digit is tender to palpation and there is pain with ambulation.
- A subungual hematoma is pathognomonic for a distal phalanx fracture and may require decompression.

20.9.3 Diagnostics/ Classification

- Plain radiographs are sufficient for diagnosis.
- These injuries are typically classified according to location, indicating which

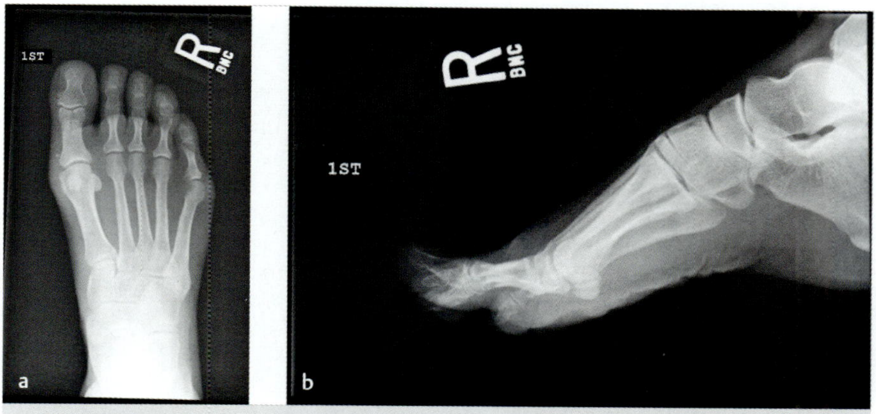

Fig. 20.9 (a,b): Hallux fracture demonstrating intra-articular extension into the interphalangeal joint. Lateral x-ray shows some extension at the fracture.

phalanx is involved and whether or not there is intra-articular extension (▶ Fig. 20.9a, b).

- There is no clear consensus on the acceptable amount of deformity that is acceptable in phalanx fractures.[47]

20.9.4 Conservative Management

- The vast majority of these fractures are managed conservatively in a post-op shoe or CAM boot.
- Buddy taping is often used for external splinting, but is not without complications, with up to 45% having skin irritation from tape adhesive, and noncompliance with taping in 65% of patients.[48]

20.9.5 Surgical Intervention

- Surgery is infrequent, with no clear radiographic parameters to guide decision-making.
- Some will advocate for fixation if there is significant rotational deformity or shortening, with the hallux being fixed more commonly than the lesser toes.
- Intra-articular extension is not necessarily an indication for surgery, as a delayed interphalangeal fusion is often technically easier to perform and has acceptable outcomes.
- Open fractures should be adequately debrided, but do not always need fixation.
- Lacerations of the nail bed or just proximal to the nail bed should be treated as an open fracture and debrided and reduced, with or without provisional pin fixation.[39]

20.9.6 Rehabilitation

- These injuries are typically treated with weight bearing as tolerated in a post-op shoe.
- Patients advance to regular shoe wear and activity as tolerated, generally over 3 to 6 weeks.

20.10 Key Testing Facts

Pilon Fracture Key Points	• Initial soft-tissue management is critical. • These are best managed in a staged fashion with delayed ORIF. • Early fibula fixation is controversial, and should be avoided if you are not the definitive treating surgery. • CT scan is critical in operative planning.
Ankle Fracture Key Points	• Ankle fractures are the most commonly treated orthopaedic injury. • Medial clear space widening on injury films or stress views indicates deltoid incompetence. • There is no consensus regarding when to treat or the appropriate method of treatment for posterior malleolar fractures or syndesmosis instability.
Calcaneal Fractures Key Points	• Most common tarsal bone fracture. • High incidence of wound dehiscence has led to less invasive techniques. • Posttraumatic subtalar arthritis is prevalent, but outcomes are better with initial ORIF when compared to nonoperative treatment.
Peritalar Dislocations Key Points	• Rare injury; typically occurs medially from high-energy trauma. • Closed reduction is often necessary and needs to be done emergently. • Bony injuries are common and need be evaluated with postreduction CT scan. • Block to reductions medially is typically extensor retinaculum or extensor digitorum brevis muscle and laterally is posterior tibialis tendon or flexor digitorum longus
Chopart Dislocations Key Points	• Rare injury but often overlooked. • Usually requires CT scan to fully evaluate. • Closed reductions are difficult, often requiring open reductions. • Open reduction and stable internal fixation and/or external fixation is required with displacement of fractures and instability.
Talus Fractures Key Points	• Fractures occur in the head, neck, or body, and are often associated with dislocations of the subtalar, talonavicular, and/or tibiotalar joints. • Tenuous blood supply of the talus creates high rates of osteonecrosis after fractures (primarily neck fractures) with higher rates associated with increased displacement. • Decreasing osteonecrosis rates is more associated with reduction accuracy more than surgical timing; ORIF is the mainstay of the treatment for any displacement. • Posttraumatic arthritis is associated with 90% of displaced talus fractures.
Lisfranc Injuries Key Points	• Lisfranc injury is a dislocation and possible fractures at the TMT joints. • Injuries should be divided into high- and low-energy injuries—the type of injury effects treatment. • Injuries are usually treated surgically unless deemed stable on weight-bearing X-rays. • Treatment of Lisfranc injuries is controversial, consisting of ORIF or primary arthrodesis.

Metatarsal Fractures Key Points	• Most metatarsal fractures can be managed with protected weight bearing in a CAM boot. • Intramedullary screw fixation of zone 2/3 fifth metatarsal fractures leads to earlier radiographic healing and quicker return to sports.
Phalanx Fractures Key Points	• Phalanx fractures are common injuries that are predominantly managed nonoperatively. • Nail bed lacerations are treated as open fractures and subungual hematomas may require decompression.

References

[1] Barei DP, Nork SE. Fractures of the tibial plafond. Foot Ankle Clin. 2008; 13(4):571–591

[2] Liporace FA, Yoon RS. Decisions and staging leading to definitive open management of pilon fractures: where have we come from and where are we now? J Orthop Trauma. 2012; 26(8):488–498

[3] Crist BD, Khazzam M, Murtha YM, Della Rocca GJ. Pilon fractures: advances in surgical management. J Am Acad Orthop Surg. 2011; 19(10):612–622

[4] Kurylo JC, Datta N, Iskander KN, Tornetta P, III. Does the fibula need to be fixed in complex pilon fractures? J Orthop Trauma. 2015; 29(9):424–427

[5] Clare MP. A rational approach to ankle fractures. Foot Ankle Clin. 2008; 13(4):593–610

[6] Aigner R, Salomia C, Lechler P, Pahl R, Frink M. Relationship of prolonged operative time and comorbidities with complications after geriatric ankle fractures. Foot Ankle Int. 2017; 38(1):41–48

[7] Orr JD, Kusnezov NA, Waterman BR, Bader JO, Romano DM, Belmont PJ, Jr. Occupational outcomes and return to running following internal fixation of ankle fractures in a high-demand population. Foot Ankle Int. 2015; 36(7):780–786

[8] Kwon JY, Gitajn IL, Walton P, Miller TJ, Appleton P, Rodriguez EK. A cadaver study revisiting the original methodology of Lauge-Hansen and a commentary on modern usage. J Bone Joint Surg Am. 2015; 97(7):604–609

[9] Kortekangas TH, Pakarinen HJ, Savola O, et al. Syndesmotic fixation in supination-external rotation ankle fractures: a prospective randomized study. Foot Ankle Int. 2014; 35(10):988–995

[10] Herscovici D, Jr, Scaduto JM, Infante A. Conservative treatment of isolated fractures of the medial malleolus. J Bone Joint Surg Br. 2007; 89(1): 89–93

[11] Koval KJ, Egol KA, Cheung Y, Goodwin DW, Spratt KF. Does a positive ankle stress test indicate the need for operative treatment after lateral malleolus fracture? A preliminary report. J Orthop Trauma. 2007; 21(7):449–455

[12] Weber M, Burmeister H, Flueckiger G, Krause FG. The use of weightbearing radiographs to assess the stability of supination-external rotation fractures of the ankle. Arch Orthop Trauma Surg. 2010; 130 (5):693–698

[13] Minihane KP, Lee C, Ahn C, Zhang LQ, Merk BR. Comparison of lateral locking plate and antiglide plate for fixation of distal fibular fractures in osteoporotic bone: a biomechanical study. J Orthop Trauma. 2006; 20(8):562–566

[14] Drijfhout van Hooff CC, Verhage SM, Hoogendoorn JM. Influence of fragment size and postoperative joint congruency on long-term outcome of posterior malleolar fractures. Foot Ankle Int. 2015; 36(6):673–678

[15] Hartwich K, Lorente Gomez A, Pyrc J, Gut R, Rammelt S, Grass R. Biomechanical analysis of stability of posterior antiglide plating in osteoporotic pronation abduction ankle fracture model with posterior tibial fragment. Foot Ankle Int. 2017; 38(1):58–65

[16] O'Connor TJ, Mueller B, Ly TV, Jacobson AR, Nelson ER, Cole PA. "A to p" screw versus posterolateral plate for posterior malleolus fixation in trimalleolar ankle fractures. J Orthop Trauma. 2015; 29(4):e151–e156

[17] Bartoníček J, Rammelt S, Tuček M. Posterior malleolar fractures: changing concepts and recent developments. Foot Ankle Clin. 2017; 22(1):125–145

[18] Swords MP, Sands A, Shank JR. Late treatment of syndesmotic injuries. Foot Ankle Clin. 2017; 22(1): 65–75

[19] Song DJ, Lanzi JT, Groth AT, et al. The effect of syndesmosis screw removal on the reduction of the distal tibiofibular joint: a prospective radiographic study. Foot Ankle Int. 2014; 35(6):543–548

[20] Hsu AR, Lareau CR, Anderson RB. Repair of acute superficial deltoid complex avulsion during ankle fracture fixation in National Football League players. Foot Ankle Int. 2015; 36(11):1272–1278

[21] Kocadal O, Yucel M, Pepe M, Aksahin E, Aktekin CN. Evaluation of reduction accuracy of suture-button and screw fixation techniques for syndesmotic injuries. Foot Ankle Int. 2016; 37(12):1317–1325

[22] Jackson JB, III, Jacobson L, Banerjee R, Nickisch F. Distraction subtalar arthrodesis. Foot Ankle Clin. 2015; 20(2):335–351

[23] Swords MP, Penny P. Early fixation of calcaneus fractures. Foot Ankle Clin. 2017; 22(1):93–104

[24] Epstein N, Chandran S, Chou L. Current concepts review: intra-articular fractures of the calcaneus. Foot Ankle Int. 2012; 33(1):79–86

[25] Kiewiet NJ, Sangeorzan BJ. Calcaneal fracture management: extensile lateral approach versus small incision technique. Foot Ankle Clin. 2017; 22 (1):77–91

[26] Clare MP, Crawford WS. Managing complications of calcaneus fractures. Foot Ankle Clin. 2017; 22(1): 105–116

[27] Radnay CS, Clare MP, Sanders RW. Subtalar fusion after displaced intra-articular calcaneal fractures: does initial operative treatment matter? J Bone Joint Surg Am. 2009; 91(3):541–546

[28] Bibbo C, Anderson RB, Davis WH. Injury characteristics and the clinical outcome of subtalar dislocations: a clinical and radiographic analysis of 25 cases. Foot Ankle Int. 2003; 24(2):158–163

[29] Rammelt S, Goronzy J. Subtalar dislocations. Foot Ankle Clin. 2015; 20(2):253–264

[30] Rammelt S, Schepers T. Chopart injuries: when to fix and when to fuse? Foot Ankle Clin. 2017; 22(1): 163–180

[31] Swords MP, Schramski M, Switzer K, Nemec S. Chopart fractures and dislocations. Foot Ankle Clin. 2008; 13(4):679–693, viii

[32] Fortin PT, Balazsy JE. Talus fractures: evaluation and treatment. J Am Acad Orthop Surg. 2001; 9(2): 114–127

[33] Grear BJ. Review of talus fractures and surgical timing. Orthop Clin North Am. 2016; 47(3):625–637

[34] Early JS. Talus fracture management. Foot Ankle Clin. 2008; 13(4):635–657

[35] Lewis JS, Jr, Anderson RB. Lisfranc injuries in the athlete. Foot Ankle Int. 2016; 37(12):1374–1380

[36] Coetzee JC. Making sense of lisfranc injuries. Foot Ankle Clin. 2008; 13(4):695–704, ix

[37] Eleftheriou KI, Rosenfeld PF. Lisfranc injury in the athlete: evidence supporting management from sprain to fracture dislocation. Foot Ankle Clin. 2013; 18(2):219–236

[38] Coss HS, Manos RE, Buoncristiani A, Mills WJ. Abduction stress and AP weightbearing radiography of purely ligamentous injury in the tarsometatarsal joint. Foot Ankle Int. 1998; 19(8):537–541

[39] Armagan OE, Shereff MJ. Injuries to the toes and metatarsals. Orthop Clin North Am. 2001; 32(1): 1–10

[40] Torg JS, Balduini FC, Zelko RR, Pavlov H, Peff TC, Das M. Fractures of the base of the fifth metatarsal distal to the tuberosity. Classification and guidelines for non-surgical and surgical management. J Bone Joint Surg Am. 1984 Feb;66(2):209–14

[41] Bowes J, Buckley R. Fifth metatarsal fractures and current treatment. World J Orthop. 2016; 7(12): 793–800

[42] Fetzer GB, Wright RW. Metatarsal shaft fractures and fractures of the proximal fifth metatarsal. Clin Sports Med. 2006; 25(1):139–150, x

[43] Aynardi M, Pedowitz DI, Saffel H, Piper C, Raikin SM. Outcome of nonoperative management of displaced oblique spiral fractures of the fifth metatarsal shaft. Foot Ankle Int. 2013; 34(12): 1619–1623

[44] O'Malley M, DeSandis B, Allen A, Levitsky M, O'Malley Q, Williams R. Operative treatment of fifth metatarsal jones fractures (zones II and III) in the NBA. Foot Ankle Int. 2016; 37(5):488–500

[45] Solan M, Davies M. Nonunion of fifth metatarsal fractures. Foot Ankle Clin. 2014; 19(3):499–519

[46] Huh J, Glisson RR, Matsumoto T, Easley ME. Biomechanical comparison of intramedullary screw versus low-profile plate fixation of a jones fracture. Foot Ankle Int. 2016; 37(4):411–418

[47] Eves TB, Oddy MJ. Do broken toes need follow-up in the fracture clinic? J Foot Ankle Surg. 2016; 55 (3):488–491

[48] Won SH, Lee S, Chung CY, et al. Buddy taping: is it a safe method for treatment of finger and toe injuries? Clin Orthop Surg. 2014; 6(1):26–31

21 Circular External Fixation in Foot and Ankle Surgery

Austin T. Fragomen and S. Robert Rozbruch

Abstract

External fixation has been an invaluable tool in treating pathology of the foot and ankle. Circular fixators allow for dynamic movement including gradual correction of deformities and contractures and bone lengthening. Circular fixators are ideal for achieving optimal stability, eradicating infection by removing the need for internal hardware at the operative site, allowing for early weight bearing, and executing the gradual correction of multiple complex deformities, providing an ideal environment for soft-tissue tolerance and osteogenesis. The hardware has evolved since the time of Ilizarov, but the principles of limb stability and tissue regeneration are unchanged. Certain conditions affecting the foot and ankle lend themselves to treatment with external fixation including distal tibial deformity, complex pilon fracture, ankle equinus contracture, salvage of failed total ankle replacement, posttraumatic ankle osteoarthritis, and Charcot's neuroarthropathy. These conditions will be discussed in greater detail and the benefits of circular fixation reviewed.

Keywords: circular external fixation, Ilizarov, deformity, nonunion, malunion, ankle distraction, complex ankle arthrodesis.

21.1 General Introduction

- External fixation has been an invaluable tool in treating pathology of the foot and ankle:[1,2]
  - Dynamic movement allows for gradual correction of deformities and contractures.
  - Spanning of a joint provides stability yet allows for motion.
  - Avoidance of internal fixation is advantageous in the setting of infection.
  - Stability is enhanced with gradual compression of fusions and nonunions.
- It is ideal for the following:
  - Achieving optimal stability.
  - Eradicating infection by removing the need for hardware at the operative site.
  - Allowing for early weight bearing.
  - Executing the gradual correction of multiple complex deformities, providing an ideal environment for soft-tissue tolerance and osteogenesis.

21.2 Diagnostics

- Anteroposterior (AP) and lateral radiographs lack the ability to interconnect the complex relationship between hindfoot, midfoot, and forefoot in many circumstances.
- Weight-bearing radiographs are essential, and the Saltzman view of the hindfoot has been helpful in uncovering hindfoot deformity.
- Computed tomography (CT) scan has been a tremendous asset for preoperative planning of deformity correction:
  - This can be done classically or as a weight-bearing study.
  - Define the integrity of the joints of the foot and ankle, the position of these joints relative to one another (and therefore the apex of any deformity), and the percentage of healing at an osteotomy or fusion site.
  - CT scan findings and physical examination help us understand the combined rotational and angular deformities affecting multiple joints.

- The proper technique for frame application is the foundation for frame stability and is the key to achieving success.
- *Universal principles* of stable frame application include the following:
  - Smaller rings are more stable.
  - Increasing the diameter of pins and wires increases rigidity of the fixation elements.
  - Spreading fixation improves stability.
  - Multiplanar fixation provides rigidity.
  - More fixation increases stability.
  - The use of additional rings improves stability.[3]
- Safe zones for passage of Ilizarov wires requires thoughtful study of cross-sectional anatomy.

Certain conditions lend themselves to treatment with external fixation. The most common pathologies, their characteristics, and nuanced treatments have been the following sections.

21.3 Distal Tibial Deformity

21.3.1 Etiology and Pathophysiology

- Deformity of the distal aspect of the tibia, whether posttraumatic, congenital, or secondary to a growth plate disturbance, places the ankle and subtalar joints at an oblique angle introducing abnormal stress often leading to ankle osteoarthritis.
- Supramalleolar osteotomy (SMO) is an effective method for correcting this deformity and preventing arthritis.[4,5]
- If arthritis is present, then the procedure will often reduce ankle pain or allow for subsequent ankle replacement surgery.

21.3.2 Symptoms

- Ankle pain and dysfunctional gait.

21.3.3 Diagnostics and Classification

- Radiographs and a CT scan or magnetic resonance imaging (MRI) of the ankle are warranted to understand the deformity and establish the presence and severity of ankle and subtalar joint osteoarthritis.
- The coronal plane, sagittal plane, and axial plane all have a translation and angulation direction and magnitude.
- The AP X-ray will reveal varus and valgus deformities.
- Lateral X-ray shows apex anterior and apex posterior angulation.
- Long-standing X-ray will allow for the measurement of axial translation (leg length discrepancy or LLD).
- Prone physical examination (thigh–foot axis).
- CT version study reveals internal and external rotational (torsional) deformity.
- Many deformities are out of the plane of the standard AP and lateral X-rays (oblique plane), but modern technology has produced the hexapod external fixator.
  - It allows simplifying the planning of deformity correction and think about the direction in the normal coronal and sagittal planes we are comfortable with.
- Radiographs also show the level of the deformity and allow for osteotomy planning (▶ Fig. 21.1 and ▶ Fig. 21.2).

21.3.4 Surgical Intervention

- The SMO is the mainstay of treatment for distal tibial deformity.
- It is created in the metaphyseal region where the blood supply of the bone is reliable.
- Although internal fixation is the most common method for bony stabilization after SMO, external fixation is the most versatile method for carrying out the reduction of the bone after osteotomy.[6,7,8,9,10]

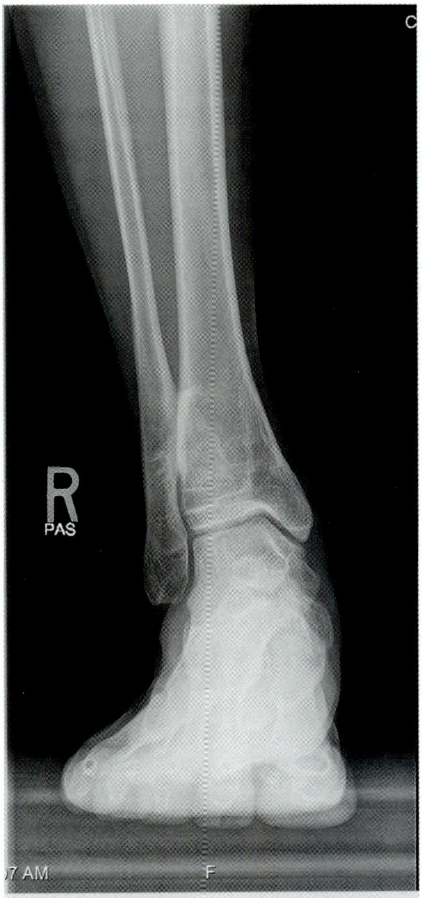

Fig. 21.1 This anteroposterior (AP), weight-bearing radiograph shows a varus deformity of the distal tibia with no apparent joint involvement.

- External fixators can gradually correct the deformity over the course of weeks taking advantage of the powerful healing produced by distraction osteogenesis.
- Soft tissue including nerves are at risk with large deformity correction, and the use of gradual correction with external fixation mitigates this risk (▶ Fig. 21.3).
- The bone can be corrected in multiple planes simultaneously and translated appropriately to keep the tibial axis aligned with the ankle joint, a necessary maneuver for the correction of larger magnitude deformities (▶ Fig. 21.4 and ▶ Fig. 21.5).
- Length can also be added to the correction using this method reestablishing equal limb lengths. The frame is typically worn for 3 to 4 months and removed once bony consolidation is seen on radiographs.
- If osteoarthritis of the ankle is also present, then the joint can be addressed simultaneously and distracted with the addition of a foot ring to allow for some cartilage regeneration and subchondral remodeling.[11]

21.4 Complex Pilon

21.4.1 Etiology and Pathophysiology

- Treatment for pilon fractures includes the following:
  - Early, provisional stabilization with pin-to-bar external fixation.
  - A period of soft-tissue recovery.
  - Staged open reduction with internal plate and screw fixation.
- Some injuries including severe soft-tissue compromise, metaphyseal bone loss, and comminution beyond salvage are too complex to fit into that treatment protocol. These are better treated definitively with external fixation.[12,13]

21.4.2 Diagnostics and Classification

- The best evaluation of a pilon fracture is done after traction has been placed on the injured limb.
- The limb should be spanned with a simple pin-to-bar frame and then reevaluated with radiographs and CT scan.

21.4.3 Surgical Intervention

- A limited, percutaneous open reduction is helpful for reconstructing the articular surface.

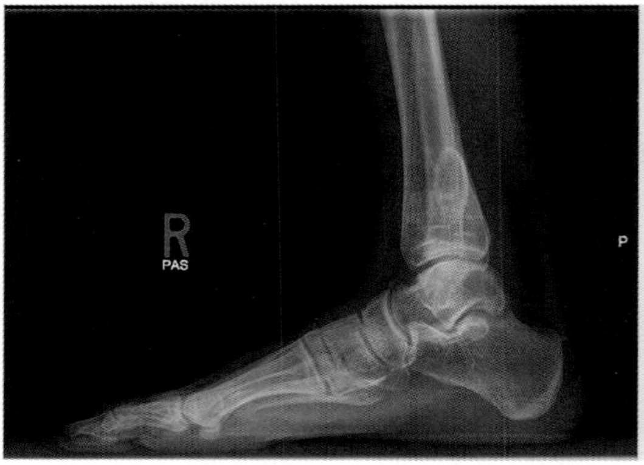

Fig. 21.2 A lateral film of the same patient shows a subtle loss of tibial tilt resulting in a block to dorsiflexion.

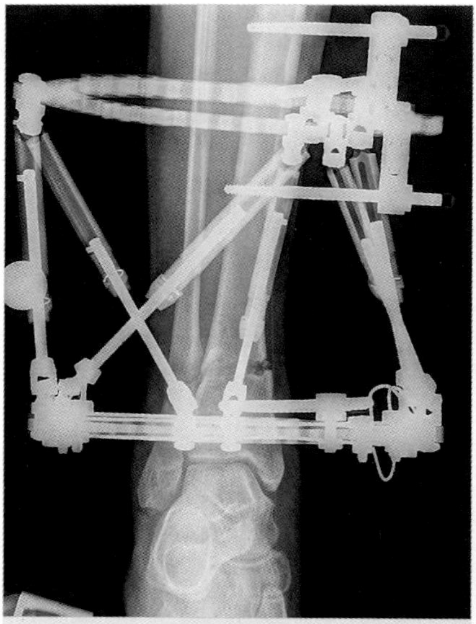

Fig. 21.3 This postosteotomy radiograph demonstrates the distal fragment being translated medially through an opening wedge gradual correction osteotomy.

- This can be done through a far less soft-tissue stripping than the traditional approach since no plates need to be inserted.
- Small screws (or wires) are utilized to hold the reduction of key fragments, and then the external fixator is used to further stabilize the limb (► Fig. 21.6).

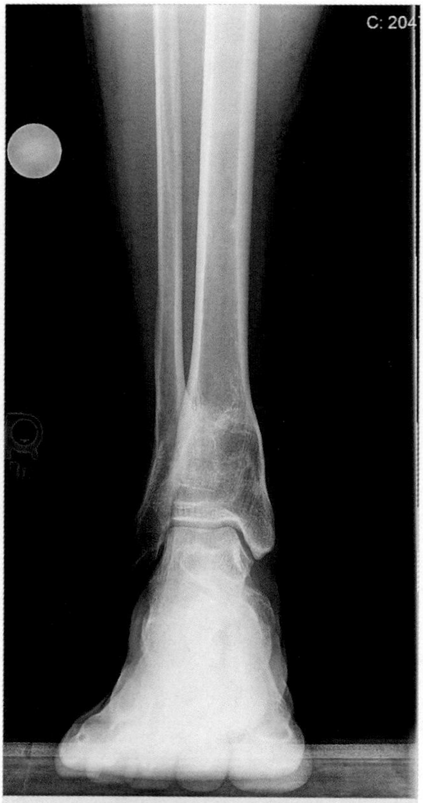

Fig. 21.4 The final anteroposterior (AP) view shows complete correction of the varus deformity. The ankle joint is located directly underneath the tibia, which required medial translation of the distal tibial fragment.

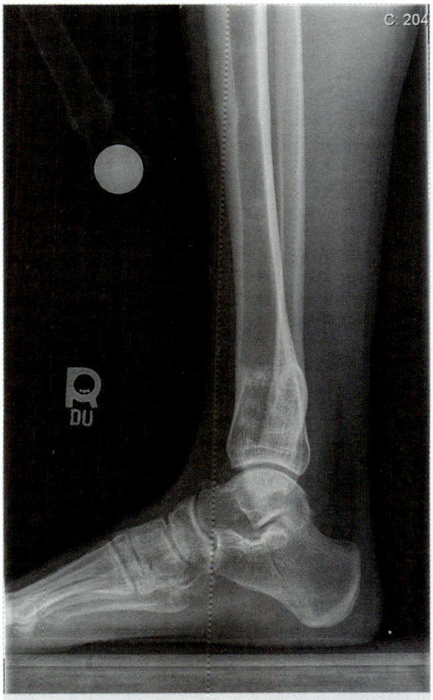

Fig. 21.5 The final lateral X-ray demonstrates restoration of the ankle joint tilt (orientation) and subtle translation of the distal tibia posteriorly in order to keep the talus underneath the tibia.

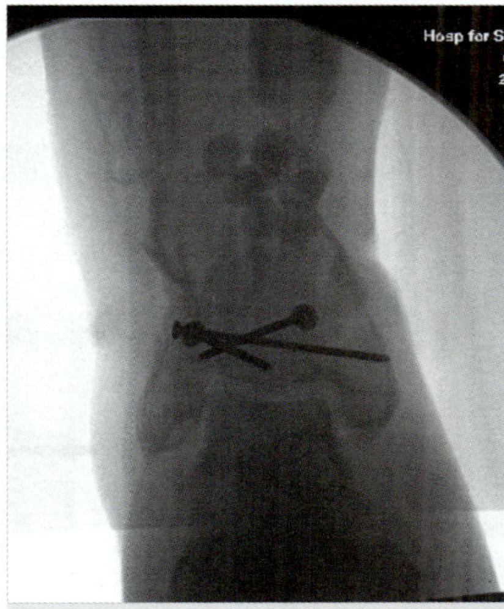

Fig. 21.6 This intra-op anteroposterior (AP) fluoroscopy shot shows the articular reduction obtained with limited internal fixation.

  - Olive wires are particularly helpful in buttressing the fragments preventing their displacement.
  - Many fine wires are inserted circumferentially around the distal fragments based on preoperative planning using the axial CT scan images.
  - The epiphyseal block is then reduced to the diaphysis by manipulating these two rings.
  - If there is a meta-diaphyseal bone defect, then this can be addressed through a proximal tibial osteotomy and distraction osteogenesis (▶ Fig. 21.7).
- The ankle can be spanned to add stability to the distal tibial fixation block.
- Spanning the ankle will prevent equinus contracture in patients with compromised dorsiflexion ability and in patients undergoing bone lengthening/transport.
- Plating the fibula is a point of contention when circular fixation has been selected as the definitive treatment.
  - An intact fibula makes manipulation of the metaphysis with diaphyseal and epiphyseal rings difficult and may increase the risk of nonunion in this setting.
  - As a rule, we advocate NOT fixing the fibula when using a circular frame for pilon fractures (▶ Fig. 21.8).
- For pilon fractures with articular destruction beyond repair, primary fusion is a reliable option.
  - External fixation is preferable if the soft-tissue sleeve is compromised.

21.5 Equinus Ankle

21.5.1 Etiology and Pathophysiology

- Equinus: joint contracture leaving the foot in plantar flexion.

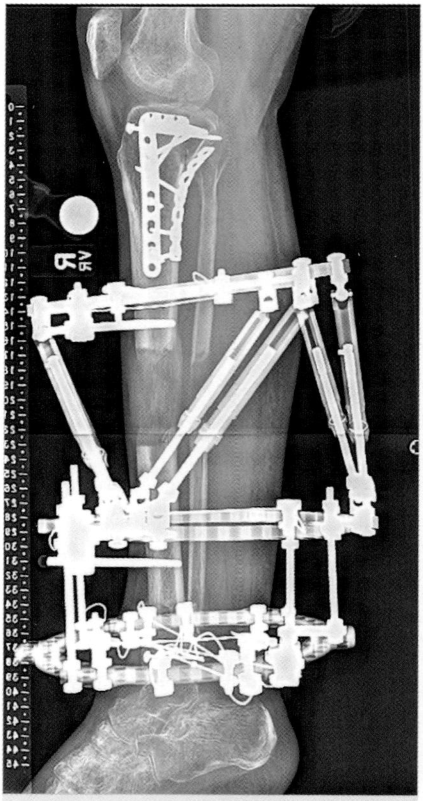

Fig. 21.7 The hexapod external fixator has been applied to reduce and compress the bone defect site and to lengthen the tibia through a mid-diaphyseal osteotomy site. Distraction osteogenesis is used to grow new bone at the lengthening site. Care is taken to ensure the fixation elements do not contact the internal fixation plates at the proximal tibia.

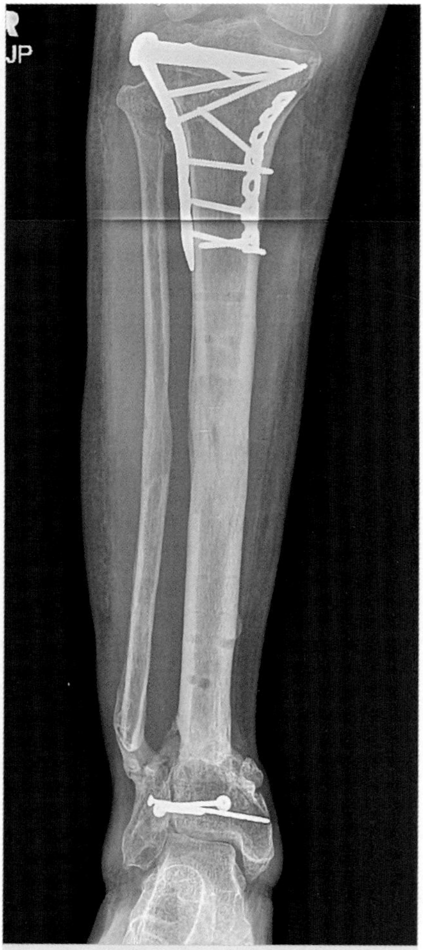

Fig. 21.8 A final anteroposterior (AP) view shows a fully healed tibia reconstruction after frame removal. The midshaft lengthening site is all autogenous bone and does not rely on internal fixation for support. The fibula was never plated in this case.

- The etiology of this deformity typically falls into one of the following categories:
  - **Neurogenic** (including postpolio, post-nerve injury, clubfoot, and spastic):
    - It is secondary to weakness of the ankle dorsiflexors relative to strong plantarflexors.
    - The posterior tibial tendon is a powerful force driving the foot into varus as well as plantar flexion in these cases.
    - Challenges in these patients are the following:
      * Preventing recurrence of the deformity after correction.
      * Not overweakening the patient causing the opposite deformity (calcaneus ankle position).

- **Posttraumatic** (ankle or pilon fracture, compartment syndrome):
  - It requires a careful assessment of the soft tissues for planning safe corridors for soft-tissue releases and for the safe placement of percutaneous fixation (wires and half pins for external fixation).

21.5.2 Symptoms

- It results in altered gait, metatarsalgia, lesser toe contractures, painful ankle osteoarthritis, difficulty with shoe wear, and ipsilateral knee hyperextension with pain.

21.5.3 Diagnostics and Classification

- Physical examination should determine the following:
  - Flexibility of the contracture.
  - Presence of spasticity.
  - An imbalance between the gastrocnemius and soleus tension.
  - The tension in the toe flexors.
  - The flexibility of varus hindfoot deformity.
  - The ability of the ankle dorsiflexor muscles to contract the soft-tissue sleeve.
  - The neurovascular status.
- Weight-bearing radiographs of the foot and ankle:
  - These are difficult to interpret due to coexisting deformities including hindfoot varus, cavus, midfoot adduction, and midfoot supination.
  - In polio, for example, patients often have midfoot cavus that looks like ankle equinus:
    - In these cases, a CT scan is very helpful.
    - A flat-topped talus needs to be recognized with imaging prior to attempting a correction as this may change the plan considerably.
  - Neurogenic equinus is often better understood after electrocardiogram-nerve conduction study (EMG-NCS) testing:
    - It will define the role for tendon transfer in preventing recurrence of the deformity after correction.
    - Posttraumatic equinus may require an MRI scan to look for muscle integrity, signs of remote compartment syndrome, and evidence of deep infection or neuromas.
- Botox injection differentiates between spasticity and true contracture.
  - Examining the deformity 2 weeks after Botox injection will reveal the true extent of the contracture and may compel the surgeon to seek a less aggressive treatment plan.

21.5.4 Surgical Intervention

- Key: The least aggressive alternative that will straighten the deformity and minimize the risk of recurrence.
- Soft-tissue lengthening is typically employed first:
  - Gastrocnemius lengthening is done if only the gastrocnemius is tight.
  - An Achilles lengthening is performed if both the gastrocnemius and soleus are tight.
  - A tendo-Achilles percutaneous lengthening is done for lesser deformities.
  - Open Z-lengthening of the Achilles is done for larger deformities.
  - The posterior tibial tendon can be released, fractionally lengthened at the musculotendinous junction, or transferred to the dorsum of the foot to assist with dorsiflexion power after the correction with external fixation.
  - If strong, the anterior tibial tendon can be split and transferred to the lateral foot to minimize inversion particularly in spastic patients.
  - The tibial nerve can be decompressed through a tarsal tunnel release, which is a safe option for large, acute contracture corrections and for patients who have undergone previous

posteromedial ankle surgery where the nerve will likely be entrapped in scar tissue.

- If there is extensive scarring, then the soft tissue can be treated with only the frame and gradual correction (▶ Fig. 21.9a, b).

- If the full correction was obtained through releases, then casting is adequate.
- If there is residual equinus, then external fixation offers a safe way to gradually correct the remainder of the contracture gradually.

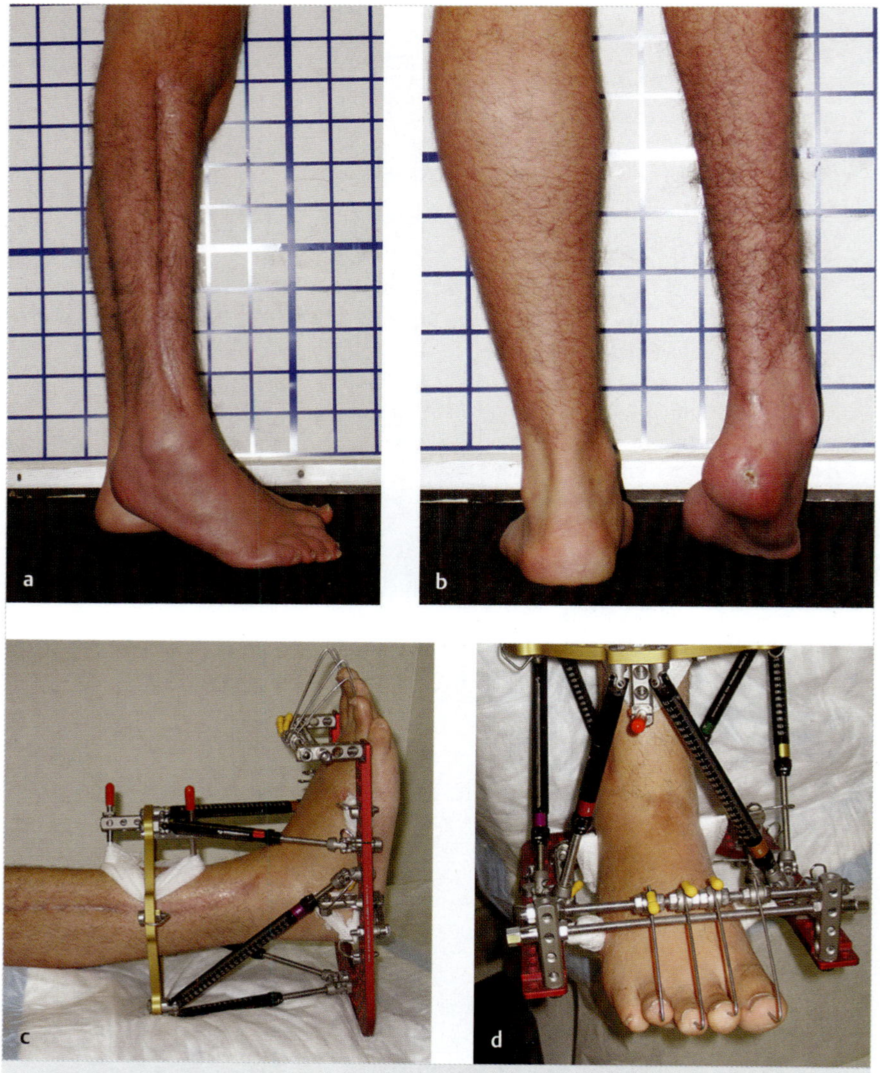

Fig. 21.9 (a) This clinical photograph shows a severe equinus deformity with soft-tissue scarring after compartment syndrome. **(b)** A photograph of the same patient from behind demonstrates the varus component of the deformity. **(c)** The external fixator was used to gradually stretch the foot and ankle into a neutral position. **(d)** The toes required pinning to prevent flexion deformity.

  - The slow stretching of the scar tissue and neurovascular structures is very well tolerated.
  - If there is a strong varus hindfoot deformity, then this needs to be corrected prior to addressing the equinus contracture:
    - Once this is done, the ankle equinus can be stretched with a minor frame adjustment (▶ Fig. 21.9c).
- The decision must be made regarding the risk of the toes contracting into a claw-toe deformity during the equinus correction:
  - If this is a likely complication, then flexor tenotomies of toes 2 to 5 or release of the flexor hallucis longus (FHL) and flexor digitorum longus (FDL) at the knot of Henry should be performed with K-wire pinning of all toes in extension (▶ Fig. 21.9d).
- Ankle fusion is another method for correcting an equinus contracture and preventing recurrence:
  - If the joint is arthritic or flaccid, then this is a good option as a primary treatment.
  - The deformity still needs to be corrected before fusion.
  - Bone can be resected from the tibia and talus to allow for an acute, tension-free correction of the contracture.
  - Ankle fusion can be fixed with either internal or external fixation.

21.6 Failed Total Ankle Replacement

21.6.1 Etiology and Pathophysiology

- Total ankle replacement has a significant failure rate of 29.3% by 10 years postsurgery.[14]
- Once an ankle prosthesis has loosened or collapsed, the implant needs to be removed, leaving a large bone defect.
  - The majority requires hindfoot fusion.
  - Most foot surgeons have chosen to insert a femoral head allograft into the defect and stabilize it with an intramedullary (IM) ankle arthrodesis nail despite high rates of collapse and nonunion.[15]
  - Our approach with bone defects in and about the ankle has been to shorten the defect to fusion and lengthen the proximal tibia.[16,17,18]

21.6.2 Symptoms

- Pain is the dominant complaint of people with failed ankle replacement.

21.6.3 Diagnostics and Classification

- Weight-bearing radiographs will show subsidence and loosening of the implant.
- CT scan provides greater detail of bony defects.
- MRI can demonstrate signs of infection provided that metal suppression sequencing can be implemented.

21.6.4 Surgical Intervention

- Circular fixation provides the ability to acutely or gradually shorten the defect, attaining contact between cut surfaces of the ankle and allowing for a reliable fusion.[19]
- The talus is typically so compromised that a subtalar fusion is needed to prevent further talar collapse (▶ Fig. 21.10).
- In cases with minimal talus, a tibiocalcaneal fusion is pursued.
  - Limb shortening of 3 cm can be anticipated,
  - Framing can compress fusion site and lengthen the proximal tibial osteotomy site[16,20] (▶ Fig. 21.11).
  - For larger discrepancies, alternative methods can be used such as lengthening and then nailing (LATN) to enhance the healing rate and reduce the time in the frame.[21,22]

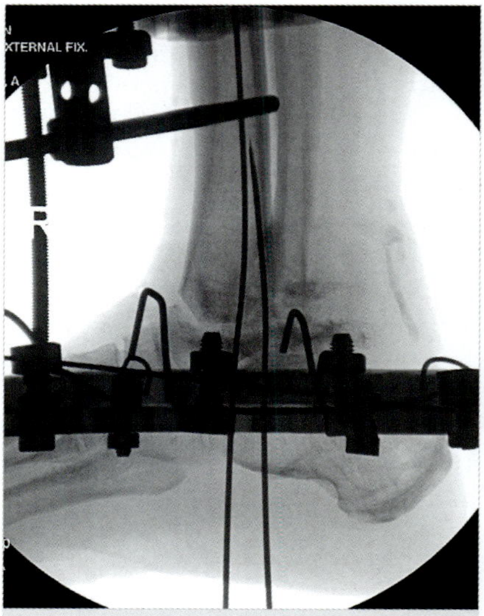

Fig. 21.10 The total ankle implant has been removed, and the thin talus remnant was retained. The defect had to be shortened gradually along the axial K-wires until the tibia docked with the talus. The subtalar joint was prepared for fusion as well.

  - The magnetic internal lengthening nail[23,24] can also be used in lieu of the proximal ring to provide a more comfortable lengthening experience (▶ Fig. 21.12).

21.7 Ankle: Posttraumatic Osteoarthritis

21.7.1 Etiology and Pathophysiology

- Posttraumatic osteoarthritis of the ankle is a common condition whose treatment continues to be suboptimal.
- Fusion causes complete immobilization of the ankle with gait disturbance and excessive loading of the adjacent foot joints eventually leading to further arthritic pain.

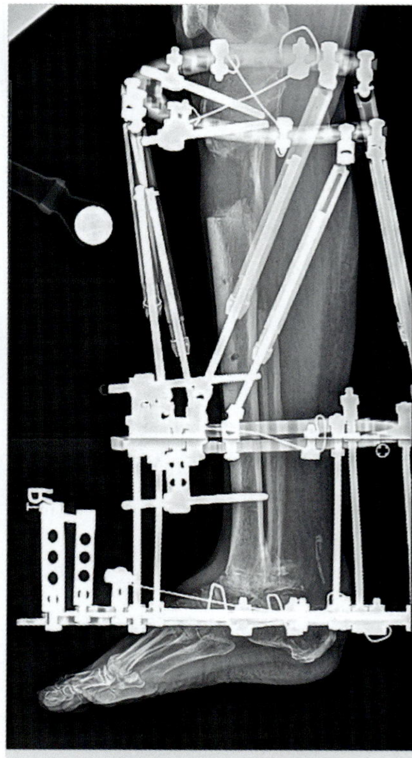

Fig. 21.11 In this lateral radiograph, the ankle fusion is seen, compressed between the foot ring and the central ring. There is a proximal tibia lengthening site with newly regenerated bone seen starting to grow between the cut ends. (The *white circle* in the picture is a calibration ball.)

- Ankle replacement arthroplasty is a poor alternative in younger patients where it has a limited life span.
- Ankle distraction arthroplasty offers a joint preservation approach to reduce arthritic ankle pain and improve patient function.[25,26,27]
- An external fixator is used to place traction across the tibiotalar joint, while allowing articulated range of motion, over the course of 3 months.
- Patients enjoy reduced pain for many years.[28]
- The success is thought to be a result of a combination of reduced subchondral

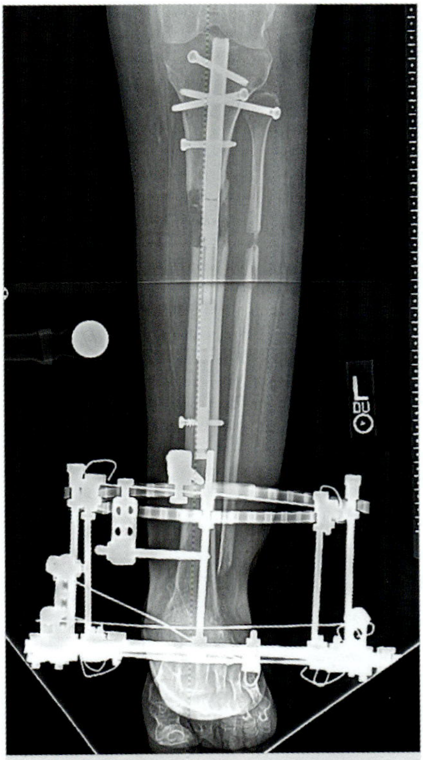

Fig. 21.12 This alternative approach utilizes the external fixator for the complex ankle fusion while taking advantage of the newer internal lengthening intramedullary (IM) nail to achieve the distraction osteogenesis for limb length equalization.

sclerosis, remodeling of subchondral cysts, and thickening of articular surface reparative cartilage.[29,30]

21.7.2 Symptoms

- Posttraumatic ankle arthritis causes pain and stiffness.
- The pain is particularly severe when staring up from a resting position and after many hours of weight-bearing activity.
- Stiffness is similarly worse in the morning and decreases throughout the day.

21.7.3 Diagnostics and Classification

- Usually posttraumatic:
  - The trauma typically takes two forms:
    - A fracture with or without deformity of the ankle and tibia:
      - Typically, more symmetrical in the coronal plane and tends to involve the anterior portion of the joint.
    - Repetitive ankle sprains:
      - Almost always asymmetric with varus intra-articular alignment and severe medial joint wear.
    - Surgical hardware may be present that can contribute to the pain and can complicate further surgery.

21.7.4 Surgical Intervention

- Ankle distraction arthroplasty spans across the ankle joint. Distraction applied between these rings results in a widening of the ankle joint space.[31]
- A distraction gap of 6 mm is thought to be adequate to prevent contact between the tibial and talar surfaces during weight bearing while in the frame.[32]
- Many adjuvant procedures can be performed in the same surgical setting including the following: removal of hardware, arthroscopy, arthrotomy, osteophyte excision, deltoid release/mobilization of the medial or lateral gutters, microfracture, bone marrow aspirate injection, bone grafting subchondral cysts, Achilles' tendon lengthening, gastrocnemius recession, and tarsal tunnel release.
- A modest amount of acute distraction (< 4 mm) can be applied acutely in the operating room but it is safest to apply at the rate of 1 mm/d starting from the first postoperative day.
- Weight-bearing radiographs demonstrate when the desired joint space has been achieved (▶ Fig. 21.13).

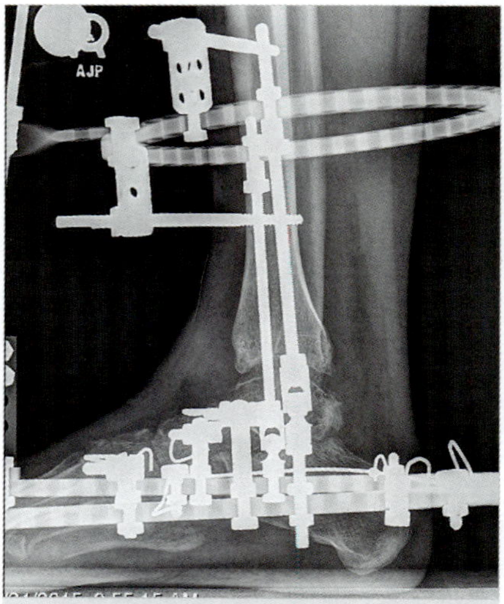

Fig. 21.13 This lateral X-ray shows a two-ring, hinged, ankle frame with a distracted arthritic ankle demonstrating a 6-mm gap in the ankle joint space.

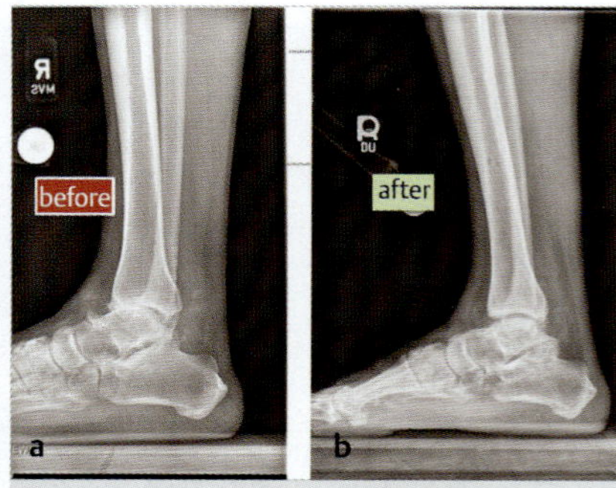

Fig. 21.14 **(a)** The before radiograph shows anterior talar subluxation and advanced asymmetric joint wear. **(b)** The after radiograph, taken 1 year after completion of treatment, shows improved joint symmetry and a large widening of the joint space on a weight-bearing film.

- The frame we use is articulated, and ankle range of motion exercises are initiated soon after surgery.
- The external fixator is maintained for 3 months and then removed under anesthesia (▶ Fig. 21.14 and ▶ Fig. 21.15).
- SMO can be performed concurrently with distraction to correct the underlying tibial deformity that is contributing to the ankle arthritis.

21.8 Charcot Ankle, Hindfoot, and Midfoot Deformity

21.8.1 Etiology and Pathophysiology

- Charcot's neuroarthropathic collapse of the hindfoot and/or midfoot, typically the result of diabetic neuropathy, continues to present challenges to orthopaedic foot specialists.

21.8.2 Symptoms

- Patients rarely have pain but instead notice a new onset foot deformity and crepitus postcollapse.
- Deformity often leads to skin ulceration that can be limb threatening.
- Shoe wear becomes a challenge from swelling and deformity, and instability can be difficult to control even with custom-molded boots due to skin irritation.

21.8.3 Diagnostics and Classification

- Radiographs and CT scan will demonstrate bony pathology.
- CT helps clarify the full extent of the bony damage.
- MRI will help determine if there is osteomyelitis present under an ulcerative site.

21.8.4 Surgical Intervention

- The goal is to correct the deformity and fuse the involved joints.

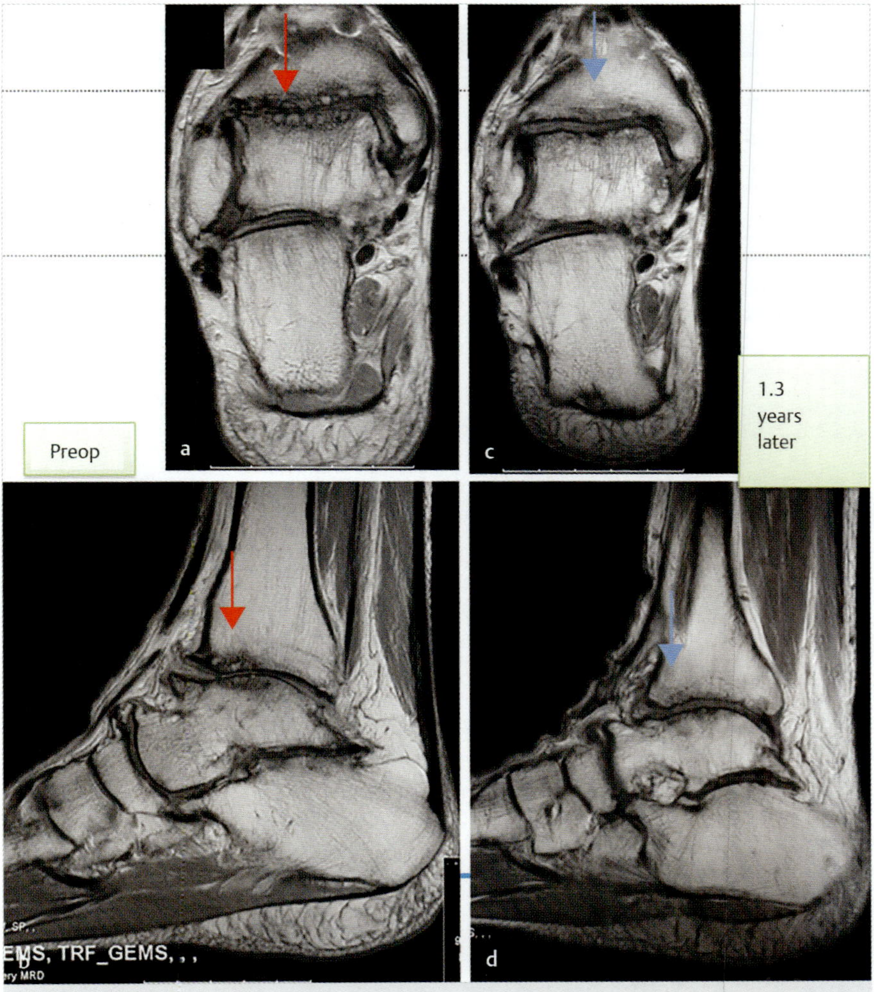

Fig. 21.15 The presurgery **(a)** coronal and **(b)** sagittal magnetic resonance (MR) images show subchondral cysts and joint space narrowing with cartilage loss. **(c,d)** The postsurgical MR images taken 1.3 years after frame removal show filling of the cysts and soft-tissue interposition (reparative cartilage) in the joint space.

- Surgery can be performed using either internal or external fixation.
- External fixation offers the ability to create a highly stable construct with sustained compression across the fusion site (▶ Fig. 21.16).
- Specific strategies in Charcot include the use of all-wire frames to avoid damage to the pathologic bone, the addition of extra rings and points of fixation to avoid pin loosening, and the use of adjuvant internal fixation at the time of frame removal to protect the fusion site. For example, an ankle arthrodesis IM nail can be inserted to prevent refracture of a tibiotalocalcaneal tibio-talo-calcaneal (TTC) fusion immediately following removal of the external fixator. We recommend using an antibiotic-coated IM nail in that circumstance.

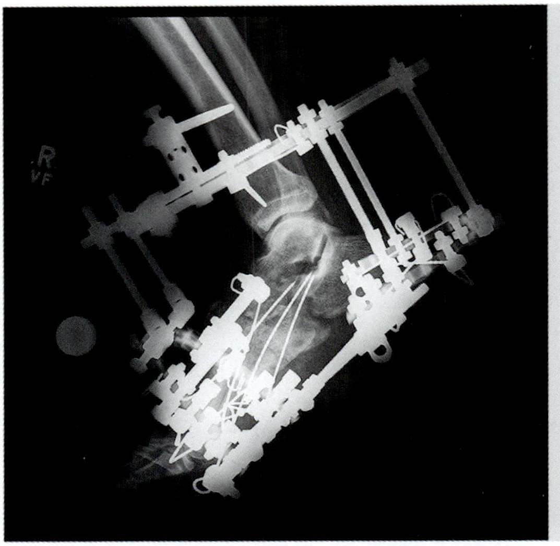

Fig. 21.16 This lateral radiograph postmidfoot reconstruction and arthrodesis for Charcot's collapse shows a circular external fixator stabilizing the foot. The ankle needs to be spanned with fixation to establish a stable hindfoot (and to correct any equinus contracture), the foundation for the reduction and stabilization of the forefoot.

21.9 Rehabilitation for Ex Fix

- In most circumstances, the patient is allowed weight-bearing ambulation.
- The percentage of weight recommended needs to be prescribed by the treating physician.
- Range of motion to adjacent joints is important staring early in the postoperative period.
- Therapy begins in the hospital and continues on an outpatient basis.[33]
- Excessive walking and joint stretching can irritate the pin sites and lead to inflammation.
- Once inflamed, the treatment is to temporarily limit rehabilitation, continue local pin care, and complete a short course of oral antibiotics. Prophylactic antibiotics have not been shown to be useful.[34]

21.10 Postoperative Care Ex Fix

- All patients treated with external fixation are at some risk of venous thromboembolic (VTE) complications and are treated with anticoagulants.
- Enoxaparin 40 mg is started 2 days postsurgery and continued for 2 weeks:
  - It can be extended longer for immobile patients.
- Pin care is performed daily and consists of showering, followed by cleaning the pin sites with diluted hydrogen peroxide and then wrapping with sterile gauze.
- Follow-up visits range from every 2 weeks (during a frame adjustment period) to monthly (during the consolidation period) and include radiographs of the entire frame to assess for bony healing as well as signs of pin loosening.

21.11 Key Testing Facts

- Origin of the deformity. One must distinguish between metaphyseal deformity and intra-articular deformity. Metaphyseal deformity can be corrected entirely through the osteotomy. Any contribution of joint wear to the total deformity should be corrected with great caution through the metaphysis since the bone is not the true location of the joint line deformity.
- Location for the osteotomy. In the case of a malunion, in particular, the healed fracture site is often sclerotic, poorly vascularized, and suboptimal for osteotomy healing. An adjacent site, often slightly distal to the malunion, will serve as a superior location for osteotomy with improved osteogenic potential.
- Osteotomy translation. The surgeon must decide if translation is needed at the osteotomy site. This can be planned preoperatively and accomplished through gradual (or acute) movement of the rings.
- Articular reduction. It is very difficult to achieve a reduction of the articular surface percutaneously without a limited open window since traction alone will not realign the fracture fragments. If possible use small incisions working through the fracture lines to improve the reduction and stabilize these fragments either with percutaneous screws or Ilizarov wires.
- All-wire stable fixation. A minimum of five tensioned wires should be used to control the epiphyseal segment.
- Prevent recurrence. Typical methods we employ to maintain the neutral foot position are stretching and bracing (with custom AFO and night splint), ankle arthrodesis, and posterior tibial tendon transfer.
- Have an external fixator available. This is recommended for any equinus surgical correction in the event of unforeseen complications requiring gradual stretching.
- TibioCalcaneal v TibioTaloCalcanel fusion. The decision whether to retain or excise the talus is an important crossroad in this reconstructive surgery. If the talus is salvaged and then proceeds to become necrotic and collapse it can compromise the entire project.
- Consolidation. The fusion can be evaluated by CT scan when healing is expected, typically around 3 months post surgery [35]. In cases where healing is suboptimal, an IM nail can be inserted at the time of frame removal. We recommend using an antibiotic cement coated nail in these cases to prevent deep infection [36].
- Olive wires. The use of opposing olive wires is useful in achieving optimal calcaneal fixation. Olive wires can be used in the forefoot as well, but, with weight bearing, they tend to erode the bone at an accelerated pace.
- Articulated distraction. The hinges need to be aligned in an oblique plane along the axis of ankle motion.
- Distraction Gap. If joint space is lost between subsequent follow up visits then additional distraction is applied as needed post surgery.
- Delayed gratification. Maximum improvement is seen 1-2 years after frame removal and is sustained for years. The patient needs to be warned of this for expectation management.
- Non weight bearing. Many Charcot patients are overweight and have poor balance. They tend to load the operative limb excessively if not admonished against weight bearing. Most will walk on the limb unconsciously which can lead to typical problems including: pin/wire fracture, pin/wire loosening, stress fracture through a pin site, infection, loss of fixation, or ring fracture. Non-weight bearing is the best method to avoid these obstacles.
- Adjuvant internal fixation. Another strategy is to be prepared to augment the fixation of the fusion at the time of frame removal by inserting internal fixation. This can be risky with regard to infection. Coating implants with antibiotic cement can help avoid this complication [36].

References

[1] Fragomen AT, Bernstein M, eds. Trauma and foot &ankle volume. In: Rozbruch SR, Hamdy R, eds. Limb Lengthening and Reconstruction Surgery Case Atlas. Cham, Switzerland: Springer International Publishing; 2015

[2] Haleem AM, Balagadde A, Borst EW, Do HT, Fragomen AT, Rozbruch SR. Distraction osteogenesis for brachymetatarsia: clinical results and implications on the metatarsophalangeal joint. J Limb Lengthening Reconstr. 2015; 1:29–37

[3] Fragomen AT, Rozbruch SR. The mechanics of external fixation. HSS J. 2007; 3(1):13–29

[4] Horn DM, Fragomen AT, Rozbruch SR. Supramalleolar osteotomy using circular external fixation with six-axis deformity correction of the distal tibia. Foot Ankle Int. 2011; 32(10):986–993

[5] Rozbruch SR, Fragomen AT. Percutaneous supramalleolar osteotomy using the Ilizarov/Taylor spatial frame. In: Maffulli N, Easley M, eds. Minimally Invasive Surgery of the Foot and Ankle. London: Springer; 2011:363–395

[6] Rozbruch SR, Fragomen AT, Ilizarov S. Correction of tibial deformity with use of the Ilizarov-Taylor spatial frame. J Bone Joint Surg Am. 2006; 88 Suppl 4:156–174

[7] Rozbruch SR. Reconstruction of the ankle after trauma. In: Rozbruch SR, Ilizarov S, eds. Limb Lengthening and Reconstruction Surgery. New York, NY: Informa Healthcare USA Inc.; 2007

[8] Rozbruch SR. Percutaneous supramalleolar osteotomy using the Ilizarov/Taylor spatial frame. In: Scuderi GR, Tria AJ, eds. Minimally Invasive Surgery in Orthopaedics. New York, NY: Springer; 2010

[9] Fragomen AT, Rozbruch SR. Supramalleolar osteotomy with external fixation: perspective 1. In: Easley ME, Wiesel SW, eds. Operative Techniques in Foot and Ankle Surgery. Philadelphia, PA: Lippincott Williams Wilkins; 2010

[10] Rozbruch SR. Percutaneous supramalleolar osteotomy using the Ilizarov/Taylor spatial frame. In: Scuderi GR, Tria AJ, eds. Minimally Invasive Surgery in Orthopaedics. 2nd ed. Cham: Springer International Publishing; 2015

[11] Rozbruch SR. Posttraumatic reconstruction of the ankle using the Ilizarov method. HSS J. 2005; 1(1): 68–88

[12] Schottel PC, Muthusamy S, Rozbruch SR. Distal tibial periarticular nonunions: ankle salvage with bone transport. J Orthop Trauma. 2014; 28(6):e146–e152

[13] Tellisi N, Deland JT, Rozbruch SR. Gradual reduction of chronic fracture dislocation of the ankle using Ilizarov/Taylor spatial frame. HSS J. 2011; 7(1):85–88

[14] Brunner S, Barg A, Knupp M, et al. The Scandinavian total ankle replacement: long-term, eleven to fifteen-year, survivorship analysis of the prosthesis in seventy-two consecutive patients. J Bone Joint Surg Am. 2013; 95:711–717

[15] Jeng CL, Campbell JT, Tang EY, Cerrato RA, Myerson MS. Tibiotalocalcaneal arthrodesis with bulk femoral head allograft for salvage of large defects in the ankle. Foot Ankle Int. 2013; 34(9): 1256–1266

[16] McCoy TH, Goldman V, Fragomen AT, Rozbruch SR. Circular external fixator-assisted ankle arthrodesis following failed total ankle arthroplasty. Foot Ankle Int. 2012; 33(11):947–955

[17] Rozbruch SR, Buksbaum JR, Fragomen AT, Borst EW, DeMille P. Oxygen consumption testing and self-reported outcomes following limb salvage with tibiocalcaneal or tibio-talo-calcaneal fusion. J Limb Lengthening Reconstr. 2016; 2:69–75

[18] Fragomen AT, Meyers KN, Davis N, Shu H, Wright T, Rozbruch SR. A biomechanical comparison of micromotion after ankle fusion using 2 fixation techniques: intramedullary arthrodesis nail or Ilizarov external fixator. Foot Ankle Int. 2008; 29 (3):334–341

[19] Fragomen AT, Borst E, Schachter L, Lyman S, Rozbruch SR. Complex ankle arthrodesis using the Ilizarov method yields high rate of fusion. Clin Orthop Relat Res. 2012; 470(10):2864–2873

[20] Tellisi N, Fragomen AT, Ilizarov S, Rozbruch SR. Limb salvage reconstruction of the ankle with fusion and simultaneous tibial lengthening using the Ilizarov/ Taylor spatial frame. HSS J. 2008; 4(1):32–42

[21] Rozbruch SR, Kleinman D, Fragomen AT, Ilizarov S. Limb lengthening and then insertion of an intramedullary nail: a case-matched comparison. Clin Orthop Relat Res. 2008; 466(12):2923–2932

[22] Bernstein M, Fragomen AT, Sabharwal S, Barclay J, Rozbruch SR. Does integrated fixation provide benefit in the reconstruction of posttraumatic tibial bone defects? Clin Orthop Relat Res. 2015; 473(10): 3143–3153

[23] Fragomen AT, Rozbruch SR. Lengthening and deformity correction about the knee using a magnetic internal lengthening nail. SICOT J. 2017; 3(25):1–10

[24] Kirane YM, Fragomen AT, Rozbruch SR. Precision of the PRECICE internal bone lengthening nail. Clin Orthop Relat Res. 2014; 472(12):3869–3878

[25] Bernstein M, Reidler J, Fragomen A, Rozbruch SR. Ankle distraction arthroplasty: indications, technique, and outcomes. J Am Acad Orthop Surg. 2017; 25(2):89–99

[26] Tellisi N, Fragomen AT, Kleinman D, O'Malley MJ, Rozbruch SR. Joint preservation of the osteoarthritic ankle using distraction arthroplasty. Foot Ankle Int. 2009; 30(4):318–325

[27] Fragomen AT, Rozbruch SR. Distraction arthroplasty for ankle osteoarthritis. In: Kocaoglu M, Tsuchiya H, Eralp L, eds. Advanced Techniques in Limb Reconstruction Surgery. Berlin: Springer; 2015

[28] Greenfield S, Matta KM, McCoy TH, Rozbruch SR, Fragomen A. Ankle distraction arthroplasty for ankle osteoarthritis: a survival analysis. Strateg Trauma Limb Reconstr. 2019; 14(2):65–71

[29] Intema F, Thomas TP, Anderson DD, et al. Subchondral bone remodeling is related to clinical improvement after joint distraction in the treatment of ankle osteoarthritis. Osteoarthritis Cartilage. 2011; 19(6):668–675

[30] Smith NC, Beaman D, Rozbruch SR, Glazebrook MA. Evidence-based indications for distraction ankle arthroplasty. Foot Ankle Int. 2012; 33(8):632–636

[31] Inda JI, Blyakher A, O'Malley MJ, Rozbruch SR. Distraction arthroplasty for the ankle using the Ilizarov frame. Tech Foot Ankle Surg. 2003; 2(4): 249–253

[32] Fragomen AT, McCoy TH, Meyers KN, Rozbruch SR. Minimum distraction gap: how much ankle joint space is enough in ankle distraction arthroplasty? HSS J. 2014; 10(1):6–12

[33] Rozbruch SR, Fragomen AT. Tibial/Femoral Osteotomy. In: Green A, Hayda R, eds. Orthopaedic Postoperative Rehabilitation. Rosemont, IL: American Academy of Orthopaedic Surgeons; 2017

[34] Fragomen AT, Miller AO, Brause BD, Goldman V, Rozbruch SR. Prophylactic postoperative antibiotics may not reduce pin site infections after external fixation. HSS J. 2017; 13(2):165–170

22 Foot and Ankle Tumors

Benjamin Jong, Michael Russell, John Yanik, Jocelyn Compton, and Benjamin J. Miller

Abstract

Like all areas of the body, soft tissues and bony structures of the foot and ankle can give rise to tumors and tumorlike lesions. Proper identification and prompt appropriate treatment is essential for maximizing patient outcomes. In this chapter, we will review the initial presentation and suggested workup for these conditions. We will then review the most common benign and malignant tumors of bone and soft tissue, and briefly discuss their associated treatments.

Keywords: tumor, neoplasm, benign, malignant, sarcoma

22.1 Introduction: Basics of Musculoskeletal Tumors

22.1.1 Initial Presentation

- Very commonly an incidental finding on radiographs obtained for other purposes:
  - Stable imaging on radiographs over time reassuring feature for benign pathology.
- Insidious onset of pain without trauma with enlarging bone or soft-tissue mass concerning for possible malignant potential.

22.1.2 Initial imaging

- *Plain radiographs*:
  - Indicated for all bone tumors; can be helpful but not absolutely necessary in soft-tissue tumors.[1]
- *Magnetic resonance imaging (MRI)*:
  - With and without contrast to better evaluate the mass.
  - Best subsequent study if there is a concern for malignancy.
  - Demonstrates intramedullary extension and soft-tissue component.
  - *Indications in bone tumors:* Periosteal reaction, soft-tissue mass, poorly defined borders, cortical breakage, and concern for malignancy.
  - *Indications in soft-tissue tumors*: Large (> 5 cm), growing, deep to the fascia, and painful.[1]
- *Computed tomography (CT)*:
  - *Site of concern:* If contraindication to MRI or need to assess bony integrity.
  - *Staging of chest/abdomen/pelvis:* If concern for metastatic disease of bone (unusual in the distal lower extremity).[1]
- *Bone scan*:
  - Helpful to determine if a lesion is active or inactive.
  - Difficult to differentiate between benign and malignant entities in isolation.
  - Indicated only if there is a specific question or concern, not routinely.[1]
- *Other advanced imaging (e.g., positron emission tomography [PET] scan)*:
  - Leave to the discretion of the treating oncology service after confirmation of malignancy.[1]

22.1.3 Biopsy Principles

- Refer to a sarcoma center prior to biopsy if there is any concern for sarcoma.[2]
- Done in line with the anticipated surgical incision to allow for track excision during definitive treatment of sarcoma.
- Four biopsy options:
  - *Fine-needle aspiration*:
    - Provides only cells, no structure.
    - Typically not adequate for diagnosis of bone and soft-tissue tumors.
  - *Core needle biopsy*:
    - Provides cells and structure.

- Done under local anesthesia as an outpatient.
- Most common biopsy technique for soft-tissue tumors.
- *Incisional biopsy*:
  - Standard of care for diagnostic accuracy.
  - Requires an operation but allows for a frozen section to confirm diagnostic material.
- *Excisional biopsy*:
  - En bloc resection of the mass performed without knowledge of diagnosis.
  - Use with care but may be appropriate for small, superficial tumors and tumors with characteristic features (e.g., schwannoma).

22.1.4 Margins

- Planned margin depends on underlying histology.[3]
- *Enneking classification*:
  - Intralesional: resection through the tumor itself.
    - Benign bone tumors.
    - Metastatic disease of bone.
  - Marginal: complete resection through reactive zone surrounding tumor:
    - Sarcoma, often with adjuvant radiation.
    - Benign soft-tissue tumors.
  - Wide: complete resection with a cuff of normal tissue:
    - Sarcoma.
  - Radical: complete compartmental resection (i.e., entire bone or muscle from origin to insertion):
    - Rarely performed.
- *Residual tumor (R) classification*:
  - R0: negative:
    - Includes Enneking marginal, wide, and radical.
  - R1: microscopically positive.
  - R2: macroscopically positive (i.e., gross residual disease).

22.2 Malignant Bone Tumors

22.2.1 General Principles/Initial Management of Malignant Bone Tumors of the Foot

- Clinical history and physical examination, including review of systems for constitutional symptoms.
- Imaging should begin with radiographs of the foot and ankle with a low threshold to image the entire limb. This should be followed in most cases by MRI.
- Biopsy tracts should be carefully planned in discussion with the treating orthopaedic oncologist, and should either be performed by the treating surgeon, according to the plan of the treating surgeon, or by a radiologist in consultation.
- The biopsy should be planned with the aim of obtaining an accurate tissue diagnosis while avoiding compromising the final resection and/or limb salvage surgery.

22.2.2 General Principles of Surgical Management of Malignant Bone Tumors of the Foot

- Wide surgical margins where possible.
- Neoadjuvant/adjuvant therapy dependent on tissue diagnosis.
- Amputation versus limb salvage is primarily dependent on the ability to obtain sufficient surgical margins, but also dependent on patient age, comorbidities, preferences, and predicted function of salvage versus amputation.

22.2.3 Osteosarcoma

- Presentation:
  - More commonly in long bones, particularly about the knee; rarely

found in the distal tibia, fibula, or bones of the foot (< 4% of all osteosarcomas).
  - Bimodal age distribution, with the first peak in adolescents/young adults and the second peak in the elderly.
- Pathology:
  - Primary bone forming tumor.
  - Malignant atypical spindle cells with neoplastic bone formation (osteoid).
  - Typically aggressive with metastatic potential.
- Imaging:
  - *Radiographs:* Increasing density within or around bone with aggressive periosteal reaction, osteolysis, and cortical destruction.
  - *MRI:* Ossific matrix seen with associated heterogenous soft-tissue mass representative of hemorrhage and necrosis. MRI depicts the intra-/extraosseous extent of the tumor most accurately.
  - Potential for skip lesions necessitates full limb radiographs/MRI.
- Surgical intervention/treatment:
  - Wide resection and chemotherapy (neoadjuvant and adjuvant):
    - Amputation common for malignancy in the distal tibia, ankle, and foot.
  - MAP (methotrexate, Adriamycin, cisplatin) first line (▶ Fig. 22.1).

22.2.4 Ewing's Sarcoma

- Presentation:
  - Second-most common malignant bone tumor in children.
  - Eighty percent of patients are under 20 years old.
  - Constitutional symptoms (weight loss, fever, and anorexia) common.
  - Male-to-female ratio of 1.5:1.
  - Rarely occurs in the foot. When it does occur, calcaneus, talus, and metatarsals are most commonly involved.
- Pathology:
  - Associated with chromosomal translocation (t11:22) in 85% of cases.
  - Small round-cell tumor of bone and soft tissue with neuroectodermal differentiation.
  - Highly aggressive tumor with a predilection for local tissue invasion and lung metastasis.
- Imaging:
  - Radiographs: Bones appear "moth eaten" with marked osteolysis. Classic "onion skin" periosteal reaction more common in diaphyseal bones.
  - In the foot, bony destruction tends to be more pronounced than elsewhere in the body and there is a lesser tendency to have a large soft-tissue mass.
  - Associated soft-tissue mass may be seen both on radiographs and MRI.

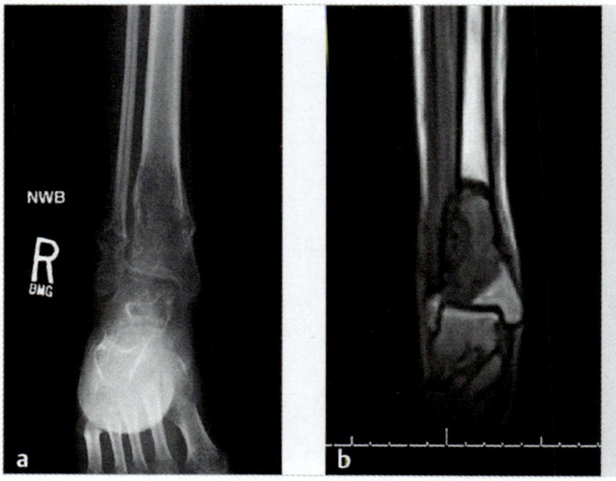

Fig. 22.1 (a,b) Radiograph and T1 magnetic resonance imaging (MRI) of osteosarcoma in the distal tibia of a 17-year-old adolescent girl. Below knee amputation and chemotherapy were required.

- Surgical intervention/treatment:
  - Mainstay of treatment is wide resection and chemotherapy.
  - Vincristine, Adriamycin, and cyclophosphamide (VAC) ± ifosfamide and etoposide (IE) first line.
  - Radiotherapy may be considered if poor response to chemotherapy or inadequate surgical margins obtained (▶ Fig. 22.2).

22.2.5 Chondrosarcoma

- Presentation:
  - Rare in the foot and ankle in comparison to other sites, representing less than 5% of all chondrosarcomas.
  - However, one of the most common malignant tumors when considering only the foot and ankle. Lesions will typically involve the distal tibia, distal fibula, tarsal bones, and metatarsal bones.
  - Peak prevalence occurs between fourth and sixth decade of life.
  - Patients with hereditary multiple exostoses, Ollier disease, or Maffuci syndrome are at higher risk of developing chondrosarcomas.

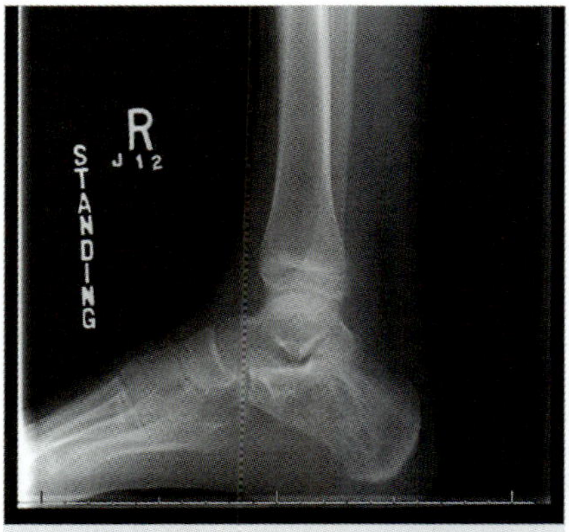

Fig. 22.2 Ewing's sarcoma of the calcaneus in a 13-year-old adolescent boy. This patient ultimately required chemotherapy, below knee amputation, and treatment of lung metastasis.

- Pathology:
  - Cartilage/stroma producing malignant cells.
  - May arise de novo or in previously benign cartilaginous lesions (osteochondromas, enchondromas).
- Imaging:
  - Radiographs and CT show mixed lytic and sclerotic lesions, with sclerosis representing calcified chondroid matrix.
  - May also see endosteal scalloping indicating cortical destruction with soft-tissue mass.
  - MRI will reveal lobulated masses with marrow replacement.
- Surgical intervention/treatment:
  - Wide surgical excision is the mainstay of treatment.
  - Chemotherapy and radiation therapy are typically ineffective (▶ Fig. 22.3).

22.3 Benign Bone Tumors

22.3.1 Tumors of Bone

- Osteoid osteomas:
  - Small lesions, less than 1.5 cm in size. Most commonly seen in the second and third decades of life. More common in males; predominantly affect the lower extremities including the foot and ankle.
  - Characterized by pain that is worse at night and relieved by aspirin and nonsteroidal anti-inflammatory drugs (NSAIDs).
  - Diagnosis often based on clinical examination and X-ray imaging or a CT scan showing a round or oval well-circumscribed lucent lesion with a central nidus (▶ Fig. 22.4).
  - Conservative management consists of anti-inflammatory medications for

pain. If patients can tolerate this definitively, the lesion often heals within 3 to 4 years.
- Surgical interventions consist of guided percutaneous radiofrequency ablation of the lesion or open en bloc resection:
  - En bloc resection is associated with a lower recurrence rate, but higher rates of iatrogenic fracture or need for supplemental stabilization (▶ Fig. 22.4).

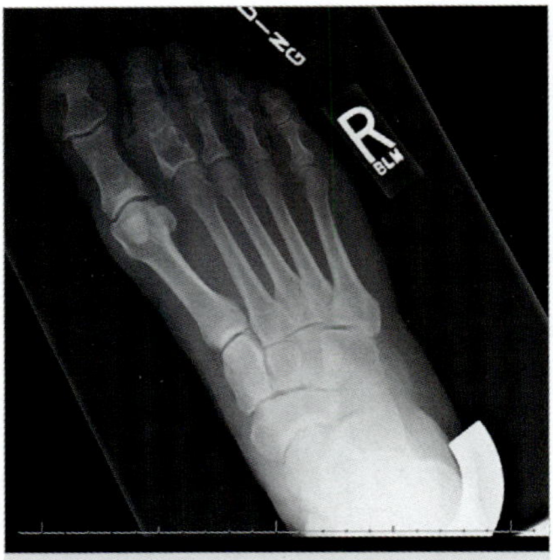

Fig. 22.3 Chondrosarcoma of the second proximal phalanx in a 56-year-old man with a history of curettage and grafting of an enchondroma at the same site 10 years prior. The patient returned due to new-onset swelling. Aggressive features were noted on magnetic resonance imaging (MRI), and following amputation of the second toe, the pathology returned as grade II chondrosarcoma.

- Osteoblastomas:
  - Slow-growing lesions; 2 to 10 cm in size; most common in males aged 10 to 30 years. Make up less than 1% of all bone tumors. In the extremities, generally found in the femur and tibia but can be found in the foot and ankle.
  - Generally present with progressive dull pain. Can cause swelling, warmth, and altered gait depending on the size, location, and presence of surrounding muscle atrophy.
  - X-rays are often variable and nondiagnostic. The lesions are commonly radiolucent but may be sclerotic or mixed.
  - Treatment is usually curettage and bone grafting. Recurrence rate roughly 10 to 20%.

22.3.2 Tumors of Cartilage

- Enchondroma:
  - A benign proliferation of hyaline cartilage within the intramedullary canal, often in the metaphysis/metadiaphysis. Occur in all age groups. Males and females are equally affected.
  - Generally asymptomatic, often found incidentally on X-rays.
  - In the foot and ankle, they are generally found in the phalanges.[4]
  - Appear as well-defined lytic lesions on X-ray; may develop intralesional calcifications over time (often described as "stippled," "punctate," or "popcorn").
  - Important to differentiate enchondromas from low-grade

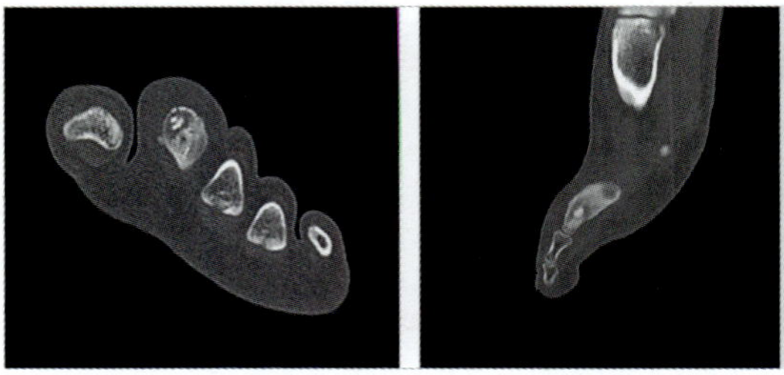

Fig. 22.4 Computed tomography (CT) scan of an osteoid osteoma in the second proximal phalanx. Note the well-circumscribed lucent lesion with a central nidus.

chondrosarcomas; consider an MRI for painful lesions or lesions with atypical radiographic appearance (cortical break, scalloping > 50%, large noncalcified areas).
 - Multiple enchondromas:
   - *Ollier's disease:* A rare nonhereditary entity also known as multiple enchondromatosis. There is a 25% risk of sarcomatous transformation by age 40 years.
   - Maffucci's syndrome: Multiple enchondromas with overlying soft-tissue hemangiomas. Sarcomatous transformation thought to be inevitable over time.
 - Treatment for isolated enchondromas is observation. If a lesion grows or becomes symptomatic, consideration should be given for sarcomatous transformation.
- Chondroblastoma:
 - Rare neoplasm that occurs more commonly (2:1) in males; usually presents in patients younger than 25 years of age. Represents less than 1% of all primary bone tumors.
 - In the lower extremities, most commonly found in the distal femur, femoral apophysis, proximal tibia, calcaneus, or talus.
 - Presents with progressive pain.
 - Characteristically located in the epiphysis or apophysis. Fifty percent cross the growth plate. Appear as round or oval lytic lesions with a well-defined sclerotic border on X-ray.
 - The natural history is slow progressive enlargement and associated destruction of bone.
 - Treatment usually consists of curettage with or without bone grafting. There is a 10 to 15% local recurrence rate. Care must be taken to protect the grown plate during surgery.
- Chondromyxoid fibroma:
 - Very rare neoplasm. Most commonly presents in the second and third decade of life. Less than 0.5% of all primary bone tumors; described as the least common benign cartilaginous lesion.
 - Seventy-five percent occur in the lower extremities; proximal tibia is the most common location. Reports of foot and ankle involvement range from 10 to 31%.[5] Appear as lytic lesions with scalloped, sclerotic, and lobulated margins (▶ Fig. 22.5).
 - Diagnosis usually by histology; shows areas of chondroid, myxoid, and fibrous tissues.
 - Treatment consists of curettage and bone grafting. Recurrence occurs in 12.5 to 20% of cases; patients should be monitored for recurrence for 3 to 5 years postoperatively (▶ Fig. 22.6).
- Osteochondroma:
 - Most common benign bony lesion. Usually found in children at times of rapid growth.

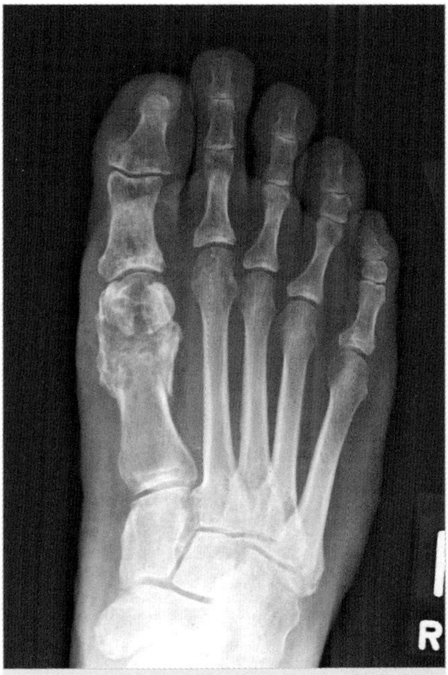

Fig. 22.5 Chondromyxoid fibroma in the first metatarsal.

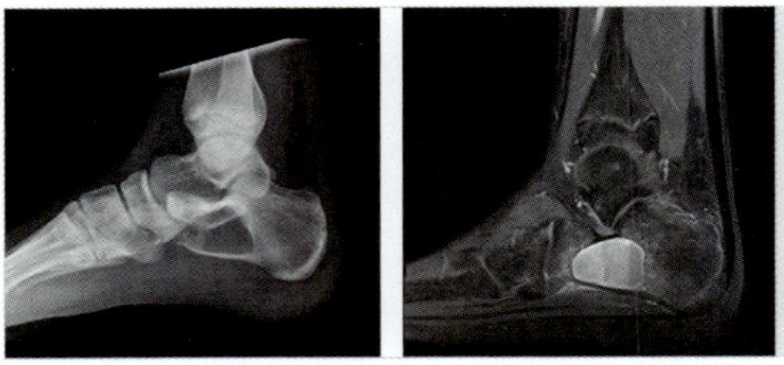

Fig. 22.6 Imaging of a unicameral bone cyst located within the calcaneus. Although not necessary to make the diagnosis, the magnetic resonance imaging (MRI) shows a single well-defined fluid-filled cavity.

- In the foot and ankle, it has been reported as representing approximately 12% of all benign bone tumors.[6]
- On imaging, it appears as a bony outgrowth with a cartilaginous cap that is generally < 1.5 cm thick; lesions with thicker caps raise suspicion for chondrosarcomatous transformation. Malignant transformation occurs in 1% of solitary lesions.
- Lesions are asymptomatic. Generally discovered incidentally or due to pain from irritation of surrounding soft tissues. Ninety percent of lesions are solitary and isolated.
- *Multiple hereditary exostoses (MHE):* Mutation in the ETX1 gene (chromosome 8q24) or EXT2 gene (chromosome 11p11) leading to formation of multiple osteochondromas. Autosomal dominant. Malignant degeneration is thought to occur in 5% of MHE cases.
- Treatment consists of observation for asymptomatic lesions and excision of larger symptomatic lesions. Complete removal of the cartilaginous cap is important to prevent recurrence, which occurs less than 2% of the time.

22.3.3 Other

- Giant cell tumor of bone:
  - A benign but locally aggressive tumor. Most commonly presents in the third and fourth decades of life. Slight male predominance (1.5:1).
  - Typically benign but can metastasize to the lungs in approximately 3% of patients.
  - In the feet, they are usually found in the metatarsals as opposed to the tarsals/phalanges.
  - Clinically, patients usually present with localized pain. Appear as eccentric lytic lesions on X-ray; usually in the subchondral or epiphyseal portion of the bone. Cortical thinning can occur. Patients may present with pathologic fracture.
  - In more aggressive appearing lesions, telangiectatic osteosarcoma should be considered.
  - Treatment consists of curettage and filling of the defect. Depending on size, location, and amount of bony destruction, some lesions may necessitate resection/reconstruction.
  - Adjuvants should be used intraoperatively. Recurrence rates are generally 5 to 17%. Recurrences should be treated in the same manner as primary tumors.
- Aneurysmal bone cyst (ABC):
  - A benign but locally destructive blood-filled cyst that generally occurs in patients younger than 20 years. Slight female predominance.
  - Symptoms generally include mild pain and swelling.
  - Plain X-rays show radiolucent eccentric destructive lesions that may push on and expand the cortex and periosteum. MRI shows multiloculated fluid-filled cavities, which help

distinguish this entity from a unicameral bone cyst (UBC).
  - Treatment is curettage and bone grafting. Recurrence occurs in 10 to 34% of cases; more common in young patients. Recurrence treated with repeat curettage and grafting.
  - Rarely occurs in bones of the feet.
- UBC:
  - Common benign lesions; usually found in long bone metaphyses in children. Male predominance (2:1).
  - In the foot and ankle, most commonly found in the calcaneus of adults.
  - The lesions themselves are asymptomatic. They are generally found incidentally on X-ray or due to pain from an associated pathologic or impending pathologic fracture.
  - Appear as well-defined central lytic lesions (▶ Fig. 22.6). If there is an associated pathologic fracture, X-rays may characteristically show a "fallen leaf" or "fallen fragment" sign. This is a thin fractured piece of cortex sitting in a dependent position within the cyst.
  - Treatment of asymptomatic lesions is observation only. In the calcaneus, open curettage and bone grafting of symptomatic lesions is the most effective treatment (▶ Fig. 22.6).[7]
- Nonossifying fibroma:
  - This is a very common metaphyseal fibrous defect that often presents in the first two decades of life. It may be present in up to 30 to 40% of children.
  - It represents 5.6% of benign bony foot and ankle tumors.[6]
  - It is usually painless and discovered incidentally. It may present with a pathologic fracture.
  - Plain radiographs reveal well-defined lobulated or "bubbly" lesions (▶ Fig. 22.7); with time, the lesions usually regress and become sclerotic. They often start in the metaphysis but appear to migrate toward the diaphysis as the bone grows.

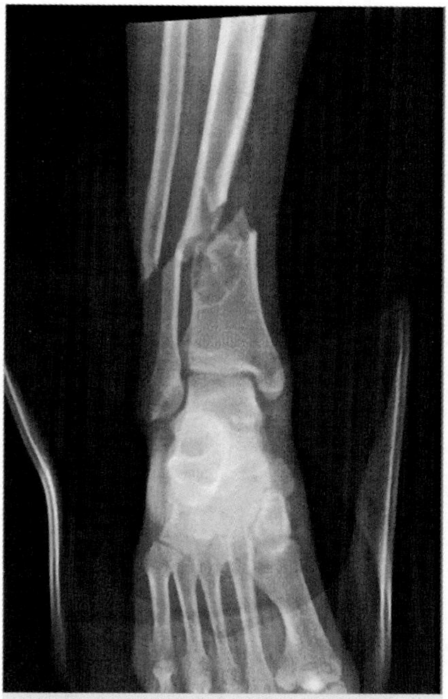

Fig. 22.7 A patient who presented with a pathologic open distal tibia fracture through a nonossifying fibroma. Although pathologic fractures can be treated nonoperatively, this patient underwent curettage and bone grafting with open reduction and internal fixation due to the open nature of his injury.

  - Histology shows spindle cells in a whorled pattern.
  - Treatment is observation for asymptomatic lesions. Pathologic fractures can also frequently be treated nonoperatively. Recurrence is rare.
- Fibrous dysplasia:
  - This is a common developmental abnormality of bone that may involve one bone (monostotic) or several bones (polyostotic). No gender predilection is observed. It can be associated with McCune–Albright syndrome or Mazabraud's syndrome. It can involve any bone in the body.
  - Pain is generally the presenting feature. They may, however, be found

incidentally. Patients may also note deformity or present with a pathologic fracture.
  - Imaging shows irregular, well-defined, "bubbly," lesions with a sclerotic appearing rim. Occasionally, biopsy is needed to make the final diagnosis.
  - Surgical treatment is generally avoided due to a high recurrence rate. Lesions presenting with deformity or pathologic fracture are best treated with cortical allograft or intramedullary fixation in the case of long bones.
- Osteofibrous dysplasia (Campanacci's disease):
  - A rare lesion that is most commonly found in the tibia and distal fibula. Usually presents in the first and second decades of life. Has loose associations with neurofibromatosis type 1 (NF1) and trisomy 7, 8, 12, and 22.
  - Lesions are often asymptomatic; pain may occur due to high stress or pathologic fracture. The tibia is often enlarged and bowed anteriorly.
  - As in fibrous dysplasia, imaging often shows well-defined, "bubbly," lesions with a sclerotic appearing rim. Anterior bowing and tibial enlargement may be present, which is a finding that can mimic adamantinoma.
  - Some argue that osteofibrous dysplasia is a precursor to adamantinoma. Diagnosis can often be made on examination and with plain radiographs; however, a biopsy may be performed to confirm the diagnosis and rule out adamantinoma.
  - Treatment consists of monitoring asymptomatic lesions. Pathologic fractures are often treated nonsurgically. Surgery is rare and usually only preformed to correct deformity.
- Langerhans cell histiocytosis:
  - A non-neoplastic proliferation of Langerhans-type histiocytes, a large cell with an indented nucleus and abundant eosinophilic cytoplasm. Cells stain positive for S100.
  - Occurs more frequently before the age of 21 years, but can be discovered later in life as well.
  - Slightly more common in males when it presents before the age of 21 years. For those presenting after the age of 21 years, the male-to-female ratio is 3:1.
  - Localized pain is generally the chief complaint. Imaging can vary, but generally shows one or multiple lytic lesions. Consider a skeletal survey to identify additional lesions. More common in the axial skeleton and long bones.
  - A biopsy confirms the diagnosis and rules out more aggressive lesions.
  - Conservative management with observation is preferred; isolated lesions generally resolve spontaneously. Curettage and grafting may be performed for pain or pathologic fracture after the diagnosis has been firmly established. Cortical steroid injections and low-dose radiation have also been used to effectively treat these lesions. Low rate of recurrence.
- Bizarre periosteal osteochondromatous proliferation (Nora's lesion):
  - Very rare osteochondromatous growth that can appear to have malignant features, despite its benign nature.
  - In the foot, it is usually found in the metatarsals.
  - Affects males and females equally.
  - Usually presents in the second and third decades of life.
  - Presents as a rapidly growing sometimes painful mass.
  - Plain radiographs show spiculated or irregular lesions arising from, but not affecting, the cortex. A CT scan confirms absence of cortical involvement, differentiating it from osteochondroma.

  - As it may be confused with malignant lesions, a biopsy often confirms the diagnosis.
  - Treatment is excision. Recurrence in up to 51% of cases; treat with repeat excision.

22.3.4 Non-neoplastic

- Synovial cyst (ganglion cyst):
  - Common benign outpouchings of the joint capsule that contain synovial fluid; can rarely extend and become intraosseous. Can form anywhere a joint or tendon is present.
  - Usually present as painless soft masses, but can cause irritation of soft tissues or pain on intraosseous extension.
  - Plain X-rays will show a lytic lesion in the case of intraosseous cysts. An MRI is not required to make the diagnosis but may be obtained; it will show a homogeneous, well-defined fluid-filled mass that does not enhance on postcontrast series.
  - Treatment consists of resection of overlying soft tissues and curettage of symptomatic intraosseous lesions. Recurrence is rare.
- Infection:
  - Osteomyelitis can mimic tumors.
  - Whenever a biopsy or pathologic analysis of a musculoskeletal neoplasm is preformed, tissues should be sent for Gram stain and culture.
  - Rarely, malignant changes can occur at sites of chronic infection. Squamous cell carcinoma and fibrosarcoma have been reported.

22.4 Malignant Soft-Tissue Tumors

22.4.1 Initial Management of Soft-Tissue Malignancy

- Initial workup with clinical history and examination.
- Imaging of choice is lesion specific; however, MRI commonly aids in diagnosis.
- Complex anatomy of the foot and ankle may render tissue biopsy more difficult.
- Biopsy should avoid contamination of healthy tissues, tendon sheaths, and neurovascular bundles.
- Up to 10% of sarcoma biopsies result in change in management.
- Site and trajectory of biopsy may be performed by a radiologist in conjunction with consultation with the orthopaedic oncologist who will be resecting the tumor.

22.4.2 Surgical Management

- Sarcomas should be treated with wide margins when possible.
- Limb salvage surgery is often possible, which is an important consideration when performing biopsy.
- Amputation often offers good function and potential cure for many soft-tissue malignancies.
- After soft-tissue resection, may opt for healing by secondary intention versus local flap, skin graft, or other reconstruction options.

22.4.3 Skin Cancers

- **Malignant melanoma**:
  - Most common tumor to metastasize to skin in men.
  - In one study, it accounted for 18.6% of all malignant soft-tissue tumors in the foot and ankle (Toepfer et al 2016).
  - Although localization to the lower extremity may confer better outcomes, specific localization to the foot has poorer prognostic outcomes.
  - Acral lentiginous may be the most common type of melanoma.
  - Subungual melanoma carries a worse prognosis.

- Associated with fair complexion, repeated sun exposure, tanning booth use, and family history of melanoma.
- Melanoma may be indicated by lesions with **A**symmetry, **B**order irregularity, **C**olor variegation, **D**iameter greater than 6 mm, **E**volution/**E**nlargement (▶ Fig. 22.8).
- Differential diagnosis includes atypical nevi, seborrheic keratosis, and dermatofibromas.
- Pathology: Melanocytic atypia with nuclear pseudoinclusions; presence of invading lymphocytes is a good prognostic finding.
- American Joint Committee on Cancer (AJCC) depth and mitotic rates are important prognostic variables:
  - Ulceration is a clinical indicator of increased mitotic rate in microscopic examination.

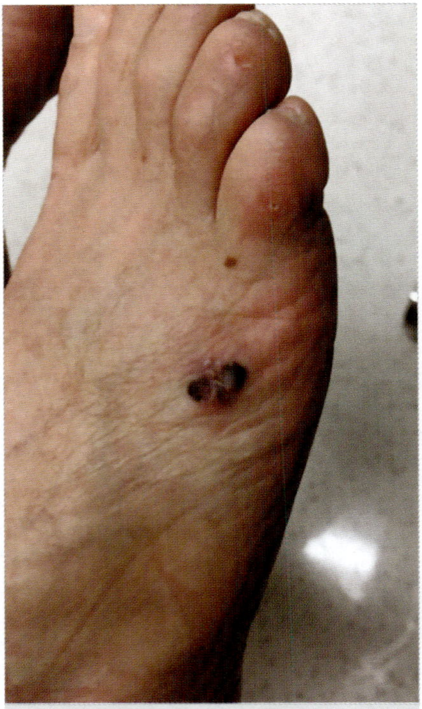

Fig. 22.8 A 55-year-old woman with malignant melanoma (stage III) treated with wide excision and primary closure.

- Regional lymph nodes are the most common site of initial metastasis.
- Surgical treatment: wide excision with consideration of sentinel lymph node biopsy for depth greater than 1.0 mm.
- Seventy-five percent cure rate with wide excision; 50% of recurrences occur in the first year after wide excision.
- Adjuvant therapy based on predicted relapse; the only approved therapy is interferon-A2b (▶ Fig. 22.8).

- **Squamous cell carcinoma**:
  - Among most common human malignancies, but only approximately 5% occurs in the foot and ankle.
  - White plaque with possible induration, hemorrhage, and ulceration (▶ Fig. 22.9).
  - Nonhealing ulceration or chronically draining sinus that does not respond to topical treatments should raise concern (Marjolin's ulcer).

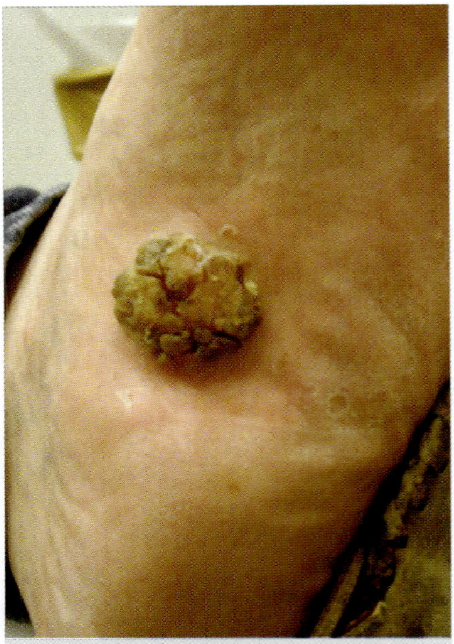

Fig. 22.9 A 60-year-old man with left plantar foot squamous cell carcinoma, initially treated with wide excision and fasciocutaneous flap, however with local recurrence requiring eventual amputation.

  - Associated with chronic osteomyelitis, human papilloma virus, local trauma, and genetic conditions.
  - Differential diagnosis includes basal cell carcinoma, cutaneous granulomas, periungual verrucae, osteomyelitis, tinea pedis, and keratoacanthomas.
    - High rate of unplanned total excision without appropriate margins:
    - MRI indicated for lesions greater than 2 cm wide or 4 mm deep indicated in order to avoid incomplete excision.
    - Pathology: Abundant pink cytoplasm with keratinization; may be well or poorly differentiated.
  - Surgical management includes wide excision ± lymph node biopsy.
  - Metastatic potential correlates with duration of symptoms and involvement of lymph nodes.
- **Dermatofibrosarcoma protuberans**:
  - Presentation: slow-growing, painless mass in adolescent and young adults.
  - Pathology: storiform fascicles of spindle cells, mild mitotic activity with + CD34 staining.
  - Can be locally aggressive and may recur after local excision.
  - MRI is the preferred imaging modality.
  - Most commonly found in the trunk and abdomen but can involve the extremities more infrequently.

22.4.4 Soft-Tissue Sarcomas

- **Clear cell sarcoma**:
  - Presentation: slow-growing, painful soft-tissue mass most common in young females.
  - Lower extremity, including the foot and ankle, is the most common musculoskeletal site affected:
    - More likely to occur in tendons and muscle aponeuroses than in bone.
  - MRI shows relatively benign lesion in contrast with its aggressive nature.
  - Pathology: neural crest cells with melanocytic differentiation.
  - Wide local excision, radical excision, or amputation are all surgical possibilities.
  - Up to 60% 5-year survival rate after complete excision.
  - Tumor size and necrosis are prognostic indicators of 5-year survival.
  - MRI is the imaging modality of choice:
    - May be misleading.
    - Tissue biopsy is necessary for diagnosis.
  - Pathology: "packeting" of tumor cells with clear cytoplasm and large nuclei with central nucleoli.
- **Synovial sarcoma**:
  - Young adults with slow-growing, painful multinodular mass in periarticular tissues:
    - Does not originate from synovium and is rarely intra-articular.
    - Name originated from histologic appearance similar to synovial tissue.
  - A "great mimicker" of many benign processes.
  - Considered a high-grade sarcoma.
  - SS18-SSX fusion oncogene.
  - Can occur at almost any anatomic site, but rare in the skin and within the joint or bursa.
  - Marked predilection for the lower extremity and most common sarcoma in the foot and ankle.
  - Fifty percent of patients have metastatic disease (tendency to metastasize to lung).
  - Thirty percent have radiographic calcifications; MRI is the imaging modality of choice (T2 shows heterogeneity of signal and halo of hyperintensity indicating reactive edema).
  - Pathology: hypercellular array of small uniform spindle cells (monophasic, more common); fibroblastlike spindle cells forming glandlike structures (biphasic, less common); + epithelial differentiation markers.

- Fifty percent to 60% 5-year survival rates; subcentimeter lesions of the foot have a better prognosis.
- Treat with wide surgical excision (including radical resection of the involved compartments), radiotherapy, and chemotherapy (sensitive to alkylating agents).

- **Angiosarcoma**:
  - Rare tumor of older males (70–80 years); variable in appearance.
  - More invasive than immediately apparent, and thus prone to incomplete excision.
  - Cutaneous angiosarcoma is clinically aggressive; may be associated with chronic lymphedema.
  - Most commonly found in the scalp and face.
  - MRI is imaging modality of choice with diffuse hypointense T1 signal and hyperintense T2 signal.
  - Pathology: atypical endothelial cells with spindle cell proliferation and vascular markers.
  - High propensity for local recurrence.
  - Surgical resection in combination with radiation therapy, chemotherapy, and immunotherapy offers best results.

22.5 Benign Soft-Tissue Tumors

22.5.1 Lipoma

- Most common soft-tissue tumor and composed almost entirely of adipocytes. Typically mobile, rubbery mass that is encapsulated and located in the subcutaneous tissue. Can be found anywhere in the body including the foot and ankle.
- Usually painless but can compress nearby nerves causing pain.
- Lipomas that rapidly grow, are painful, or not freely mobile; may be further imaged and considered for removal. Other removal indications are primarily cosmetic.
- Homogeneous appearance on MRI, consistent with fat, implies benign lipoma or atypical lipomatous tumor (formerly called well-differentiated liposarcoma).
- Surgical removal is via local resection of the encapsulated mass with an attempt at marginal margins (► Fig. 22.10).

22.5.2 Hemangioma: Infantile Variant

- Benign vascular neoplasm comprising endothelial cells, pericytes, and vascular progenitor cells and are GLUT1 positive.
- Typically presents within the first year of life as a small red macule that gradually increases in size.

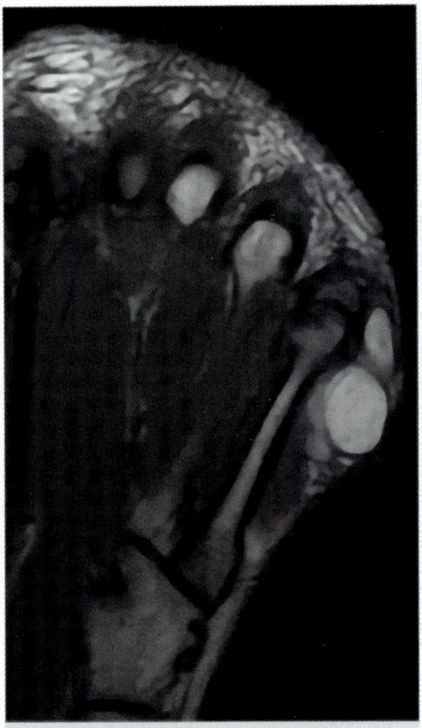

Fig. 22.10 A 46-year-old man with lipoma lateral to the fifth metatarsal (MT) on T1 magnetic resonance imaging (MRI). It was treated with local surgical resection.

- Can occur anywhere in the body but most common on the face and scalp.
- Vast majority of lesions (70%) will resolve within the first 7 years of life.
- Must consider angiosarcoma in differential diagnosis, but this would typically have a much larger soft-tissue component.
- Treatment is typically for cosmetic and functional purposes and consists of medical management with propanol as the first-line agent. Secondary treatment options include corticosteroids, laser resections, and surgery as a last-line resort.
- Congenital variant has similar pathogenesis and treatment but is fully formed at birth.

22.5.3 Schwannoma

Giant Cell Tumor of Tendon Sheath (aka Focal-Type Tenosynovial Giant Cell Tumor)

- Originates from tendon sheath or bursa and is characterized by histiocytes, multinucleated giant cells, and mononuclear cells with hemosiderin deposits.
- Vast majority occur in the hand and wrist, but it is estimated that 3 to 5% originate in the foot and ankle.[8]
- Typically is painless in presentation and do not interfere with range of motion.
- Appear as homogenous, hypoechoic, and solid mass on ultrasound.
- MRI shows extra-articular synovial origination in close proximity or enveloping a tendon.
- Integral resection with minimal margins typically performed with the option for hydrogen peroxide lavage.
- Important to differentiate from pigmented villonodular synovitis (PVNS).
  - Histologically identical, dependent on extent of disease (PVNS is a diffuse-type tenosynovial giant cell tumor involving an entire joint).
- Arises from Schwann cells present in the peripheral nervous system. These cells are responsible for producing myelin, which insulates peripheral nerves.
- More common in the upper extremities and rare in the lower extremities.
- Due to cellular makeup; always present on periphery of nerve.
- Typically asymptomatic but can begin to cause pain as schwannoma grows and compresses nerve (Tinel's sign on examination).
- Extremely low malignant potential.
- Local resection indicated for schwannomas causing motor symptoms or pain.
- Extremely fine resection necessitated due to intimate involvement with neurovascular structures.

22.5.4 Neurofibromas

- Arise from the fascicles of neuron cells and comprised of Schwann cells, fibroblasts, and perineural cells.
- Solitary lesions not typically associated with NF, but multiple neurofibromas or plexiform lesions typically due to NF1.
- Several variants, but localized intraneural neurofibroma is most common.
- Typically present as enlarging painless flesh-colored mass that can eventually progress to pain or neurological dysfunction. Can occur in any part of the body.
- Extremely rare malignant transformation of less than 5% that occurs in larger masses.
- Differentiated from schwannomas in that they are not encapsulated and infiltrate between the nerves.
  - Resection requires resection of the affected nerve.
- Surgical resection with complete excision of involved nerve typically indicated for symptomatic, isolated neurofibromas.
  - May not be possible in major nerves if a significant functional consequence is anticipated.

- Nonsurgical treatment for diffuse lesions, those associated with NF1, or asymptomatic.

22.5.5 Nodular Fasciitis

- Typically develops as a result of local trauma.
- Presents as firm and painless, rapidly growing subcutaneous mass. Can mimic malignant sarcoma.
- Most common in the forearm and the lower extremities, including the foot and ankle.
- Spindle cell lesion composed of fibroblasts and myofibroblasts with positive vimentin staining on histochemistry.
- Best diagnosed with MRI, followed by core needle biopsy.
- If no concerns for malignancy, can be managed conservatively.
- Complete marginal excision indicated if symptomatic or if there are concerns for malignancy.
- Very rare recurrence rates.

22.5.6 Plantar Fibromatosis

- A benign hyperproliferative disease of the plantar aponeurosis.[9]
- Composed of spindle-shaped fibrous cells with large amount of collagen.
- Tendency for local recurrence and infiltrative growth, but they never metastasize.
- Deep and superficial variants, with deep typically growing at a much faster rate.
- Plantar aponeurosis most common location in lower extremity and common bilaterally.
- Typically presents as one or multiple hard, subcutaneous lesions in the medial aponeurosis.
- Typically asymptomatic until large enough to cause pain by mass effect or invasion of local structures.
- First-line treatment is conservative with shoe inserts, anti-inflammatories, and activity modifications.
- Additional nonoperative considerations include hormonal therapy, corticosteroid injections, collagenase injections, and radiation. Minimally invasive percutaneous ultrasonic emulsification has also been described.[9]
- Surgical excision with wide margins reserved for symptomatic cases. Requires resection of the plantar fascia with functional consequences and high recurrence rates, so should be avoided if possible.

22.5.7 Pigmented Villonodular Synovitis

- Condition where joint synovium thickens and overgrows with accompanying hemosiderin deposits.
- Most commonly occurs in the knee but can affect any synovial joint in the body.
- PVNS involves the foot and ankle less than 10% of the time.[10]
- Localized PVNS involves only isolated aspects of the joint and responds better to treatment than complete joint involvement in diffuse PVNS.
- Uncertain etiology but typically presents with isolated joint pain and swelling that is intermittent in nature but gradually worsens.
- MRI reveals synovial hypertrophy.
- Synovectomy via either arthroscopy or open procedure typical treatment of choice with possible total joint arthroplasty for more advanced cases.
- Relatively high recurrence rates of up to 20% in one meta-analysis[11] (▶ Fig. 22.11).

22.5.8 Synovial Chondromatosis

- Metaplasia of synovium with resulting transformation into cartilage that subsequently detaches and becomes a loose body within the joint.
- Most commonly affects the knee but can affect all synovial lined joints including the foot and ankle.

- Typically presents with swelling, pain, and restricted range of motion of the affected joint.
- X-rays show radiopaque loose body with MRI serving as an additional modality for soft-tissue evaluation.
- Loose body removal with additional synovectomy via arthroscopic or open approach is the treatment of choice.
- Arthroplasty or fusion can be additionally considered if resulting osteoarthritis has developed.

22.5.9 Glomus Tumors

- Believed to arise from arteriovenous anastomoses.
- Histologically appear as endothelial cells surrounded by epithelioid and glomus cells.
- Much more commonly arise in the hand but can arise in the foot.
- Most commonly occur in solitary fashion the subungual region but can also be multiple or familial in nature and outside of the subungual region.
- Patients typically present with intense pain isolated to a small region, sensitivity to cold, and paroxysmal pain.
- MRI serves as the best diagnostic imaging but can still miss smaller masses.

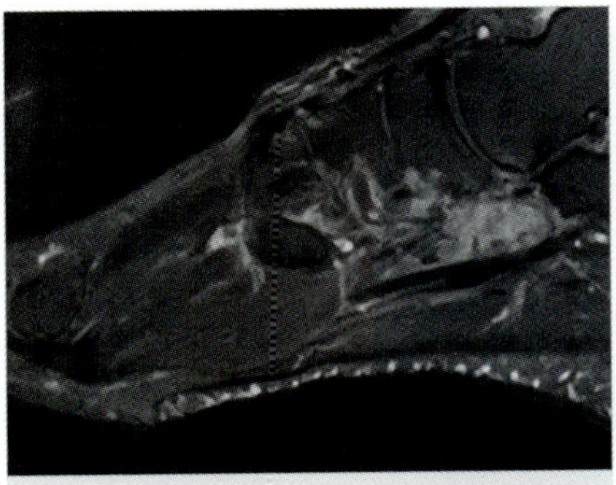

Fig. 22.11 A 47-year-old man with pigmented villonodular synovitis (PVNS) shown on T2 magnetic resonance imaging (MRI). It was treated with local surgical excision.

- Surgical excision with narrow margins serves as the definitive treatment.

22.5.10 Epidermal Inclusion Cysts

- Typically arise secondary to trauma to the pilosebaceous unit but can occur in hair-free regions.
- More common in the upper extremities but can occur in the foot and ankle.
- Histologically lined by keratin containing squamous epithelial tissue.
- Patients typically present with a painless, slowing-growing mass but some can experience pain due to mass effect.
- Best diagnosed clinically as a firm, cystic mass intradermally or subcutaneously.
- MRI can aid in surgical planning for larger masses.
- Surgical excision is appropriate for larger masses causing patient distress or cosmetic issues (▶ Fig. 22.12).

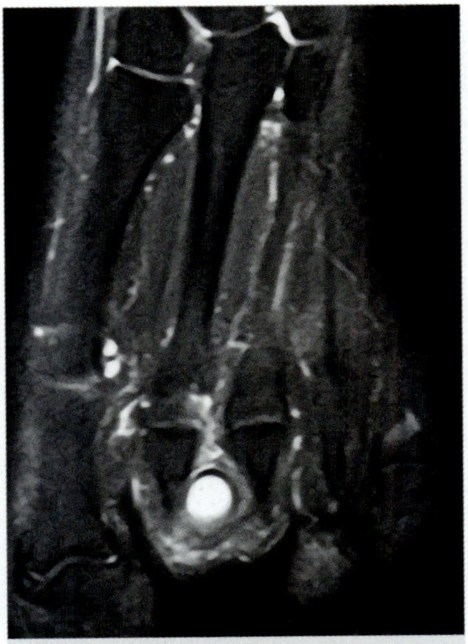

Fig. 22.12 A 36-year-old woman with epidermal inclusion cyst between second and third toes shown on T2 magnetic resonance imaging (MRI). It was treated with surgical excision.

22.6 Key Testing Facts

General principles	
Imaging	
X-ray	• Indicated for all bone tumors; may be helpful for some soft-tissue tumors
MRI	• Best next study if concern for malignancy/soft-tissue tumor suspected
CT	• Used for staging of chest/abdomen/pelvis and to evaluate bony integrity
Biopsy	
	• If suspecting malignancy, refer to sarcoma center prior to biopsy—any biopsy of a sarcoma must be performed in consultation with the treating surgeon/ sarcoma team as any biopsy tract must be planned with the definitive surgery in mind • Both cells and histology (tissue structure) are usually required for diagnosis—thus, fine needle aspirations = frequently not adequate
Margins	
	• Planned resection margins are dependent on histology • Intralesional: through the tumor itself • Marginal: complete resection through reactive zone surrounding tumor • Wide: complete resection with cuff of normal tissue • Radical: complete compartmental resection
Malignant bone tumors	
Presentation	• Varies, but frequently swelling or enlarging mass or change in known benign mass, may or may not be painful • Constitutional symptoms are possible • Age varies depending on specific pathology
Diagnostics	• Generally begin with radiographs of the foot and ankle, often the entire limb • Followed with MRI in most cases • Biopsy as per guidance of sarcoma center—should not be performed with consulting sarcoma center. • Careful screening for metastasis (IE, CT of the chest/abdomen/pelvis)
Treatment	• Wide surgical margins are commonly planned • Neoadjuvant/adjuvant treatment is dependent on pathology • Treatment of metastases is dependent on pathology
Benign bone tumors	
Presentation	• Variable depending on pathology and anatomic location • Frequently painless and slow growing • Presentation is dependent on local destruction/mass effect of tumor
Diagnostics	• Generally begin with radiographs of the foot and ankle; X-rays can be diagnostic • Low threshold to MRI if there is any concern for malignancy • Biopsy (in consultation with sarcoma center) if imaging is unclear
Treatment	• Depending on pathology and anatomic location • Marginal resections are frequently adequate • Need for surgery is often based on pain and whether tumor is causing local destruction of tissue

Malignant soft-tissue tumors	
Presentation	• Highly variable depending on pathology—skin cancers can be seen, or may present with nonhealing ulcers • Soft-tissue sarcomas may present as slow-growing, painful masses
Diagnostics	• MRI is frequently helpful in diagnosis • Biopsies should be performed carefully to avoid contamination of healthy structures • Careful screening for metastasis, especially in lesions with high metastatic potential (IE, melanoma)
Treatment	• For primary tumor site, wide margins • Treatment of metastases is dependent on pathology
Benign soft-tissue tumors	
Presentation	• Generally present as slow-growing, painless masses—however, may cause local symptoms due to tissue destruction, mass effect, or specific pathology (IE, glomus tumor)
Diagnostics	• MRI is often the most helpful in diagnosis and characterization of lesion • Formal biopsy prior to surgery may or may not be required based on radiographic imaging
Treatment	• Generally, resection is reserved for lesions that are symptomatic, causing unacceptable local tissue destruction, or cosmetically unfavorable • Marginal resection typically adequate (notable exception: fibromatosis)

Abbreviations: CT, computed tomography; IE, ifosfamide and etoposide; MRI, magnetic resonance imaging.

References

[1] Musculoskeletal Tumor Society. Systematic Literature Review on the Use of Imaging Prior to Referral to a Musculoskeletal Oncologist. Rosemont, IL: Musculoskeletal Tumor Society; 2018

[2] Crago AM, Brennan MF. Principles in management of soft tissue sarcoma. Adv Surg. 2015; 49(1):107–122

[3] Jawad MU, Scully SP. In brief: classifications in brief: Enneking classification: benign and malignant tumors of the musculoskeletal system. Clin Orthop Relat Res. 2010; 468(7):2000–2002

[4] Singer AD, Datir A, Tresley J, et al. Benign and malignant tumors of the foot and ankle. Skeletal Radiol. 2016; 45(3):287–305

[5] Sharma H, Jane MJ, Reid R. Chondromyxoid fibroma of the foot and ankle: 40 years' Scottish bone tumour registry experience. Int Orthop. 2006; 30(3):205–209

[6] Toepfer A, Harrasser N, Recker M, et al. Distribution patterns of foot and ankle tumors: a university tumor institute experience. BMC Cancer. 2018; 18 (1):735

[7] Levy DM, Gross CE, Garras DN. Treatment of unicameral bone cysts of the calcaneus: a systematic review. J Foot Ankle Surg. 2015; 54(4): 652–656

[8] Chen YU, Yu XC, Xu SF, Wang B. Giant cell tumor of the tendon sheath originating from the ankle capsule: a case report and literature review. Oncol Lett. 2016; 11(5):3461–3464

[9] Espert M, Anderson MR, Baumhauer JF. Current concepts review: plantar fibromatosis. Foot Ankle Int. 2018; 39(6):751–757

[10] Brien EW, Sacoman DM, Mirra JM. Pigmented villonodular synovitis of the foot and ankle. Foot Ankle Int. 2004; 25(12):908–913

[11] Guo Q, Shi W, Jiao C, Xie X, Jiang D, Hu Y. Results and recurrence of pigmented villonodular synovitis of the ankle: does diffuse PVNS with extra-articular extension tend to recur more often? Knee Surg Sports Traumatol Arthrosc. 2018; 26(10): 3118–3123

Suggested Readings

Malignant Bone Tumors

Mascard E, Gaspar N, Brugières L, Glorion C, Pannier S, Gomez-Brouchet A. Malignant tumours of the foot and ankle. EFORT Open Rev. 2017; 2(5):261–271

Rhee JH, Lewis RB, Murphey MD. Primary osseous tumors of the foot and ankle. Magn Reson Imaging Clin N Am. 2008; 16(1):71–91, vi

O'Connor MI, Pritchard DJ. Ewing's sarcoma. Prognostic factors, disease control, and the reemerging role of surgical treatment. Clin Orthop Relat Res. 1991(262): 78–87

Murari TM, Callaghan JJ, Berrey BH, Jr, Sweet DE. Primary benign and malignant osseous neoplasms of the foot. Foot Ankle. 1989; 10(2):68–80

Benign Bone Tumors

Azar FM, Beaty JH, Canale ST. Campbell's Operative Orthopaedics. Philadelphia, PA: Elsevier; 2017

Cannada LK. OKU 11: Orthopaedic Knowledge Update. Rosemont, IL: American Academy of Orthopaedic Surgeons; 2014

DiCaprio MR, Enneking WF. Fibrous dysplasia. Pathophysiology, evaluation, and treatment. J Bone Joint Surg Am. 2005; 87(8):1848–1864

Lee EH, Shafi M, Hui JHP. Osteoid osteoma: a current review. J Pediatr Orthop. 2006; 26(5):695–700

Levy DM, Gross CE, Garras DN. Treatment of unicameral bone cysts of the calcaneus: a systematic review. J Foot Ankle Surg. 2015; 54(4):652–656

Mahajan S, Chandra R, Mohan Lal Y. "Nora lesion": bizarre parosteal osteochondromatous proliferation. J Clin Orthop Trauma. 2012; 3(2):119–121

Schwartz HS, Menendez LR. OKU: Orthopaedic Knowledge Update. Rosemont, IL: American Academy of Orthopaedic Surgeons; 2007

Schwartz HS, Zimmerman NB, Simon MA, Wroble RR, Millar EA, Bonfiglio M. The malignant potential of enchondromatosis. J Bone Joint Surg Am. 1987; 69(2): 269–274

Malignant Soft-Tissue Tumors

Deenik W, Mooi WJ, Rutgers EJ, Peterse JL, Hart AA, Kroon BB. Clear cell sarcoma (malignant melanoma) of soft parts: a clinicopathologic study of 30 cases. Cancer. 1999; 86(6):969–975

Dzwierzynski WW. Managing malignant melanoma. Plast Reconstr Surg. 2013; 132(3):446e–460e

Papagelopoulos PJ, Mavrogenis AF, Badekas A, Sim FH. Foot malignancies: a multidisciplinary approach. Foot Ankle Clin. 2003; 8(4):751–763

Sanlorenzo M, Osella-Abate S, Ribero S, et al. Melanoma of the lower extremities: foot site is an independent risk factor for clinical outcome. Int J Dermatol. 2015; 54(9):1023–1029

Schaffer JV, Bolognia JL. The clinical spectrum of pigmented lesions. Clin Plast Surg. 2000; 27(3):391–408, viii

Thacker MM, Potter BK, Pitcher JD, Temple HT. Soft tissue sarcomas of the foot and ankle: impact of unplanned excision, limb salvage, and multimodality therapy. Foot Ankle Int. 2008; 29(7):690–698

Thway K, Fisher C. Synovial sarcoma: defining features and diagnostic evolution. Ann Diagn Pathol. 2014; 18 (6):369–380

Benign Soft-Tissue Tumors

Biswas D, Marnane CN, Mal R, Baldwin D. Extracranial head and neck schwannomas: a 10-year review. Auris Nasus Larynx. 2007; 34(3):353–359

Carpenter B. Neurofibroma of the anterior leg: a case report. Foot Ankle Online J. 2012; 5(6):2

Dahlin LB, Besjakov J, Veress B. A glomus tumour: classic signs without magnetic resonance imaging findings. Scand J Plast Reconstr Surg Hand Surg. 2005; 39(2): 123–125

Gibbons CL, Khwaja HA, Cole AS, Cooke PH, Athanasou NA. Giant-cell tumour of the tendon sheath in the foot and ankle. J Bone Joint Surg Br. 2002; 84(7):1000–1003

Knight DM, Birch R, Pringle J. Benign solitary schwannomas: a review of 234 cases. J Bone Joint Surg Br. 2007; 89(3):382–387

Kukreja S. A case report of synovial chondromatosis of the knee joint arising from the marginal synovium. J Orthop Case Rep. 2013; 3(1):7–10

Kuru I, Oktar SO, Maralcan G, Yaycioğlu S, Bozan ME. Familial glomus tumor encountered in the same finger and localization in four family members. Acta Orthop Traumatol Turc. 2005; 39(4):365–368

Luis LR, Jr, Kaoru GR, Shemuel PB, Mills JL, Sr. Lower extremity glomus tumors: comprehensive review for surgeons. Vascular. 2008; 16(6):326–332

Murphey MD, Smith WS, Smith SE, Kransdorf MJ, Temple HT. From the archives of the AFIP. Imaging of musculoskeletal neurogenic tumors: radiologic-pathologic correlation. Radiographics. 1999; 19(5):1253–1280

Nigam JS, Bharti JN, Nair V, et al. Epidermal cysts: a clinicopathological analysis with emphasis on unusual findings. Int J Trichology. 2017; 9(3):108–112

Pehlivan M, Özbay PO, Temur M, Yılmaz Ö, Gümüş Z, Güzel A. Epidermal cyst in an unusual site: a case report. Int J Surg Case Rep. 2015; 8C:114–116

Reilly KE, Stern PJ, Dale JA. Recurrent giant cell tumors of the tendon sheath. J Hand Surg Am. 1999; 24(6): 1298–1302

Robbin MR, Murphey MD, Temple HT, Kransdorf MJ, Choi JJ. Imaging of musculoskeletal fibromatosis. Radiographics. 2001; 21(3):585–600

Sethuraman G, Yenamandra VK, Gupta V. Management of infantile hemangiomas: current trends. J Cutan Aesthet Surg. 2014; 7(2):75–85

Sharma R, Gaillard F. Lipoma. Radiopaedia.org2018

Skandhan A, St-Amant M. Neurofibroma. Radiopaedia. org2018

Spinelli N, Khorassani N. Nodular fasciitis: an uncommon disease with common medical management challenges at a remote naval hospital. Mil Med. 2013; 178(9): e1051–e1054

Weinreb I, Shaw AJ, Perez-Ordoñez B, Goldblum JR, Rubin BP. Nodular fasciitis of the head and neck region: a clinicopathologic description in a series of 30 cases. J Cutan Pathol. 2009; 36(11):1168–1173

Zheng JW, Zhang L, Zhou Q, et al. A practical guide to treatment of infantile hemangiomas of the head and neck. Int J Clin Exp Med. 2013; 6(10):851–860

23 Pediatric Disorders of the Foot and Ankle

Ian S. MacLean, David Zhu, Charles P. Hannon, and Monica Kogan

Abstract

Pediatric disorders of the foot and ankle are a diverse set of conditions with etiologies and treatment options that range over a wide spectrum. Some pathologies occur in isolation and are not indicative of any greater underlying problem. These may resolve on their own with conservative treatment or persist but without significant effect on the child's development and activity. Others are strongly associated with genetic, developmental, or neuromuscular disorders that should immediately receive referral for a multidisciplinary evaluation. A thorough history and physical examination is critical for appropriate diagnosis and treatment. Bracing and casting are the mainstays of treatment for pediatric foot and ankle conditions. However, some conditions require significant reconstructive efforts.

Keywords: clubfoot, congenital talipes equinovarus, metatarsus adductus, pes cavus, tarsal coalition, talipes calcaneovalgus, juvenile bunions, Kohler's disease, flexible pes planus, toe walking, accessory navicular, congenital hallux varus, syndactyly, polydactyly, curly toe, overlapping toe

23.1 Clubfoot: Congenital Talipes Equinovarus

23.1.1 Etiology and Pathophysiology

- Incidence of clubfoot varies widely with respect to race and geography with it being more commonly seen in areas such as the South Pacific.[1,2]
- Male predominance is 2:1.
- Bilateral disease occurs in 50% of cases.
- Approximately 25% of patients have a positive family history.
- Pathogenesis is multifactorial and is likely due to both environmental and genetic factors. Chromosomal, viral, and vascular etiologies have also been proposed.
- High incidence of genetic anomalies associated with clubfoot including neural tube defects, trisomy 18, and congenital heart defects.
- Secondary etiologies, such as neuromuscular disorders (e.g., arthrogryposis, spinal muscular atrophy, and spina bifida), can lead to clubfoot, which is more complex and more difficult to treat than idiopathic clubfoot.

23.1.2 Symptoms

- Gross deformity noted at birth or on prenatal ultrasound.

23.1.3 Diagnostics and Classification

- Physical exam findings[3]:
  - Foot deformity (▶ Fig. 23.1): hindfoot equinovarus, midfoot cavus, and forefoot adduction.
    - Hindfoot equinus is rigid and resists passive correction.
  - Small calf and foot:
  - Shortened tibia.
  - Medial and posterior foot skin creases. Depth of creases may correlate with severity of deformity.
- Imaging findings:
  - Imaging is often unnecessary, but may be used to confirm the clinical diagnosis or help rule out associated anomalies.
  - Radiographs:
    - Anteroposterior (AP) view:
      - Talocalcaneal angle less than 20 degrees (normal: 20–40 degrees).

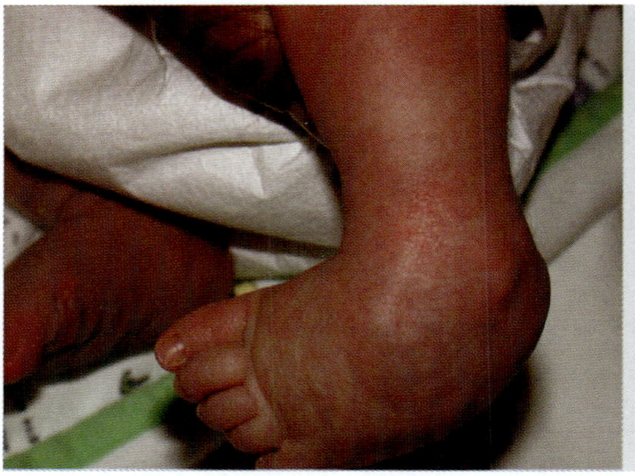

Fig. 23.1 Clubfoot demonstrating hindfoot equinovarus, midfoot cavus, and forefoot adduction.

        * *Talus:* first metatarsal angle less than 0 degrees (normal: 0–20 degrees)
        * Hindfoot parallelism.
        * Lateral:
        * Talar neck is medially rotated, shortened, plantarflexed.
        * *Turco view:* dorsiflexion lateral:
        * Hindfoot parallelism between the talus and the calcaneus.
        * Talocalcaneal angle less than 35 degrees.
        * Flat talar head.
    - Ultrasound:
        - May be used for prenatal diagnosis as early as 12 weeks.
        - High false-positive rate.
        - When diagnosis is made prenatally, genetic testing is recommended given the high incidence of associated genetic anomalies.
- Classification[4]:
    - *Dimeglio's classification:* based on a 20-point score:
        - Deformity evaluated based on four components with attempted reduction of the foot:
            * Degree of sagittal plane equinus.
            * Degree of coronal plane varus.
            * Degree of axial plane calcaneopedal internal rotation.
            * Degree of axial plane forefoot adduction relative to the hindfoot.
            * Each component is scored from 1 to 4.

Reducibility	Points
90–45 degrees	4
45–20 degrees	3
20–0 degrees	2
0 to –20 degrees	1

        - Additional points given for the presence of the following:
            * Medial crease.
            * Posterior crease.
            * Cavus.
            * Poor muscle condition.

Grade	Type	Score
I	Benign	< 5
II	Moderate	5 to < 10
III	Severe	10 to < 15
IV	Very severe	15–20

23.1.4 Conservative Management

- First-line treatment for all clubfeet regardless of severity.
- Ponseti's method[5]:
    - Reducing the talonavicular joint by externally rotating the forefoot around the talus.
    - After the talonavicular joint is reduced, the foot is dorsiflexed to neutral.
    - Achilles tenotomy may be performed to allow for neutral dorsiflexion.

- Order of correction (CAVE):
  - Midfoot cavus.
  - Forefoot adductus.
  - Hindfoot varus.
  - Hindfoot equinus.
- Long leg plaster cast with minimal padding should be used and changed every week for the first 6 weeks, then every 2 weeks until the age of 4 to 6 months.
- After successful casting, must wear foot abduction orthosis (FAO) 23 hours a day for 3 months and then for 14 to 16 hours a day until the age of 3 or 4 years.[6]
- Ninety percent success rate with outcomes equal to or better than those of patients treated surgically.[7,8]
- Up to 70% of patients may require a percutaneous Achilles tenotomy to get the foot to dorsiflex to neutral.

23.1.5 Surgical Intervention

- Surgical intervention is reserved for failed conservative management, when the foot fails to attain anatomic or neutral positioning after 3 to 6 months of treatment, or when recurrence occurs and the child is too old to attempt repeat casting.[9]
- Several reported releases in the literature including wide circumferential release as well as more localized posteromedial soft-tissue release and tendon lengthening[10]:
  - Posteromedial soft-tissue release realigns the navicular on the talus moving it away from the medial malleolus.
  - Medial release includes takedown of the abductor hallucis muscle and the talonavicular capsule often with a posterior tibial tendon lengthening.
  - Posterior release involves the Achilles tendon and the posterior tibiotalar joint capsule. It may also involve the posterior subtalar joint and associated structural ligaments.
- The authors' preferred method is the Ponseti technique with serial casting and percutaneous Achilles tenotomy to correct equinus, if needed.

23.1.6 Rehabilitation

- FAO should be used after conservative management to prevent relapse.
- Daily duration and total length of use are not well defined and are often surgeon preference. Many suggest 23 h/d for the first 3 months, followed by nighttime and naptime bracing for up to 2 years.

23.2 Metatarsus Adductus

23.2.1 Etiology and Pathophysiology

- Medial deviation of the forefoot on the hindfoot with a neutral or slightly valgus heel (▶ Fig. 23.2).
- Occurs in 0.1% of all births with equal frequency in females and males.
- Bilateral in approximately 50% of cases.
- Increased incidence seen with males, late pregnancy, first pregnancy, and twin pregnancies.
- Multiple etiologies proposed, including the following: packing defect in utero; sleeping position (e.g., prone with hips and knees forefoot adducted) after birth; anatomic differences including muscle imbalance with tight anterior tibial tendon; and abnormal development of the medial cuneiform.
- Associated with developmental dysplasia of the hip (DDH) and torticollis.

23.2.2 Symptoms

- Parents complain of cosmesis issue or intoeing during the first year of life.

23.2.3 Diagnostics and Classification

- Physical examination findings:
  - Metatarsus adductus:
    - C-shaped foot with concave medial border and convex lateral border
    - Medial soft-tissue crease indicates rigid deformity.
    - Pressure sites in shoe wear may include the medial border of the first metatarsophalangeal joint (MTPJ) or a prominent lateral border at the base of the fifth metatarsal.
    - Normal hindfoot and subtalar motion.
  - Complex skew foot:
    - Tarsometatarsal adductus, talonavicular lateral subluxation, and also includes the hindfoot valgus.
- Imaging findings:
  - Radiographs are not necessary in infants with metatarsus adductus, but may be indicated for children above the age of 4 or 5 years with unresolved deformity and pain.
  - In older children, radiographs will demonstrate forefoot adduction, medial deviation at the tarsometatarsal joint, and neutral or valgus heel.
- Bleck's classification (▶ Fig. 23.3):
  - Based on coronal heel bisector line. With increasing adduction, the heel bisector line is displaced toward the fifth toe.
  - Normal:
    - Heel bisector line through the second and third toe webspace.
  - Mild:
    - Heel bisector line through the third toe.
  - Moderate:
    - Heel bisector line through the third and fourth toe webspace.

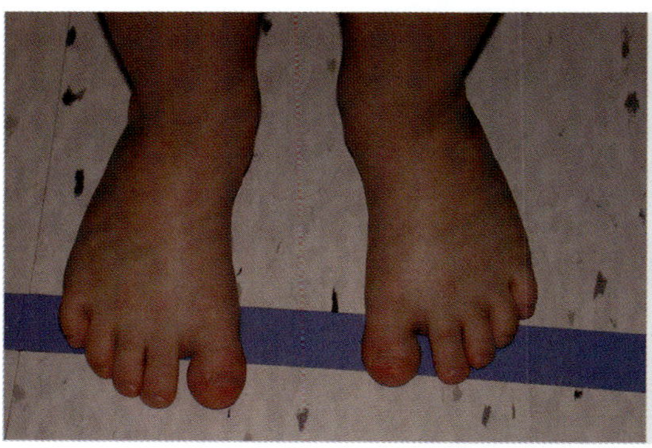

Fig. 23.2 Clinical photograph of metatarsus adductus demonstrating medial deviation of the forefoot on the hindfoot.

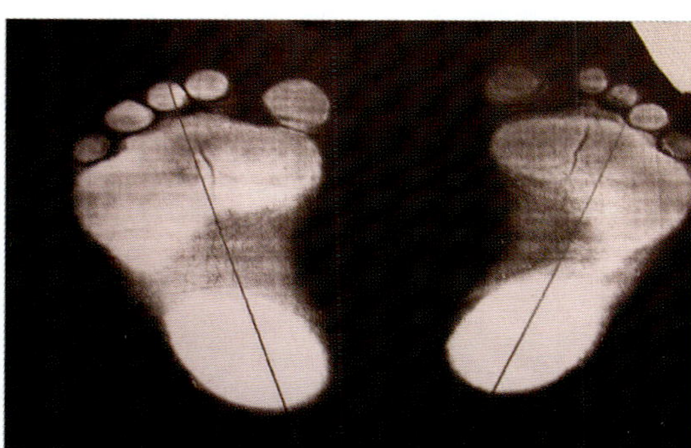

Fig. 23.3 Mild (bisector through the third toe) and moderate (bisector through the third and fourth web-spaces) metatarsus adductus using the Bleck classification.

- Severe:
  - Heel bisector line through the fourth and fifth toe webspace.
  - Convex lateral border of the foot.

23.2.4 Conservative Management

- Approximately 85% of patients with metatarsus adductus will resolve spontaneously without treatment.[11,12]
- Mild/flexible metatarsus adductus may not require any specific treatment.
- Casting indicated for rigid or persistent deformity:
  - Casts should be above the knee with the knee flexed.
  - Correction typically takes up to 6 to 8 weeks.

23.2.5 Surgical Intervention

- Rarely indicated.[13]
- Patients younger than 5 years:
  - Release abductor hallucis, tarsometatarsal capsulotomy, and metatarsal osteotomy.
- Patients older than 5 years:
  - May require proximal osteotomies of the lesser metatarsals.

23.3 Pes Cavus

23.3.1 Etiology and Pathophysiology

- Rare in children younger than 3 years, but may develop as the child grows.[14]
- Etiologies may be attributed to the brain, spinal cord, peripheral nerves, or to muscular or structural foot problems:
  - Central nervous system:
    - Cerebral palsy (CP) and hemiplegia.
  - Spinal deformities:
    - Myelodysplasia, diastematomyelia, and syringomyelia (unilateral), tethered cord syndrome, or spinal tumors.
  - Peripheral nerves:
    - Hereditary sensorimotor neuropathy (HSMN), atypical polyneuritis, and neuromuscular choristoma.
- A weak tibialis anterior and peroneus brevis with strong overpull by the tibialis posterior and peroneus longus cause hindfoot cavus, forefoot equinus, and pronation.
- Nonprogressive conditions, such as CP, have spasticity of the tibialis posterior inverting the hindfoot leading to lateral column weight bearing. Forefoot equinus due to leg length discrepancy.

23.3.2 Symptoms

- Birth history, family history of Charcot–Marie–Tooth (CMT) disease, developmental delay, hand, hip, foot, bowel, or bladder symptoms.
- Ankle instability, pain under the metatarsal heads, or sensory changes.

23.3.3 Diagnostics and Classification

- Physical examination findings:
  - Determine if the hindfoot is in varus or valgus (more commonly varus).
  - The Coleman block test determines if hindfoot deformity is flexible or fixed.[15]
  - Note the apex of the cavus, which helps determine the best location for corrective osteotomy:
    - Is it due to plantar flexion of the forefoot or dorsiflexion of the calcaneus?
  - Assess for lesser toe deformities.
  - Assess rigidity of the joints and rigidity of the deformity. Is it manually correctable?
  - Assess the muscle power of all groups, especially the tibialis anterior, tibialis posterior, peroneus longus, and peroneus brevis.
  - Absent knee or ankle reflexes may represent hypertrophic CMT disease.

    - Sensory changes may include loss of vibration and position sense.
    - Skin changes may include vasomotor signs such as flushing, cyanosis, and marbling of the skin.
- Imaging findings:
    - Radiographs of the spine should be taken to assess for scoliosis, spinal dysraphism, or diastematomyelia.[16]
    - Patients with CMT disease should have a standing AP pelvis to assess for acetabular dysplasia.
    - Magnetic resonance imaging (MRI) of spinal cord for assessment of spinal cord tumor or dysraphic lesions.
    - Computed tomography (CT) of the brain to assess for occult hydrocephalus.
    - Radiographs:
        - Plantarflexed metatarsals, midfoot dorsiflexion, MTPJ dorsiflexion.
        - Calcaneus neutral dorsiflexion/ plantar flexion, medial forefoot plantarflexed, and forefoot equinus.
        - Meary's angle greater than 5 degrees (18 degrees average in CMT).
        - Calcaneal pitch less than 30 degrees (normal ~30 degrees) indicates forefoot equinus and greater than 30 degrees may indicate calcaneocavus.
        - Hibbs' angle (line between the calcaneus and the first metatarsal) typically around 90 degrees (normal < 45 degrees).
- Classification by pathology:
    - HSMN classification:
        - Based on motor nerve conduction velocity studies.
        - Types I to III found in children.
        - Type I:
            * Hypertrophic form of CMT with decreased motor nerve conduction, and spotty peripheral nerve degeneration.
            * *Type IA most common:* duplication of peripheral myelin protein 22 (PMP-22).
        - Type II:
            * Neuronal form of CMT with intact myelin sheath and mild abnormal sensory and motor conduction velocities.
        - Type III:
            * Dejerine–Sottas disease.
            * Autosomal recessive.
            * Presents in infancy and worse prognosis.
            * Marked decrease in motor conduction because of peripheral nerve demyelination.

23.3.4 Conservative Management

- Appropriate for patients with mild or nonprogressive deformity.
- Lateral column and forefoot postorthotic may be indicated for foot with a flexible hindfoot and fixed plantar flexion of the first metatarsal.
- Orthotics for more advanced cases should focus on unloading areas of high plantar pressure.
- Runners may require activity adjustment, stretching, pain management, shoe modification, flexible orthotics, and quadriceps muscle strengthening.

23.3.5 Surgical Intervention

- The goal is to obtain a mobile plantigrade foot with correction of the cavus deformity.[17,18,19]
- Procedure type depends on patient age, activity level, deformity, and underlying etiology.
- Procedures may include soft-tissue release, osteotomy, tendon transfers, and arthrodesis, and may involve the toes.
- General surgical principles include the following:
    - Must correct underlying flexible or fixed deformity:
        - Fixed deformities (ones that do not correct with the Coleman block test) typically require osteotomies.

    - Fixed hindfoot varus requires either lateral closing wedge osteotomy or lateral slide.
    - Flexible deformities typically require soft-tissue releases.
    - Plantar fascia release for minor deformity.
    - More complex deformity requires release of plantar fascia, abductor halluces, flexor digitorum brevis, quadratus plantae, and abductor digiti quinti muscles.
    - Arthrodesis indicated for severe deformity or arthritis.
    - Triple arthrodesis reserved as a salvage procedure for adolescents with fixed cavus deformity that has failed other managements.
  - Correction should be at the site of maximum deformity:
    - Closing wedge proximal metatarsal osteotomy may be used for plantarflexed fixed first ray.
    - Several types of midfoot osteotomies have been described.
  - Motion should be preserved.
  - Underlying muscle imbalance should be corrected with either tendon transfers or lengthening.

23.4 Tarsal Coalitions

23.4.1 Etiology and Pathophysiology

- Present in approximately 1% of population.[2,20,21]
- Abnormal mesenchymal segmentation leads to failure to form a normal joint.
- Most commonly calcaneonavicular or talocalcaneal:
  - Can also be talonavicular or involve the cuboid and/or cuneiforms.
- Congenital (autosomal dominant with variable penetrance) or acquired (trauma, infection).
- Associated with other congenital limb anomalies such as fibular hemimelia and proximal focal femoral deficiency.
- Restriction of subtalar motion:
  - Talocalcaneal coalitions typically cause greater motion loss than calcaneonavicular coalitions.
  - The foot is typically in external rotation and valgus in early stance and changes to internal rotation and varus in late stance and swing phase. With restriction of subtalar motion, the foot assumes a flat and valgus position.[20]
  - Normally, the calcaneus slides forward relative to talus in dorsiflexion. Without forward translation of the calcaneus in dorsiflexion, the navicular "hinges" on the talus, leading to abnormal stresses on the capsule and periosteum—thought to be the cause of talar beaking sign.[20]

23.4.2 Symptoms

- Calcaneonavicular coalition most commonly diagnosed in ages 9 to 12 years.[20,21,22]
- Talocalcaneal coalition most commonly diagnosed in ages 12 to 15 years.
- Seventy-five percent cases are asymptomatic.
- Pain with activity.
- Onset of pain corresponds to age of ossification:
  - Caused by limited subtalar motion, flatfoot, and peroneal spasticity.[23]
  - Location depends on coalition:
  - *Calcaneonavicular:* sinus tarsi, inferior fibula:
    - *Talocalcaneal:* medial foot, below the medial malleolus.
- Peroneal spasticity → calf pain.[24]
- *Typical presentation:* history of foot or ankle injury ("ankle sprain") with persistent pain.

23.4.3 Diagnostics and Classification

- Physical examination findings[20,21]:
  - Hindfoot valgus:
    - Not corrected with toe standing.

    - Reverse Coleman block test demonstrates loss of subtalar motion.
  - Forefoot abduction.
  - Rigid flatfoot.[25]
  - Deep joint pain with passive subtalar inversion:
    - Around sinus tarsi, may radiate to dorsum of foot.
- Imaging findings[20,22,26]:
  - *Radiographs:* AP, lateral, Harris view, 45-degree internal oblique view.
  - Calcaneonavicular coalition:
    - Best visualized on oblique view.
      - No further diagnostic imaging unless multiple coalitions are suspected.
      - Anteater sign on lateral view is diagnostic (▶ Fig. 23.4)[27]:
      - Elongated anterior process of the calcaneus.
  - Talocalcaneal coalition:
    - May be visible on Harris view, but best seen on CT.
    - Talar beaking on lateral view.
    - C sign (outline of talar dome + posteroinferior sustentaculum tali).
    - Dysmorphic sustentaculum tali, loss of middle facet, and talar neck shortening.
  - CT:
    - Identify shape and size of coalition:
      - Coronal slices to measure cross-sectional area of the talocalcaneal coalition relative to that of the posterior facet.
    - Identify additional coalitions:
      - Up to 20% incidence.
- Classification by anatomy:
  - Calcaneonavicular.
  - Talocalcaneal:
    - Most commonly of the middle facet of the calcaneus.
- Classification by pathology:
  - Fibrous (syndesmosis).
  - Cartilaginous (synchondrosis).
  - Osseous (synostosis).

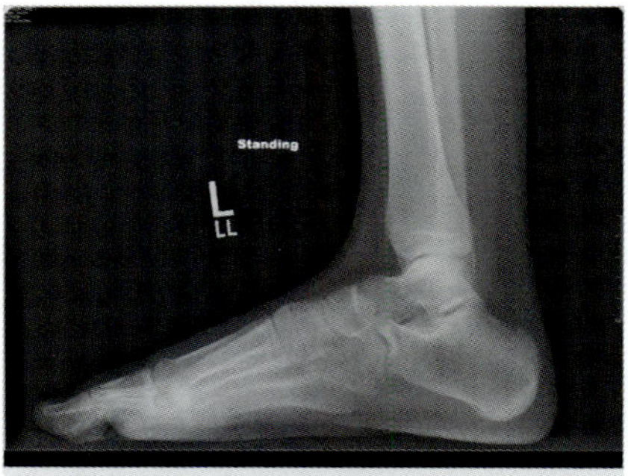

Fig. 23.4 The anteater sign (elongation of the anterosuperior aspect of the calcaneus) indicative of calcaneonavicular coalition.

23.4.4 Conservative Management

- First-line treatment.[20]
- Observation with follow-up:
  - For incidental finding without pain.
- Orthoses:
  - For mild symptoms.
  - Heel cup with medial wedge:
    - Maintain hindfoot alignment and provide medial arch support.
- Immobilization:
  - For more symptomatic cases.
  - Short-leg walking cast with slight varus mold for 2 to 4 weeks.
  - University of California Biomechanical Laboratory (UCBL) shoe orthosis.
    - Maintains hindfoot, medial arch, and lateral forefoot alignment.

23.4.5 Surgical Intervention

- Resection of coalition with interposition[20,22]:
  - For calcaneonavicular coalitions and talocalcaneal coalitions involving less than 50% of the joint.
  - Interposition graft prevents recurrence of bone formation:
    - Extensor digitorum brevis (for calcaneonavicular coalition).
    - Split flexor hallucis longus tendon (for talocalcaneal coalition).
    - Fat, bone wax.

- Triple arthrodesis:
  - For advanced coalitions (> 50% of the joint), multiple coalitions, and failed resections.
  - For coalitions associated with degenerative changes in surrounding joints.

23.4.6 Rehabilitation

- Short-leg cast and non-weight-bearing for 3 weeks.[22]
- Weight bearing as tolerated and mobilization after cast removal.

23.5 Talipes Calcaneovalgus

23.5.1 Etiology and Pathophysiology

- A packaging disorder (involving abnormal uterine positioning) rather than a structural defect.[28]
- Incidence is 1 in 1,000.
- Increased risk to subsequent children if the first child is born with a calcaneovalgus foot (1 in 20).
- More common in the following:
  - Females.
  - First-born infants.
  - Large infants.
  - Twins.

23.5.2 Symptoms

- Clinical examination reveals the following: ankle is hyperdorsiflexed, subtalar joint is everted, and the midfoot may be abducted (▶ Fig. 23.5).[28]
- The dorsal surface of the foot may be in contact with the anterolateral surface of the leg.
- Restricted plantar flexion and inversion.
- Calcaneus is palpable in the heel pad due to dorsiflexion.
- Other considerations:
  - Talipes calcaneovalgus with posteromedial tibial bowing:
    - These two conditions may occur together or separately.
    - Posteromedial tibial bowing is another packaging disorder but may lead to a future leg length discrepancy.
  - Congenital vertical talus[2,22]:
    - Calcaneus is in equinus and valgus. Forefoot is dorsiflexed at the midtarsal joint.

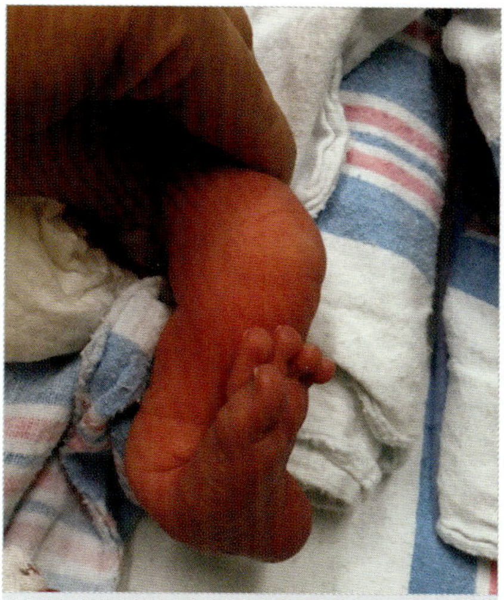

Fig. 23.5 Clinical photograph of severe talipes calcaneovalgus with posteromedial bow. The dorsal surface of the foot in contact with the anterolateral surface of the leg.

23.5.3 Conservative Management

- The natural history of the disease is excellent:[28]
  - Usually spontaneous resolution.
- Parents may perform gentle plantar flexion and inversion stretching exercises:
  - Typical resolution in 3 to 6 months.
- Serial casting indicated for more severe cases (▶ Fig. 23.6).

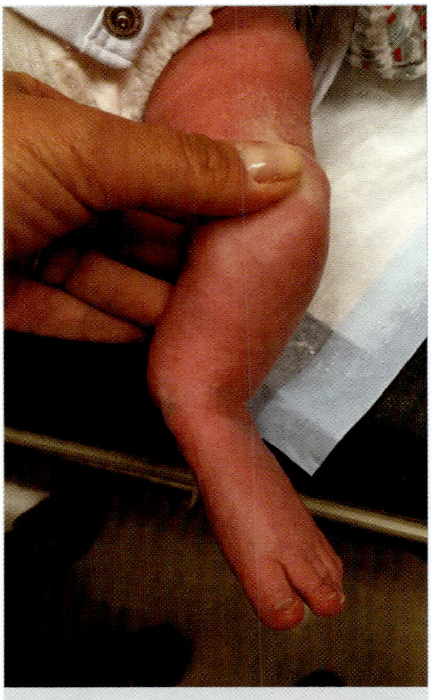

Fig. 23.6 Clinical photography showing the improvement of severe talipes calcaneovalgus after 1 week of casting.

23.6 Juvenile Bunions

23.6.1 Etiology and Pathophysiology

- The lateral deviation of the great toe and medial deviation of the first metatarsal.[2,29,30,31,32,33]
- Affects 2 to 4% of the population.
- Develops during or slightly before adolescence.
- Estimated that 40 to 50% of adult bunions actually started during childhood.
- Positive family history (usually maternal).
- May also occur as a result of muscular imbalance in neuromuscular diseases like CP.
- Female predominance.
- Usually bilateral.
- The first metatarsal–cuneiform joint is typically transverse:
  - Some children with juvenile bunions will have a medially sloping articulation.
    - This directs the first metatarsal medially.
- May also be associated with ligamentous laxity and hypermobility of the first ray.
- With development of the deformity, the adductor hallucis becomes the deforming force.

23.6.2 Symptoms

- Patients typically seek out care due to concern about cosmesis.[2,32]
- Pain, redness, or swelling over the medial eminence of the deformity.
- First MTPJ pain.
- Difficulty wearing certain shoes.
- Discomfort performing specific activities.

23.6.3 Diagnostics and Classification

- Radiographs[2,32,33,34]:
  - AP and lateral:
    - Hallux valgus angle (HVA): normal less than 15 degrees.
    - Intermetatarsal angle (IMA): normal less than 9 degrees.
    - Distal metatarsal articulator angle (DMAA): normal 0 to 8 degrees.
      - If greater than 8 degrees, the first MTPJ is considered incongruent.
- Classification—based on HVA and IMA:
  - *Mild:* HVA < 20 degrees and IMA < 13 degrees.
  - *Moderate:* 20 degrees < HVA < 40 degrees and 13 degrees < IMA < 16 degrees.
  - *Severe:* HVA > 40 degrees and IMA > 16 degrees.

23.6.4 Conservative Management

- Conservative treatment is tailored toward pain relief. It will not correct the deformity or prevent progression.[2,33,34]
- Activity modification.
- Shoes with a wide toe box.
- Toe spacers and splints.
- Delaying treatment until the child is older allows ligamentous laxity to improve and permits the resolution of flexible pes planus.
- There is a chance the deformity can progress while awaiting skeletal maturity, which must be balanced with early intervention and possible recurrence.

23.6.5 Surgical Intervention

- Should only consider surgical intervention for unrelenting pain despite conservative measures and NEVER for cosmesis alone.[32,33,34]
- Surgery should be delayed until the first metatarsal physis has closed:
  - Increased risk of failure and reoccurrence or of overcorrection into hallux varus if the surgery is done prior to skeletal maturity.
- Distal soft-tissue procedure (McBride's procedure):
  - Never performed in isolation.
  - May be used in conjunction with an osteotomy to realign an incongruent first MTPJ.
- Distal metatarsal osteotomy (Chevron's osteotomy; Mitchell's osteotomy):
  - Used in mild to moderate deformities.
- Proximal metatarsal osteotomy:
  - Wait for skeletal maturity to avoid disruption of the physis.
  - Moderate deformities.
- Double osteotomy:
  - Severe deformities:
  - Required for incongruent MTPJ (DMAA > 8 degrees).
- Metatarsal–cuneiform fusion (Lapidus' procedure):
  - May be used in skeletally mature individuals with a hypermobile first ray or as an alternative for severe deformities.
- First MTPJ fusion:
  - Indicated for symptomatic hallux valgus that affects gait and shoe ware in individuals with neuromuscular conditions.
  - Provides best correction and outcomes.[33]

23.7 Kohler's Disease

23.7.1 Etiology and Pathophysiology

- A rare, idiopathic, and self-limiting osteochondrosis of the tarsal navicular.[35,36,37]
- The natural history of Kohler's disease is benign.
  - The process typically resolves spontaneously.
  - The navicular will return to its normal architecture between 4 months and 4 years from the onset of symptoms.
  - There is no residual structural deformity or functional disability in adulthood.
- Kohler's disease is usually unilateral although there are instances of bilateral occurrence of the disease.
- Male children are affected three to five times more frequently than female children.
- Males will typically present at around 5 to 6 years of age. Females usually present a year earlier.
- The true cause of Kohler's disease is not fully known:[38]
  - Navicular ossification occurs earlier in females than in males. The average age of appearance of the ossification center in females is between 18 months and 2 years; in males between 2.5 and 3 years of age.

   ◦ One theory suggests that as the navicular is always the last tarsal bone to ossify; delayed ossification of the navicular may subject the bone to greater compressive forces:[39]
      – This pressure may produce changes ranging from flattening and increased bony density to possibly ischemia.
   ◦ Another theory proposes that avascular necrosis is responsible for Kohler's disease:
      – Compressive forces within the bone may occlude the vessels resulting in an ischemic lesion:[39]
         * The navicular has a perichondral network of five to six arteries on the nonarticular surfaces.
         * As the ossification nucleus develops, one or more penetrating branches perfuse the nucleus.
         * In the cases where the navicular develops patchy ischemia, one, but not all, of these penetrating branches is affected.
         * In some cases, only a single dorsal or plantar penetrating artery supplies the developing nucleus.
         * Occlusion of this vessel will cause more complete ischemia of the bone.
         * However, the dense perichondral ring of vessels around the navicular allows revascularization with spontaneous and complete healing.
- *Genetics:* A genetic component has not been established although there is a case report of identical twins developing bilateral Kohler's disease.[36]

23.7.2 Symptoms

- Point tenderness localized to the dorsal aspect of the midfoot is the most consistent finding on physical examination.[36]
- Tenderness may occasionally be accompanied by mild swelling and heat over the dorsum of the midfoot.
- The child may also walk with a limp.
- Duration of symptoms prior to presentation may vary ranging from a few days to a year.
- There is usually no clear history of injury or trauma to the affected foot, nor is there a history of previous or recent infections.
- All laboratory tests are normal.

23.7.3 Diagnostics

- The diagnosis of Kohler's disease is a clinical one on the basis of physical examination findings.[36]
- Radiographs will usually show findings of necrosis (▶ Fig. 23.7):

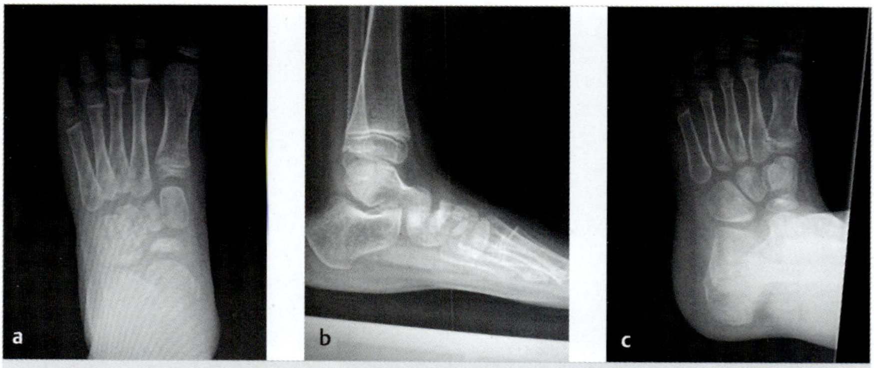

Fig. 23.7 (a–c) Radiographs of Kohler's disease showing increased radiodensity of the navicular and some loss of the trabecular pattern.

- Increased radiodensity.
- Loss of trabecular pattern.
- Fragmentation.
- Flattening of the longitudinal axis of the navicular bone.

- Radiographs should always be interpreted in the context of the physical examination findings and patient history:
  - Irregularities in navicular ossification are common and may lead to the radiographic appearance of Kohler's disease.
  - The diagnosis should not be made if clinical symptoms do not correspond with the radiographic findings.

23.7.4 Conservative Management

- Treatment is entirely symptomatic; rarely is surgery an option.[36,37,38,40]
- Treatment options include the following:
  - Hard-soled shoes.
  - Orthotics with longitudinal medial arch support.
  - Short-leg walking cast immobilization:
    - Treatment with a below-knee cast for at least 8 weeks has been shown to result in resolution of symptoms more quickly than other treatment modalities.
- The final outcome of treatment is favorable regardless of the selected therapy.
- Most patients are able to return to full activity and do not require special footwear.

23.8 Flexible Pes Planus

23.8.1 Etiology and Pathophysiology

- A flexible flatfoot is one with a medial longitudinal foot arch that is present while sitting but disappears with weight bearing.[41]
- Flexible flatfoot is the normal foot shape in the first few years of life.[42]
  - Approximately 97% of children younger than 2 years have flexible flatfeet compared with only 4% of children at the age of 10 years.
- Throughout the first decade of life, most children with flexible flatfeet will have spontaneous resolution.
- Most commonly bilateral and often familial.[43]
- Risk factors include joint laxity, male gender, and obesity.[44]
- The cause of flexible flatfeet has not been linked to any one factor. The cause is most likely multifactorial:
  - Osseous–ligamentous complex weakness:
    - The shape of the arch is largely thought to be maintained by the osseous–ligamentous complex. One common factor for loss of a normal medial arch is incompetence of the spring ligament.
  - Muscle weakness:
    - Patients with pes planus show extensor muscle weakness at rest and during the heel-contact phase of the gait cycle.
  - Limb alignment:
    - Increased tibial torsion, hindfoot malalignment, and internally rotated knees have been found to correlate with pes planus.

23.8.2 Symptoms

- Pes planus deformity is often painless and asymptomatic.[22,41]
- Children are usually brought to the physician due to parental concern.
- Symptomatic pes planus may present with a variety of complaints including the following:
  - Medial arch pain and fatigue.
  - Calluses of the medial, plantar foot—caused by localized pressure from the plantarflexed talar head.
  - Rapid shoe breakdown.
  - Recurrent ankle sprains.

23.8.3 Diagnostics and Classification

- The physician should ask about a family history of flat and/or painful feet.[22,40,41]
- General musculoskeletal examination including rotational profile of the legs.
- Assessment of ligamentous laxity using the 9-point Beighton score.
- Examination should include inspection of both feet while the patient is both sitting and standing.
  - Children should be examined from the front and back while standing.
  - An arch that is present while sitting but absent while standing is typical for a flexible pes planus deformity.
  - Having the patient perform a single-leg stand may reveal arch collapse that is not obvious with a two-leg stance:
    - The arch should reconstitute when the patient stands on tiptoes or during the "toe raising test:"
      - *Toe raising test:* The examiner dorsiflexes the great toe while the patient stands causing the arch to reconstitute due to tightening of the plantar fascia.
- Pes planus is often accompanied by hindfoot valgus, a dorsiflexed and abducted midfoot, and a pronated or externally rotated forefoot:
  - *"Too many toes" sign:* more than just the fourth and fifth toes are visible from behind (indicative of hindfoot valgus).
- Radiographs:
  - Rarely indicated if the patient is asymptomatic.
  - Should be weight bearing if obtained (► Fig. 23.8):
    - Lateral radiograph shows an apex-plantar Meary's angle (lateral talus–first metatarsal angle)—usual is 0 degrees.
    - *AP radiograph:* hindfoot and midfoot eversion and valgus demonstrated by diverging talocalcaneal axes and lateral displacement of the navicular on the talus.

23.8.4 Conservative Management

- *Asymptomatic:* best managed with observation, education, and reassurance:[22,41,45]
  - Orthotics have not been shown to alter the natural course in asymptomatic patients.
  - Most will resolve spontaneously.
- Symptomatic:
  - Best initial treatments include rest, activity modification, icing, massage, and nonsteroidal anti-inflammatory medications.
  - A home physical therapy and stretching program may be recommended if the patient has tight heel cords.
  - Orthotics may prove beneficial—in contrast to their use in asymptomatic patients.

23.8.5 Surgical Intervention

- Rarely indicated except when there is persistent pain despite exhaustion of conservative options.[22,41]

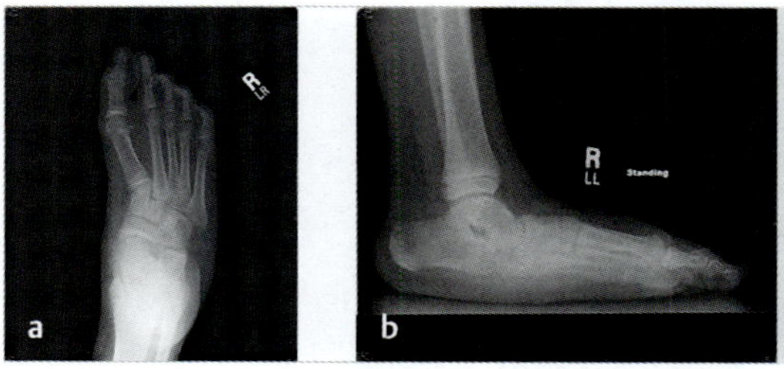

Fig. 23.8 (a,b) Anteroposterior (AP) and lateral weight-bearing radiographs demonstrating diverging talocalcaneal axes and lateral subluxation of the navicular on the talus (AP), and apex plantar Meary's angle (lateral).

- Soft-tissue procedures:
  - Achilles' tendon lengthening and tendon transfers.
  - These have high failure rates and are generally unsuccessful when performed as an isolated procedure since they do not address the underlying structural anatomy.
- Osteotomy:
  - Generally provides reliable relief of symptoms.
  - Medial displacement calcaneal osteotomy, lateral calcaneal lengthening osteotomy, triple-C (calcaneus, medial cuneiform, and cuboid) ostectomy.
- Arthrodesis:
  - Avoided in pediatric patients.

23.9 Toe Walking

23.9.1 Etiology and Pathophysiology

- Normal heel-to-toe gait should be present by age 24 months.[46]
- Idiopathic toe walking (ITW):
  - Constellation of cases without discernable etiologic abnormalities:
    - Likely genetic component.
    - Myopathic component.
  - With or without equinus contracture.
  - Electromyogram (EMG) shows abnormal gastrocnemius activation during gait (late swing phase).[47,48]
- CP:
  - *Differentiate with EMG:* CP patients show involuntary gastrocnemius coactivation with quadriceps activation (knee extension).[49]

23.9.2 Symptoms

- Lack of normal heel strike.[46]
- Weight bearing through the forefoot.

23.9.3 Diagnostics and Classification

- History[46]:
  - Detailed history of gestation, birth, development, and gait.
  - Detailed medical history—identify other potential causes:
    - CP.
    - Autism.
    - Global developmental delay.
    - Muscular dystrophy.
    - Tethered cord, spina bifida, diastematomyelia, and CMT disease.
    - Ankylosing spondylitis.
    - Limb length discrepancy.
  - Detailed family history (may be autosomal dominant pattern).
- Physical examination:
  - Inspection of the lower extremities:
    - Pelvic symmetry and leg lengths.
    - Muscle symmetry and development.
    - Range of motion of the knee and ankle:
      * Silfverskiöld's test to identify gastrocnemius or Achilles' tendon as cause of limited ankle dorsiflexion.

23.9.4 Conservative Management

- Observation[46]:
  - For patients younger than 2 years.
- Physical therapy and stretching.
- Bracing and night splints.
- Serial casting:
  - Increase dorsiflexion every 2 weeks.
  - May combine with botulinum toxin to gastrocnemius/soleus.[50]

23.9.5 Surgical Intervention

- Indicated for patients with an equinus contracture or those who have relapsed after nonoperative treatment.[46,51]
- Done by lengthening of the triceps surae muscle–tendon complex.
- Identify target (muscle or tendon) based on Silfverskiöld's test:
  - Percutaneous or open Achilles' tendon lengthening:
    - May lead to weakness and overcorrection.

- Gastrocnemius lengthening:
  - At the musculotendinous junction (Strayer's procedure).[52]
  - Midsubstance release (Baumann's procedure).[53]
  - Proximal tendon release and endoscopic procedures.[54]

23.9.6 Rehabilitation

- Six weeks in short-leg walking cast postoperatively.

23.10 Accessory Navicular

23.10.1 Etiology and Pathophysiology

- Failure of union of a secondary ossification center of the navicular.
- Normal variant present in up to 12% of population.[55]
- *Genetic:* autosomal dominant.
- Abnormal stresses through cartilage synchondrosis between accessory and navicular lead to inflammation and pain.[56]

23.10.2 Symptoms

- Usually asymptomatic.
- Medial arch pain, exacerbated by activity.
- Flatfeet.
- Posterior tibialis insufficiency:
  - Tendon insertion into navicular tuberosity.

23.10.3 Diagnostics and Classification

- Physical examination:
  - Swelling.
  - Tenderness in medial plantar foot.
- Imaging (▶ Fig. 23.9):
  - AP, lateral, and oblique views of the foot.
  - Best seen on external oblique view.[56]
- Classification by radiographic findings[55]:
  - Type 1: sesamoid in the tibialis posterior tendon.
  - Type 2: separate bone attached through synchondrosis.
  - Type 3: attached bony enlargement.

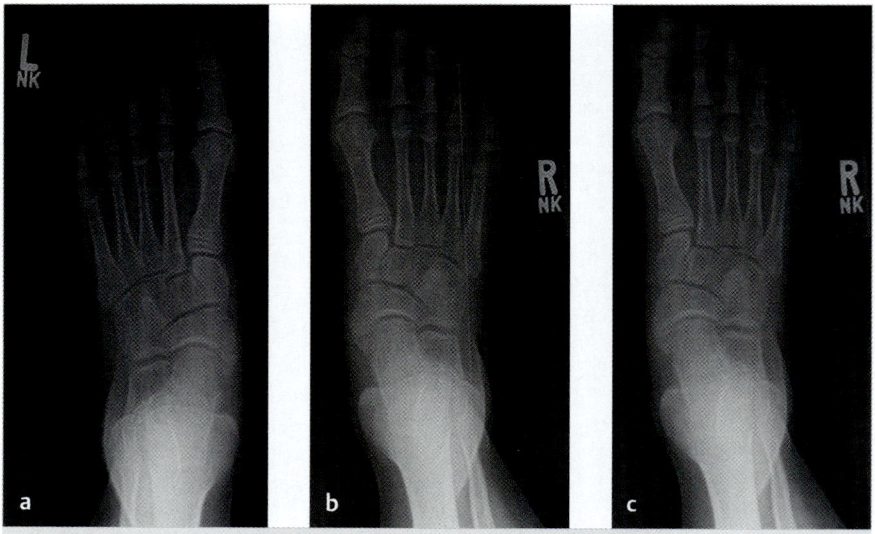

Fig. 23.9 (a-c) Anteroposterior (AP) views of the bilateral feet demonstrating bilateral accessory naviculars.

23.10.4 Conservative Management

- Activity modification.[55]
- Orthotics to decrease pressure on the medial foot:
  - Arch supports.
  - UCBL shoe orthosis.
- Symptoms usually resolve by skeletal maturity.
- If refractory, cast immobilization.

23.10.5 Surgical Intervention

- Excision (▶ Fig. 23.10)[55,57,58,59,60]:
  - Ensure adequate resection—avoid residual prominence.
  - Flatfoot correction:
    - Usually not done unless flatfoot is the primary pathology.
    - Lateral column lengthening.
    - Medial displacement calcaneus osteotomy.
- Kidner's procedure[61]:
  - Transfer of the posterior tibialis tendon:
    - Reroute under the navicular.
  - More complex procedure, with similar outcomes to excision.[59]

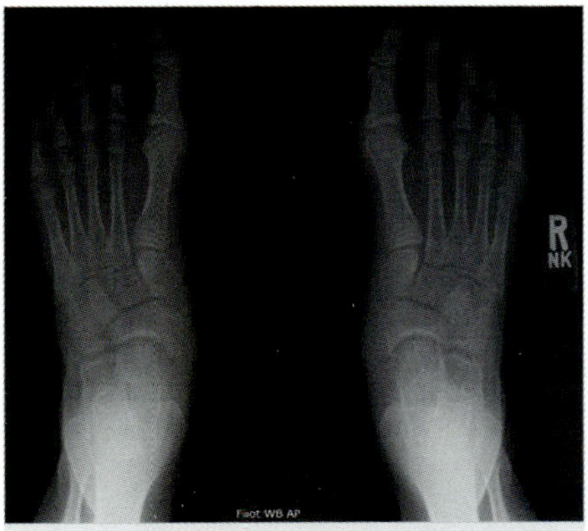

Fig. 23.10 Anteroposterior (AP) view of the bilateral feet following bilateral excision of the accessory naviculars.

23.11 Congenital Toe Disorders

23.11.1 Congenital Hallux Varus

- Fixed varus angulation of great toe due to several potential causes[62]:
  - Abductor/adductor imbalance.
  - Metatarsal morphology:
    - Longitudinal epiphyseal bracket (delta phalanx).
  - Joint morphology.
- Presents after walking age.
- Differentiate from dynamic hallux abductus:
  - Great toe deviation during ambulation.
  - Resolves with motor development; no intervention required.
- Radiographs show short, thick metatarsal.
- Surgical correction recommended—technique determined by root cause[63]:
  - Abductor hallucis release.
  - Osteotomy and arthrodesis.
  - Excision of the epiphyseal bracket.

23.11.2 Syndactyly

- Fusion of toes[64,65]:
  - Due to incomplete apoptosis during fetal development.
  - Autosomal dominant.
  - Most commonly between the second and third toes.
  - Associated with Down's syndrome and Klippel–Feil syndrome.
- Usually asymptomatic—primary complaint is cosmetic.
- Involvement of soft tissue (simple) or bone (complex):
  - Simple syndactyly usually does not require treatment.
  - Complex syndactyly treated with digit release.

23.11.3 Polydactyly

- Extra toes[66,67]:
  - Most commonly involving the lateral side of the foot.

- Due to abnormal differentiation of the apical ectodermal ridge.
- Autosomal dominant.
- Usually presents with a family history.

- Venn–Watson classification[68]:
  - Postaxial (lateral):
    - **Y**-shaped metatarsal.
    - **T**-shaped metatarsal.
    - Widened metatarsal head.
    - Metatarsal duplication.
  - Preaxial (medial):
    - Widened metatarsal head.
    - Short block metatarsal.
  - Central:
    - Duplication of the second, third, or fourth toe.
- Radiographic evaluation usually delayed until full ossification of the phalanges:
  - For surgical planning.
- Nonoperative treatment:
  - Observation if digit remains in proper alignment.
- Surgical treatment:
  - Ablation of the extra digit.
  - Usually at 9 to 12 months.

23.11.4 Curly Toe

- Usually involving the lateral three toes[69,70]:
  - Flexion and varus deformity of the interphalangeal joints.
  - Contracture of the flexor digitorum longus and brevis.
- Conservative management:
  - Usually asymptomatic; no functional deficiency.
- Operative management:
  - Flexor tenotomy.
  - For severe deformity or nail bed deformity.

23.11.5 Overlapping Toe

- Contracture of the extensor digitorum longus[69]:
  - Usually the fifth toe overlapping over the fourth toe.
  - Usually bilateral.
- Examination findings:
  - Dorsiflexion of the MTPJ.
  - Adduction and external rotation of digits.
  - Smaller nail plate.
- Conservative management:
  - Stretching.
  - Buddy tape.
- Operative management:
  - Tendon release (Butler's procedure).
  - Dorsal capsulotomy.
  - Syndactylization with the fourth toe (MacFarland's procedure).

23.12 Key Testing Facts

Clubfoot (congenital talipes equinovarus)	• Strong genetic component with positive family history and association with neural tube defects, trisomy 18, and congenital heart defects • Deformities are hindfoot equinovarus, midfoot cavus, and forefoot adduction • Ponseti's casting: order of correction (CAVE): midfoot cavus, forefoot adductus, hindfoot varus, and hindfoot equinus • Long leg cast changed every week for 6 wk, then every 2 wk until the age of 4–6 mo. The majority require an Achilles tenotomy for full dorsiflexion • After successful casting, bracing is required for 23 h/d for 3 mo and then 14–16 h/d until age 3–4 y
Metatarsus adductus	• A packaging disorder associated with developmental dysplasia of the hip and torticollis • The foot will have normal hindfoot and subtalar motion • Imaging is not necessary in infants, and the majority will resolve spontaneously • Most do not require treatment though casting may be used for rigid or persistent deformity

Pes cavus	• Numerous etiologies: may be attributable to pathology of the brain, spine, peripheral nerves, or musculature • A detailed history and physical examination are important • Additional tests including radiographs of the spine, CT brain, MRI of the spinal cord, or nerve conduction studies may be indicated depending on the differential diagnoses • Interventions vary from orthotics for simple deformities to surgical intervention • Surgical correction should be at the site of maximum deformity
Tarsal coalition	• Most common are calcaneonavicular or talocalcaneal coalitions • May lead to restriction of subtalar motion. Symptoms are typically insidious in onset • Calcaneonavicular coalition: best seen on oblique view. "Anteater sign" • Talocalcaneal coalition: may be seen on Harris view but best seen on CT. "C-sign" • Types of coalitions include fibrous, cartilaginous, and osseous • Resection of coalition with interposition for coalitions involving < 50% of the joint • Triple arthrodesis for advanced coalitions (> 50% of the joint), multiple coalitions, and failed resections
Talipes calcaneovalgus	• A packaging disorder more common in females, first-born, large infants, and twins • Deformity typically resolves spontaneously • Serial casting may be required for severe cases
Juvenile bunions	• Often a positive maternal family history • Typically presents in adolescence • Adductor hallucis is the deforming force • Conservative treatment will not correct the deformity • Surgery should never be performed for cosmesis alone
Kohler disease	• A rare, idiopathic process with a benign natural course • Much more common in males than in females • Duration of symptoms prior to presentation will vary • The diagnosis should not be made on the basis of radiographic findings in the absence of a supporting physical examination • There is no role for surgery in the treatment of Kohler's disease • The quickest resolution of symptoms occurs when treated with 8 wk of a below-knee cast
Flexible pes planus	• Flexible flatfoot is a normal finding within the first few years of life • Defined as an arch present while sitting but not while standing • Risk factors include male gender, general laxity, and obesity • If often asymptomatic although patients may have medial arch pain, foot fatigue, and calluses • Orthotics have no demonstrable benefit to asymptomatic individuals. Conversely, they may prove beneficial to individuals with symptomatic flatfeet • Surgery is rarely indicated
Toe walking	• A detailed history and physical is critical to identify secondary causes • The Silfverskiöld test is used to identify the gastrocnemius or Achilles tendon as cause of limited ankle dorsiflexion • Children younger than 2 y of age may be observed
Accessory navicular	• An autosomal dominant inheritance. Considered a normal variant • Usually asymptomatic but may cause medial arch pain and tenderness • Symptoms typically resolve by skeletal maturity

References

[1] Wynne-Davies R. Family studies and the cause of congenital club foot. talipes equinovarus, talipes calcaneo-valgus and metatarsus varus. J Bone Joint Surg Br. 1964; 46:445–463

[2] Hoffinger SA. Evaluation and management of pediatric foot deformities. Pediatr Clin North Am. 1996; 43(5):1091–1111

[3] Catterall A. A method of assessment of the clubfoot deformity. Clin Orthop Relat Res. 1991 (264):48–53

[4] Diméglio A, Bensahel H, Souchet P, Mazeau P, Bonnet F. Classification of clubfoot. J Pediatr Orthop B. 1995; 4(2):129–136

[5] Ponseti IV, Smoley EN. The classic: congenital club foot: the results of treatment. 1963. Clin Orthop Relat Res. 2009; 467(5):1133–1145

[6] Zhao D, Liu J, Zhao L, Wu Z. Relapse of clubfoot after treatment with the Ponseti method and the function of the foot abduction orthosis. Clin Orthop Surg. 2014; 6(3):245–252

[7] Harrold AJ, Walker CJ. Treatment and prognosis in congenital club foot. J Bone Joint Surg Br. 1983; 65 (1):8–11

[8] Halanski MA, Davison JE, Huang JC, Walker CG, Walsh SJ, Crawford HA. Ponseti method compared with surgical treatment of clubfoot: a prospective comparison. J Bone Joint Surg Am. 2010; 92(2): 270–278

[9] Turco VJ. Surgical correction of the resistant club foot. One-stage posteromedial release with internal fixation: a preliminary report. J Bone Joint Surg Am. 1971; 53(3):477–497

[10] Simons GW. Complete subtalar release in club feet. Part I: a preliminary report. J Bone Joint Surg Am. 1985; 67(7):1044–1055

[11] Farsetti P, Weinstein SL, Ponseti IV. The long-term functional and radiographic outcomes of untreated and non-operatively treated metatarsus adductus. J Bone Joint Surg Am. 1994; 76(2):257–265

[12] Widhe T, Aaro S, Elmstedt E. Foot deformities in the newborn: incidence and prognosis. Acta Orthop Scand. 1988; 59(2):176–179

[13] Gordon JE, Luhmann SJ, Dobbs MB, et al. Combined midfoot osteotomy for severe forefoot adductus. J Pediatr Orthop. 2003; 23(1):74–78

[14] Alexander IJ, Johnson KA. Assessment and management of pes cavus in Charcot-Marie-Tooth disease. Clin Orthop Relat Res. 1989; 246:273–281

[15] Coleman SS, Chesnut WJ. A simple test for hindfoot flexibility in the cavovarus foot. Clin Orthop Relat Res. 1977; 123:60–62

[16] De Smet AA, Asher MA, Cook LT, Goin JE, Scheuch HG, Orrick JM. Three-dimensional analysis of right thoracic idiopathic scoliosis. Spine. 1984; 9(4): 377–381

[17] Paulos L, Coleman SS, Samuelson KM. Pes cavovarus. Review of a surgical approach using selective soft-tissue procedures. J Bone Joint Surg Am. 1980; 62(6):942–953

[18] Sammarco GJ, Taylor R. Combined calcaneal and metatarsal osteotomies for the treatment of cavus foot. Foot Ankle Clin. 2001; 6(3):533–543, vii

[19] Sherman FC, Westin GW. Plantar release in the correction of deformities of the foot in childhood. J Bone Joint Surg Am. 1981; 63(9):1382–1389

[20] Vincent KA. Tarsal coalition and painful flatfoot. J Am Acad Orthop Surg. 1998; 6(5):274–281

[21] Lemley F, Berlet G, Hill K, Philbin T, Isaac B, Lee T. Current concepts review: tarsal coalition. Foot Ankle Int. 2006; 27(12):1163–1169

[22] Sullivan JA. Pediatric flatfoot: evaluation and management. J Am Acad Orthop Surg. 1999; 7(1): 44–53

[23] Page JC. Peroneal spastic flatfoot and tarsal coalitions. J Am Podiatr Med Assoc. 1987; 77(1):29–34

[24] Mosier KM, Asher M. Tarsal coalitions and peroneal spastic flat foot. A review. J Bone Joint Surg Am. 1984; 66(7):976–984

[25] Cowell HR, Elener V. Rigid painful flatfoot secondary to tarsal coalition. Clin Orthop Relat Res. 1983; 177:54–60

[26] Crim JR, Kjeldsberg KM. Radiographic diagnosis of tarsal coalition. AJR Am J Roentgenol. 2004; 182 (2):323–328

[27] Oestreich AE, Mize WA, Crawford AH, Morgan RC, Jr. The "anteater nose": a direct sign of calcaneonavicular coalition on the lateral radiograph. J Pediatr Orthop. 1987; 7(6):709–711

[28] Yu GV, Hladik J. Residual calcaneovalgus deformity: review of the literature and case study. J Foot Ankle Surg. 1994; 33(3):228–238

[29] Coughlin MJ. Roger A. Mann Award. Juvenile hallux valgus: etiology and treatment. Foot Ankle Int. 1995; 16(11):682–697

[30] Coughlin MJ, Jones CP. Hallux valgus: demographics, etiology, and radiographic assessment. Foot Ankle Int. 2007; 28(7):759–777

[31] Harb Z, Kokkinakis M, Ismail H, Spence G. Adolescent hallux valgus: a systematic review of outcomes following surgery. J Child Orthop. 2015; 9(2):105–112

[32] Lowery NJ, Wukich DK. Adolescent hallux valgus: evaluation and treatment. Oper Tech Orthop. 2009; 19(1):52–57

[33] Chell J, Dhar S. Pediatric hallux valgus. Foot Ankle Clin. 2014; 19(2):235–243

[34] Shi GG, Whalen JL, Turner NS, III, Kitaoka HB. Operative approach to adult hallux valgus deformity: principles and techniques. J Am Acad Orthop Surg. 2020; 28(10):410–418

[35] Borges JL, Guille JT, Bowen JR. Köhler's bone disease of the tarsal navicular. J Pediatr Orthop. 1995; 15(5):596–598

[36] Tsirikos AI, Riddle EC, Kruse R. Bilateral Köhler's disease in identical twins. Clin Orthop Relat Res. 2003(409):195–198

[37] Ippolito E, Ricciardi Pollini PT, Falez' F. Köhler's disease of the tarsal navicular: long-term follow-up of 12 cases. J Pediatr Orthop. 1984; 4(4):416–417
[38] Williams GA, Cowell HR. Köhler's disease of the tarsal navicular. Clin Orthop Relat Res. 1981(158):53–58
[39] Waugh W. The ossification and vascularisation of the tarsal navicular and their relation to Köhler's disease. J Bone Joint Surg Br. 1958; 40-B(4):765–777
[40] Benedetti MG, Ceccarelli F, Berti L, et al. Diagnosis of flexible flatfoot in children: a systematic clinical approach. Orthopedics. 2011; 34(2):94
[41] Carr JB, II, Yang S, Lather LA. Pediatric pes planus: a state-of-the-art review. Pediatrics. 2016; 137(3): e20151230
[42] Staheli LT, Chew DE, Corbett M. The longitudinal arch. A survey of eight hundred and eighty-two feet in normal children and adults. J Bone Joint Surg Am. 1987; 69(3):426–428
[43] Chen KC, Yeh CJ, Tung LC, Yang JF, Yang SF, Wang CH. Relevant factors influencing flatfoot in preschool-aged children. Eur J Pediatr. 2011; 170 (7):931–936
[44] Chang JH, Wang SH, Kuo CL, Shen HC, Hong YW, Lin LC. Prevalence of flexible flatfoot in Taiwanese school-aged children in relation to obesity, gender, and age. Eur J Pediatr. 2010; 169(4):447–452
[45] Jane MacKenzie A, Rome K, Evans AM. The efficacy of nonsurgical interventions for pediatric flexible flat foot: a critical review. J Pediatr Orthop. 2012; 32(8):830–834
[46] Oetgen ME, Peden S. Idiopathic toe walking. J Am Acad Orthop Surg. 2012; 20(5):292–300
[47] Eastwood DM, Dennett X, Shield LK, Dickens DR. Muscle abnormalities in idiopathic toe-walkers. J Pediatr Orthop B. 1997; 6(3):215–218
[48] Griffin PP, Wheelhouse WW, Shiavi R, Bass W. Habitual toe-walkers. A clinical and electromyographic gait analysis. J Bone Joint Surg Am. 1977; 59(1): 97–101
[49] Policy JF, Torburn L, Rinsky LA, Rose J. Electromyographic test to differentiate mild diplegic cerebral palsy and idiopathic toe-walking. J Pediatr Orthop. 2001; 21(6):784–789
[50] Brunt D, Woo R, Kim HD, Ko MS, Senesac C, Li S. Effect of botulinum toxin type A on gait of children who are idiopathic toe-walkers. J Surg Orthop Adv. 2004; 13(3):149–155
[51] Kogan M, Smith J. Simplified approach to idiopathic toe-walking. J Pediatr Orthop. 2001; 21(6):790–791
[52] Strayer LM, Jr. Recession of the gastrocnemius; an operation to relieve spastic contracture of the calf muscles. J Bone Joint Surg Am. 1950; 32-A (3):671–676
[53] Herzenberg JE, Lamm BM, Corwin C, Sekel J. Isolated recession of the gastrocnemius muscle: the Baumann procedure. Foot Ankle Int. 2007; 28 (11):1154–1159
[54] Saxena A, Widtfeldt A. Endoscopic gastrocnemius recession: preliminary report on 18 cases. J Foot Ankle Surg. 2004; 43(5):302–306
[55] Pretell-Mazzini J, Murphy RF, Sawyer JR, et al. Surgical treatment of symptomatic accessory navicular in children and adolescents. Am J Orthop. 2014; 43(3):110–113
[56] Grogan DP, Gasser SI, Ogden JA. The painful accessory navicular: a clinical and histopathological study. Foot Ankle. 1989; 10(3):164–169
[57] Tan SM, Chin TW, Mitra AK, Tan SK. Surgical treatment of symptomatic accessory navicular. Ann Acad Med Singap. 1995; 24(3):379–381
[58] Jasiewicz B, Potaczek T, Kacki W, Tesiorowski M, Lipik E. Results of simple excision technique in the surgical treatment of symptomatic accessory navicular bones. Foot Ankle Surg. 2008; 14(2):57–61
[59] Macnicol MF, Voutsinas S. Surgical treatment of the symptomatic accessory navicular. J Bone Joint Surg Br. 1984; 66(2):218–226
[60] Kopp FJ, Marcus RE. Clinical outcome of surgical treatment of the symptomatic accessory navicular. Foot Ankle Int. 2004; 25(1):27–30
[61] Cha SM, Shin HD, Kim KC, Lee JK. Simple excision vs the Kidner procedure for type 2 accessory navicular associated with flatfoot in pediatric population. Foot Ankle Int. 2013; 34(2):167–172
[62] Stanifer E, Hodor D, Wertheimer S. Congenital hallux varus: case presentation and review of the literature. J Foot Surg. 1991; 30(5):509–512
[63] Shim JS, Lim TK, Koh KH, Lee DK. Surgical treatment of congenital hallux varus. Clin Orthop Surg. 2014; 6(2):216–222
[64] Kim JH, Kim BJ, Kwon ST. Foot syndactyly: a clinical and demographic analysis. Arch Plast Surg. 2016; 43(6):559–563
[65] Kawabata H, Ariga K, Shibata T, Matsui Y. Open treatment of syndactyly of the foot. Scand J Plast Reconstr Surg Hand Surg. 2003; 37(3):150–154
[66] Phelps DA, Grogan DP. Polydactyly of the foot. J Pediatr Orthop. 1985; 5(4):446–451
[67] Miura T, Nakamura R, Imamura T. Polydactyly of the hands and feet. J Hand Surg Am. 1987; 12(3): 474–476
[68] Venn-Watson EA. Problems in polydactyly of the foot. Orthop Clin North Am. 1976; 7(4):909–927
[69] Shirzad K, Kiesau CD, DeOrio JK, Parekh SG. Lesser toe deformities. J Am Acad Orthop Surg. 2011; 19 (8):505–514
[70] Hamer AJ, Stanley D, Smith TW. Surgery for curly toe deformity: a double-blind, randomised, prospective trial. J Bone Joint Surg Br. 1993; 75(4): 662–663

24 Orthotics and Prosthetics

Keith L. Wapner

Abstract

Conservative treatment of disorders of the foot and ankle can be simple, inexpensive, and highly effective. Footwear serves to protect the foot from the outside environment and distributes forces evenly about the foot. A significant percentage of foot pathology stems from inappropriate footwear. Shoe uppers can be modified via their material makeup or by altering lacing patterns to avoid bony prominences or accommodate deformity. Outsole modifications include flares to prevent unwanted motion or rocker soles to encourage more physiologic gait patterns. Over the counter insoles, metatarsal pads as well as other appliances often provide significant relief to patients with plantar foot pain from disorders such as plantar fasciitis, Morton's neuroma, and metatarsalgia. Depending on symptom and disease severity, custom insoles may be necessary. The University of California Biomechanics Laboratory (UCBL) foot orthosis is custom made to position and immobilize the hindfoot and midfoot in patients with arthritis and tendon disorders. The more commonly applied orthoses for disorders of the ankle and foot are the molded ankle–foot orthosis (AFO) and Arizona brace. These braces cross the ankle joint and through various modifications can be tailored to the specific needs of each patient. At the conclusion of the chapter, disorders of the hindfoot and forefoot are listed and paired with orthoses utilized in their treatment.

Keywords: nonoperative treatment, orthotic, insert, insole, outsole, UCBL, ankle foot orthosis, AFO, Arizona brace

Conservative measures are an important tool in the surgeon's armamentarium:

- Simple, inexpensive, and often very effective.
    - Many disorders of the foot and ankle do not require surgery.
    - Nonoperative treatment can often provide adequate control of pain and deformity in patients unwilling or medically unfit to undergo surgery.

The main goal of footwear is to protect the foot from extrinsic environment[1]:

- Shoes also serve to decrease plantar foot pressures and shear forces while weight bearing, cushion painful areas, and support or accommodate deformity:[2,3]
    - Shoe shape and shoe size dictate proper shoe fit.[1]
    - Bulk of acquired adult forefoot pathology stems from improper shoe fit (▶ Fig. 24.1).[1]
    - Both surgical and nonsurgical treatment may be ineffective unless the patient adopts proper footwear.[3]

24.1 Footwear Anatomy

The basic parts of a shoe include the following (▶ Fig. 24.2):

- Upper: the top portion of the shoe contacting the dorsal foot:
    - Can be made from a variety of materials including mesh, nylon, and leather.
    - Heat moldable form also available to decrease shear forces in neuropathic patients:[3]
        - Different lacing stay patterns.
        - Changing lacing pattern may accommodate deformity and decrease pressure across dorsal prominences, as with midfoot arthritis:
            - Shoemakers' wand can be used to further modify a shoe to create a recessed area to decrease focal pressure against the foot.
- Outsole: the portion of the shoe in contact with the ground:

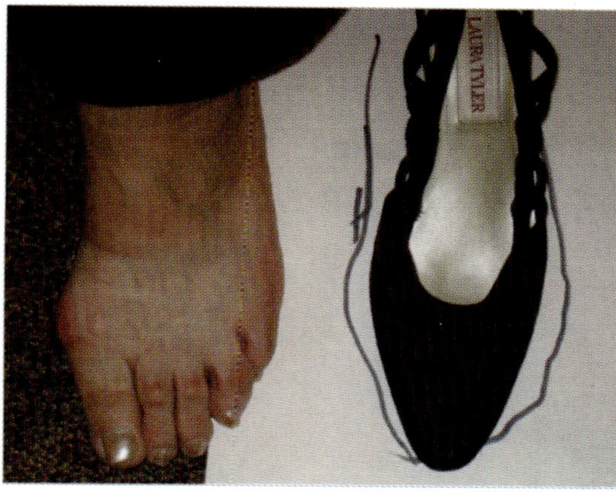

Fig. 24.1 It is often necessary to remind patients that, for daily dress, there is no other part of the body they would consider putting in a container whose shape is so drastically different than that body part.

- Newer materials improve force transmission to the foot and ankle.
- Modifications can significantly reduce plantar pressures:[4]
  - Include adding:
    - Wedges: medially or laterally to influence foot position in flexible deformities.
    - Metatarsal bars: proximal to metatarsal heads to distribute force across the midfoot instead of focally on metatarsal heads.
    - Rocker soles: allow for improved gait pattern in patients with fixed hindfoot deformity/fusion, plantar midfoot prominences, or rigid bracing.
    - The apex of the rocker should be placed proximal to the area where pressure relief is desired.[2]
    - Heel: a flared heel can be added as an outrigger provides a broader base of support.
    - Helpful in patients with fixed coronal plane deformity, subtalar arthrosis, or ankle instability.[2]
    - Heel lifts can be used to address limb length inequality.
- Insole: the portion of the shoe that interacts with the plantar weight-bearing portion of the foot:
  - Can be over the counter or custom insert.
  - Extra depth shoes more easily accept an insert and accommodate deformity.[3]

24.2 Foot Orthoses

- Foot orthoses serve to distribute force to the entire plantar surface, offload painful areas, provide shock absorption, and support or accommodate deformity using soft moldable materials.[2]
- Over-the-counter (OTC) inserts are able to accomplish many of the above goals:
  - Inexpensive and readily available.
    - Soft insoles and metatarsal pads redistribute forefoot pressures to the midfoot to alleviate pain associated with metatarsalgia, Morton's neuroma, and fat pad atrophy symptoms.[3]
    - Heel cups and inserts similarly redirect plantar heel pressures to the midfoot in patients with plantar heel pain or plantar fasciitis.[5]
  - The use of an inexpensive running shoe alone over a standard oxford shoe can significantly reduce the plantar pressures experienced[6] (▶ Fig. 24.3).
- Custom insoles can provide superior offloading to high-pressure areas in patients who have incomplete relief with OTC inserts.[7]

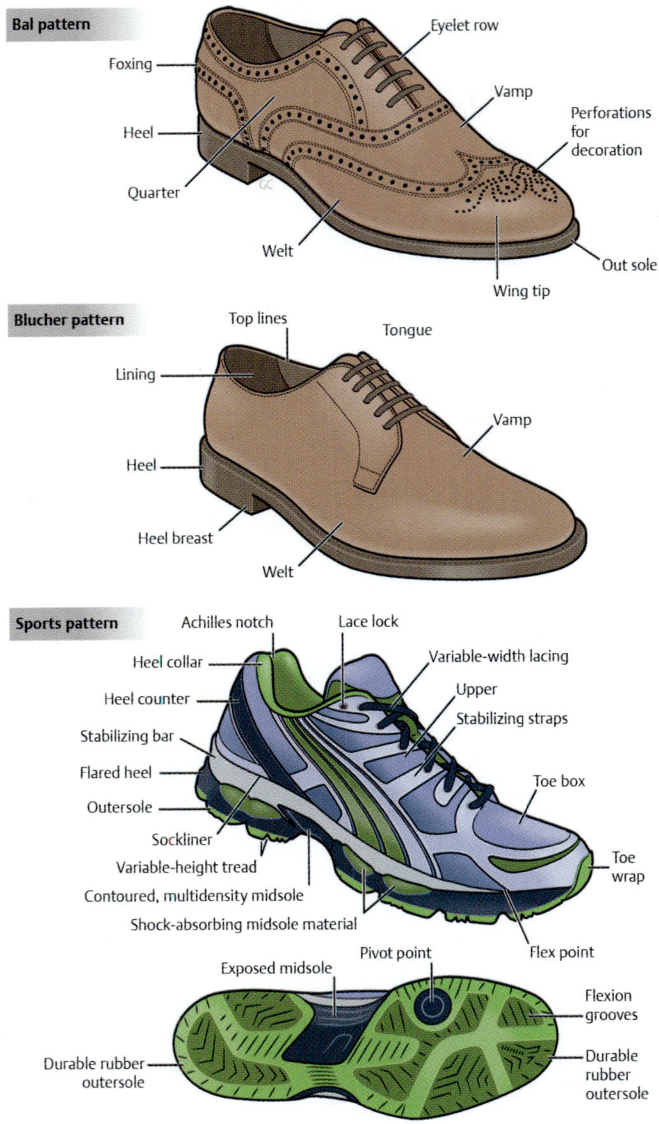

Fig. 24.2 Anatomy of the shoe.

- Improved conformity of the insole may be a more important variable in reducing plantar pressures than the choice of material for the insole.[8]
- Particularly beneficial for neuropathic and rheumatoid patients to avoid skin breakdown or ulceration (▶ Fig. 24.4).

- General types of insoles:
  - Soft: useful for impact absorption and shear reduction.
    - Particularly in patients with bony prominences or deformity.
    - Can be used to line more rigid orthoses.

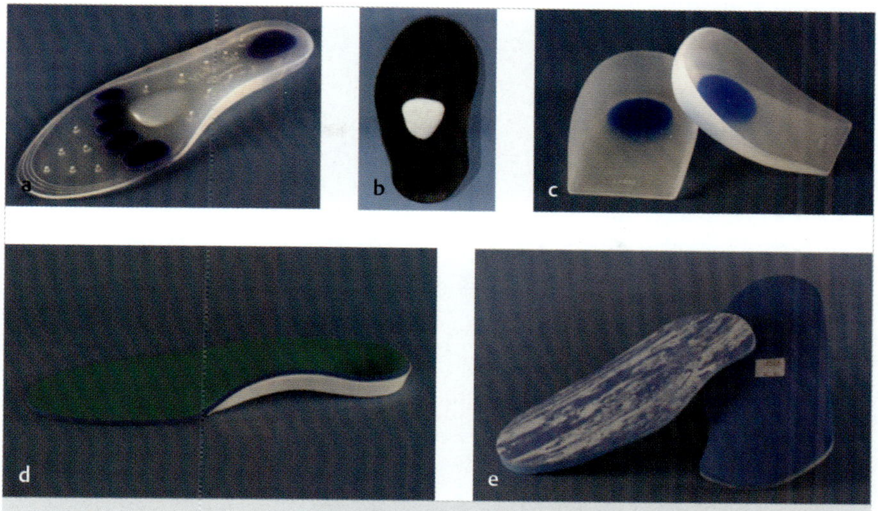

Fig. 24.3 (a–e) Various orthoses: **(a)** silicone orthotic; **(b)** metatarsal head pad; **(c)** silicone heel cup; **(d)** off the shelf full length orthotic; **(e)** custom full length insert.

    - Semirigid: also used for shock absorption but can stabilize flexible deformities.
        - Medial hindfoot posting keeps the heel out of the valgus.
        - Also helpful for midfoot arthritis.
        - Molded in situ.
        - Can be lined with softer material for shock absorption.
    - Rigid: stiffens the shoe to control or decrease motion.
        - No shock absorbing qualities.
        - Can be poorly tolerated in patients with fat pad atrophy or plantar bony prominences.[3]
- University of California Biomechanics Laboratory Orthosis (UCBL):
    - Controls flexible foot deformity by holding the hindfoot in neutral.
    - Must be molded with the hindfoot in maximally reduced position.
    - Particularly helpful for flexible flatfoot deformity

24.3 Ankle–Foot Orthoses

- Ankle–foot orthoses (AFO) can be made from double uprights attached to a shoe or from molded polypropylene.[3]
- Custom-molded polypropylene is used to create a posterior shell or incorporated into a leather lacer known as an Arizona brace.[3]
- Numerous modifications are made to target specific pathology.
- A mold is taken from a positive cast of the lower limb.
- A three-point mold can be used to control hindfoot alignment.
- Reliefs or added liners can accommodate deformity.
- The orthosis can have a hinge for ankle motion or be fixed.
- Trim lines are modified to dial in rigidity.
    - Trim lines anterior to the malleoli diminish ankle motion.
    - Those behind the malleoli allow some ankle motion but limit subtalar and transverse tarsal motion. A full foot plate can be used to limit midfoot motion.[3]

24.4 Appliances

- Various appliances are available to relieve forefoot pain, although they

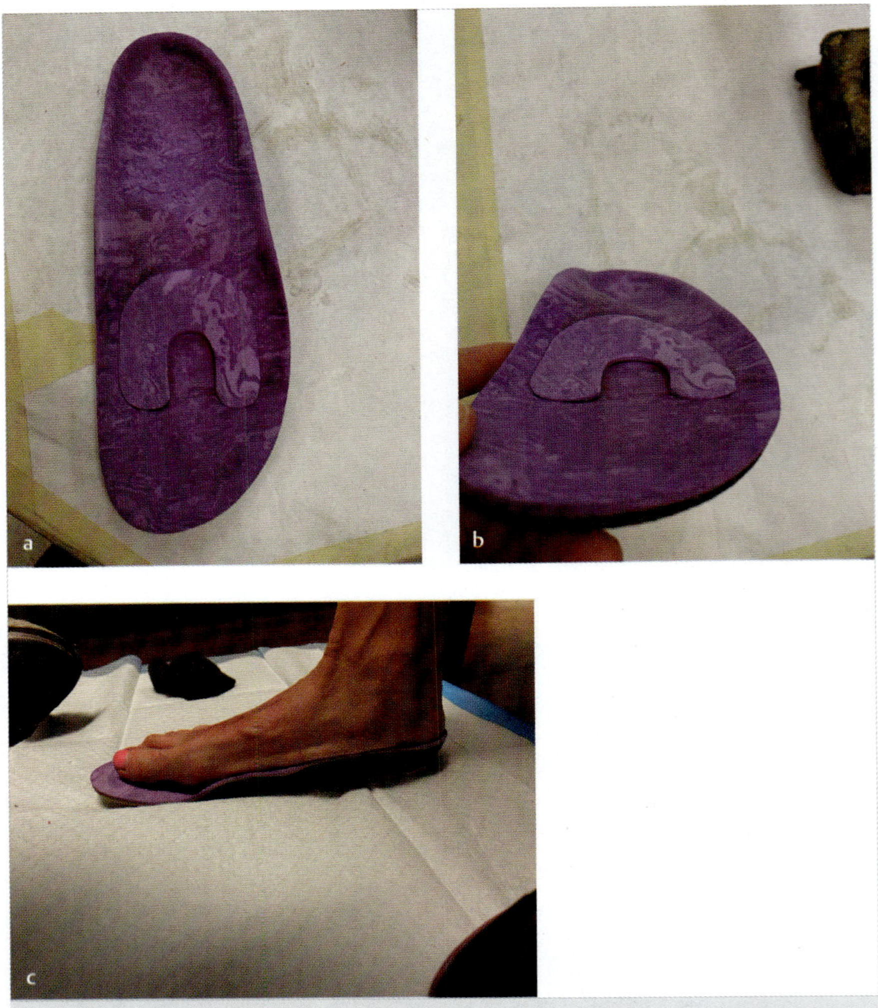

Fig. 24.4 (a–c) Custom-made inserts.

require an accommodative well-fitting shoe and do not correct deformity.[3]

- *Toe crests:* Relieve pressure at the tips of the toes from hammer and mallet deformities.
- *Corn and callus pads:* Relieve pressure points when combined with lesion paring.
- Foam or gel sleeves: Pad pressure points on toes.
- Lamb's wool: Functions as a toe separator and wicks moisture (▶ Fig. 24.5).

24.5 Treatment of Specific Disorders

- Orthoses relieve symptoms by controlling position, limiting motion, and through pressure relief, although they may not cure pathology.
- Additional symptom and gait improvement may be observed when orthoses are combined with high-quality running shoes or rocker bottom soles.[3]

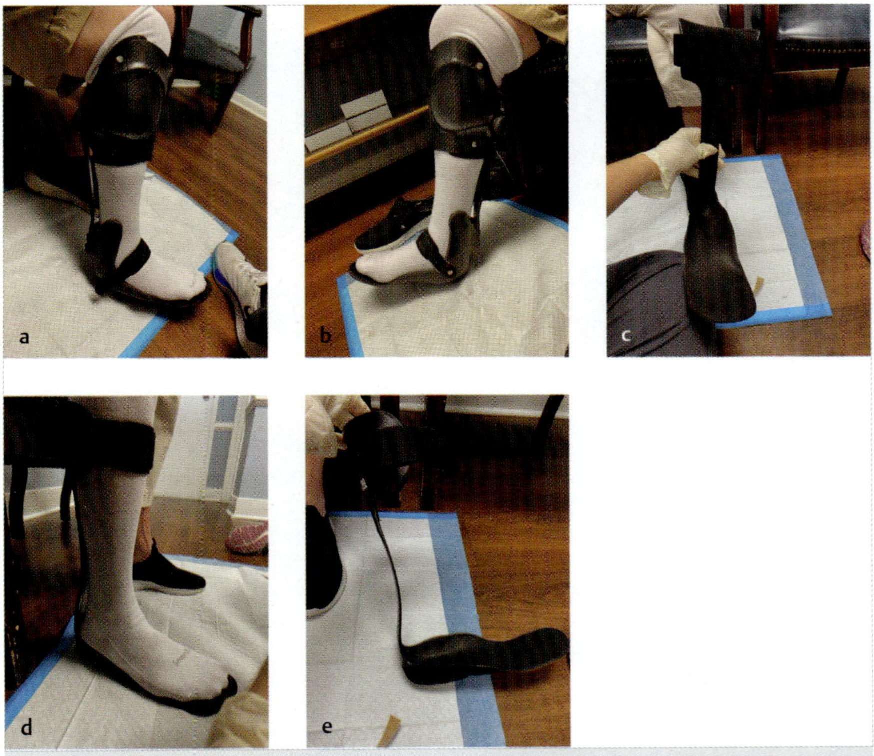

Fig. 24.5 (a–e) Custom-made ankle–foot orthoses (AFO).

24.5.1 Arthritis

- Ankle arthritis:
  - Molded AFO or Arizona brace.
- Subtalar arthritis:
  - Molded AFO or UCBL.
- Midfoot arthritis:
  - Modified shoe lacing to relieve dorsal pressure on spurs, stiff-soled shoe, carbon fiber full-length insert, UCBL, or AFO with accommodative arch support for severe cases.[9]

24.5.2 Tendon Disorders

- Tendinitis or early tendinosis:
  - Ankle stirrup brace, with healing demonstrated by resolution of pain and swelling within 6 months.[3]
- Significant tendon dysfunction:
  - Permanent ankle stirrup brace or AFO.
- Tendon rupture:
  - Permanent ankle stirrup brace or AFO.
- Chronic dysfunction with fixed deformity:
  - Molded AFO.
- Posterior tibial tendon dysfunction:
  - Stage I: cast, walking boot, or articulated AFO followed by foot orthosis.[10]
  - Stage II: ankle stirrup brace, UCBL, AFO (articulated or fixed), or Arizona brace.[10]
  - Stage III: fixed deformity treated with Arizona brace or molded AFO.

24.5.3 Heel Pain

- Chronic plantar fasciitis:
  - Soft inserts for shock absorption (such as visco heels), stiffer conforming foot orthosis to redistribute pressure away from the heel, well-padded shoes, and night splints.[5,8,11]
- Heel pad atrophy:
  - Soft inserts and well-padded shoe.

24.5.4 Great Toe Disorders

- Hallux valgus deformity:
  - Accommodate with proper wide footwear with soft upper or prestretch toe box with a shoemaker's wand; splinting may alleviate symptoms but does not prevent or correct deformity.[12]
- Hallux rigidus:
  - Accommodate dorsal exostosis in extra-depth shoe or stretched toe box, reduce hallux pressures by restricting motion with stiff sole, carbon fiber or steel insert, or custom orthosis with Morton extension, and improve gait with rocker bottom shoe.[3,13]
- Sesamoid disorders:
  - Metatarsal pad placed proximal to the sesamoids, which can be combined with soft insert with recess for sesamoids.

24.5.5 Lesser Toe Disorders

- Calluses and corns:
  - Appropriate well-padded footwear reducing pressure on prominences combined with removal of hyperkeratosis.[3,14]
- Metatarsalgia seen with plantar callosity:
  - Metatarsal pad positioned proximal to metatarsal head, either integrated in orthosis or placed directly in the shoe.
- Dorsal corn:
  - Toe sleeve or toe crest, stretching of toe box with shoemaker's wand (ball and ring stretcher), and avoidance of narrow dress shoes.
- Hammer toe and crossover toe deformity:
  - Metatarsal pad to relieve plantar pain, taping to stabilize the metatarsophalangeal joint (0.5-inch tape), toe sling, or sleeve.[3]
- Morton's neuroma:
  - Wide shoe with metatarsal pad placed proximal to the metatarsal heads and webspace to spread the metatarsals and relieve pressure on the neuroma[3] (► Fig. 24.6).
- Bunionette deformity:
  - Wide shoe or stretching of the shoe to alleviate pressure.

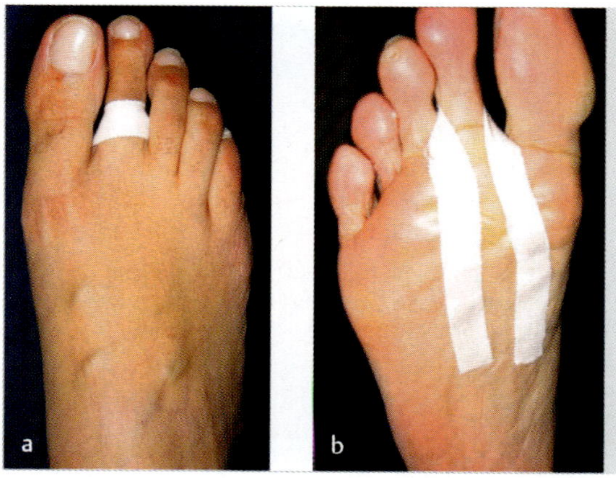

Fig. 24.6 (a, b) Taping for a cross-over toe, flexible hammertoe, or plantar plate tear.

24.6 Key Testing Facts

- Many disorders of the foot and ankle do not require surgery. Nonoperative treatment can often provide adequate control of pain and deformity in patients unwilling or medically unfit to undergo surgery.
- Foot orthoses serve to distribute force to the entire plantar surface, offload painful areas, provide shock absorption, and support or accommodate deformity, and can be soft, semi-rigid, or rigid depending on the pathology.
- AFO can be made from double uprights attached to a shoe, molded polypropylene to fit in a shoe or from molded polypropylene covered in leather to fit in a shoe. These serve to control motion and provide support.

References

[1] Janisse DJ. The art and science of fitting shoes. Foot Ankle. 1992; 13(5):257–262

[2] Janisse DJ, Janisse E. Shoe modification and the use of orthoses in the treatment of foot and ankle pathology. J Am Acad Orthop Surg. 2008; 16(3): 152–158

[3] Coughlin MJ, Saltzman CL, Anderson RB, eds. Mann's Surgery of the Foot and Ankle. Philadelphia, PA: Elsevier; 2014:121–134

[4] Cavanagh PR, Ulbrecht JS, Zanine W, Welling RL, Leschinsky D, van Schie C. A method for the investigation of the effects of outsole modifications in therapeutic footwear. Foot Ankle Int. 1996; 17 (11):706–708

[5] Bonanno DR, Landorf KB, Menz HB. Pressure-relieving properties of various shoe inserts in older people with plantar heel pain. Gait Posture. 2011; 33(3):385–389

[6] Perry JE, Ulbrecht JS, Derr JA, Cavanagh PR. The use of running shoes to reduce plantar pressures in patients who have diabetes. J Bone Joint Surg Am. 1995; 77(12):1819–1828

[7] Owings TM, Woerner JL, Frampton JD, Cavanagh PR, Botek G. Custom therapeutic insoles based on both foot shape and plantar pressure measurement provide enhanced pressure relief. Diabetes Care. 2008; 31(5):839–844

[8] Goske S, Erdemir A, Petre M, Budhabhatti S, Cavanagh PR. Reduction of plantar heel pressures: insole design using finite element analysis. J Biomech. 2006; 39(13):2363–2370

[9] Patel A, Rao S, Nawoczenski D, Flemister AS, DiGiovanni B, Baumhauer JF. Midfoot arthritis. J Am Acad Orthop Surg. 2010; 18(7):417–425

[10] Alvarez RG, Marini A, Schmitt C, Saltzman CL. Stage I and II posterior tibial tendon dysfunction treated by a structured nonoperative management protocol: an orthosis and exercise program. Foot Ankle Int. 2006; 27(1):2–8

[11] Wapner KL, Sharkey PF. The use of night splints for treatment of recalcitrant plantar fasciitis. Foot Ankle. 1991; 12(3):135–137

[12] Easley ME, Trnka HJ. Current concepts review: hallux valgus part 1: pathomechanics, clinical assessment, and nonoperative management. Foot Ankle Int. 2007; 28(5):654–659

[13] Shurnas PS. Hallux rigidus: etiology, biomechanics, and nonoperative treatment. Foot Ankle Clin. 2009; 14(1):1–8

[14] Young MJ, Cavanagh PR, Thomas G, Johnson MM, Murray H, Boulton AJ. The effect of callus removal on dynamic plantar foot pressures in diabetic patients. Diabet Med. 1992; 9(1):55–57

25 Orthobiologic Growth Factor Therapy in Foot and Ankle

Nicholas Genovese, Anthony Lin, Maximilian Muñoz, Jayenth Mayur, Ethan Krell, and Sheldon S. Lin

Abstract

Musculoskeletal injuries are painful and entail an extensive healing process. In order to expedite and aid bone and tendon healing, orthobiologics were developed. These autologously derived products accelerate recovery by inundating the injury site with growth factors and proteins. In this chapter, we review current clinical studies regarding three popular orthobiologic agents: platelet-derived growth factor, bone morphogenetic proteins, and platelet-rich plasma.

Keywords: biologics, recombinant human bone morphogenetic protein, platelet-derived growth factor, platelet-rich plasma

25.1 Platelet-Derived Growth Factor

25.1.1 Introduction

Overview

- Platelet-derived growth factor (PDGF) is a family of dimeric isoforms primarily secreted by platelets early in the trauma repair cascade.[1]
- It facilitates bone regeneration by osteogenesis, vascularization, and mesengenesis.[2]
- It binds to tyrosine kinase receptors on macrophage and perivascular mesenchymal cells.
- PDGF-BB is the isoform of greatest potential therapeutic value given that it exhibits universal affinity to all known PDGF receptor isotypes.[3,4,5,6]
- Recombinant human PDGF-BB (rhPDGF-BB) has been approved for use as an autograft alternative in hindfoot and ankle procedures in the United States, Canada, Australia, and New Zealand.[7]
- PDGF does not have any nascent osteoconductive properties, so it is a commercially available packed synthetic bone graft to act as a scaffold for bone formation.

25.1.2 rhPDGF for Ankle and Hindfoot Fusion

- The Augment Bone Graft (Stryker, Memphis, TN) is a formulation of rhPDGF-BB/beta-tricalcium phosphate (β-TCP) used for ankle, hindfoot, or midfoot arthrodesis.
- There is equivalent union rates in ankle, hindfoot, and midfoot arthrodesis compared to autologous bone graft, without risk of donor site morbidity.[3,4]
- Overall, there is no significant difference in adverse events compared to autologous bone graft.

25.1.3 Limitations/ Contraindications

- While there is the theoretical risk that rhPDGF-BB could promote tumor formation, no correlation has been found to date.[8]
- *Pregnant women:* The potential effects of rhPDGF-BB on the human fetus have not been evaluated.
- Active infection due to its proinflammatory properties.
- Individuals younger than 18 years of age or no radiographic evidence of closure of epiphyses.

25.1.4 Conclusion

- PDGF, specifically rhPDGF-BB, has been shown to be a safe effective alternative to autograft for ankle and hindfoot fusions, eliminating the pain and morbidity associated with autograft harvesting (▶ Fig. 25.1).

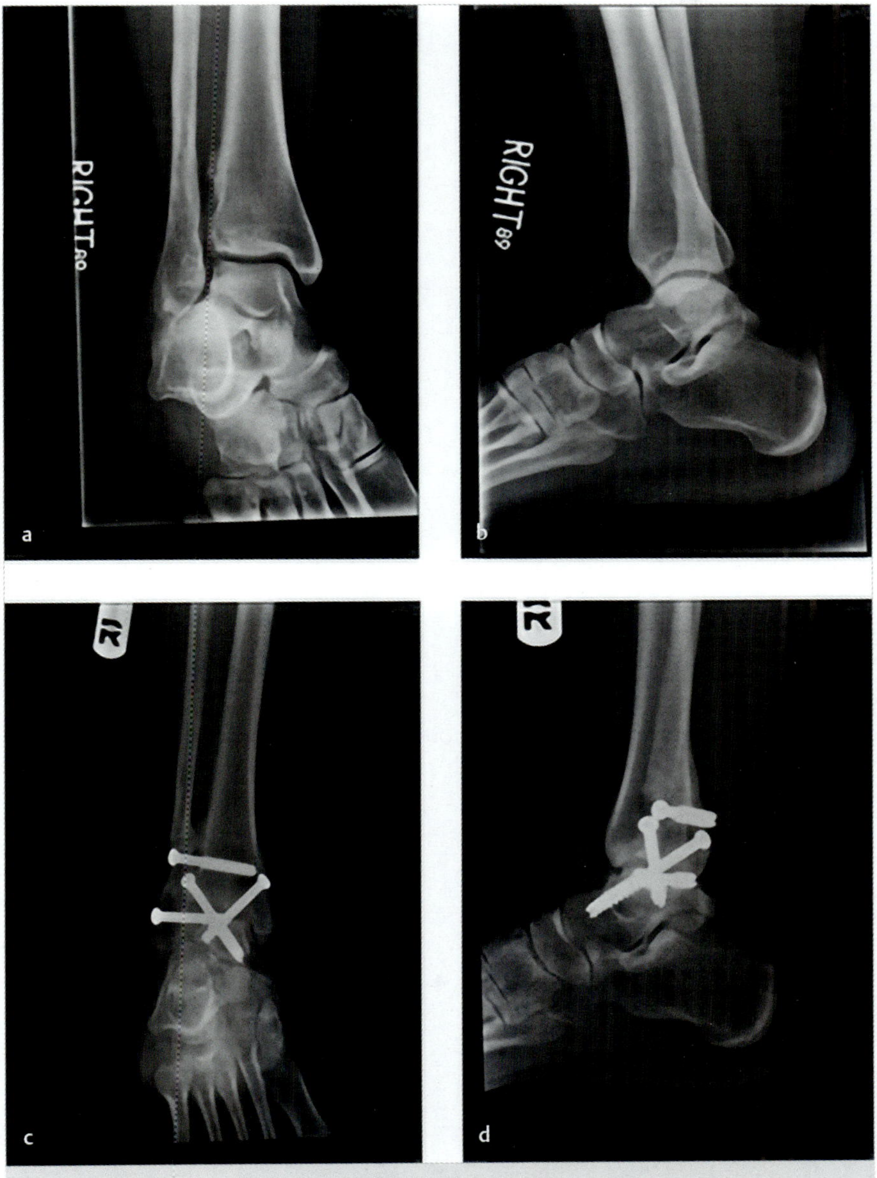

Fig. 25.1 Platelet-derived growth factor (PDGF) case study. A woman requiring ankle fusion surgery. Treatment consisted of rigid internal fixation plus recombinant human PGDF-BB and beta-tricalcium phosphate (rhPDGF-BB/β-TCP; Augment Bone Graft). Comparisons between **(a,b)** preoperative and **(c,d)** 36-week postoperative anteroposterior and lateral images of the ankle, respectively, show the extent of union.

25.2 Bone Morphogenetic Proteins

25.2.1 Introduction

- Bone morphogenetic proteins (BMPs) are part of the transforming growth factor-β (TGF-β) superfamily.
- Display osteoinductive and chondroinductive activity.[9]
- Bind to transmembrane serine-threonine kinase receptors on undifferentiated perivascular mesenchymal cells.[10,11,12]
- Two recombinant human bone morphogenetic proteins (rhBMPs)[13] have become commercially available: both rhBMP-2 (INFUSE, Medtronic, Minneapolis, MN) and rhBMP-7 (OP-1, Stryker, Kalamazoo, MI) are Food and Drug Administration (FDA) approved for aid in the bone-healing process.[14]
- rhBMP-2 approved for use in acute open tibial shaft fractures[15,16] treated within 14 days, and single-level anterior lumbar interbody fusion procedures with a lumbar tapered fusion device.
- rhBMP-7 approved by FDA under a humanitarian device exemption (HDE) as an alternative autograft in recalcitrant long bone nonunions where use of autograft is unfeasible and alternative treatments have failed.
  - Due to economic burden of production, it is currently commercially unavailable.[17]
- BMPs are also used off-label for arthrodesis, high-risk fractures, delayed unions, and nonunions in the foot and ankle.
- BMP acts as a differentiating agent and does not have any nascent osteoconductive properties, so it is commercially available as a solution that is applied to an absorbable collagen sponge, which delivers the rhBMP-2 to the implant site and acts as a scaffolding for the formation of new bone.

25.2.2 Recombinant Human Bone Morphogenetic Protein-2

- Off-label use of rhBMP-2 has been evaluated in the ankle, forefoot, midfoot, hindfoot arthrodesis, as well as revision hindfoot arthrodesis procedures.[18,19,20,21,22]
- Significantly higher union rates in high-risk ankle and hindfoot fusions compared to autologous bone graft.[18,23]
- *Hindfoot arthrodesis:* equivalent time to union compared to ABG.
- No effect on fusion rates when rhBMP-2 used as adjunct to ABG in high-foot and ankle fusions and fracture nonunions (▶ Table 25.1).[24]
- *Financial burden:* BMP-2 found to be economically favorable to treat open tibial fractures (▶ Fig. 25.2).[25]

25.2.3 Recombinant Human Bone Morphogenetic Protein-7

- Off-label use of rhBMP-7 is uncommon given its inferior osteogenic properties compared to BMP-2. To date, it has been evaluated in primary ankle and hindfoot fusions, as well as revision arthrodesis procedures of the ankle and hindfoot.
- Overall noninferior union rates compared to historical controls.[22,26]

25.2.4 Limitations/ Contraindications

- One major complication regarding the use of BMP in the extremities is the possible formation of heterotopic bone, leading to joint pain and stiffness.[26]
- Relative risk in patients with malignancies as BMP-2 and BMP-7 has been shown to stimulate tumor growth.[25]

Table 25.1 Union rates for each site of rhBMP-2 application

Site of rhBMP-2 use	No. of sites	Union rate (%)	Mean days to union (95% CI)
Tibiotalar fusion	19	89.5	124 (102–145)
Subtalar fusion	18	100	119 (103–135)
Talonavicular fusion	6	100	116 (82–149)
Calcaneocuboid fusion	6	100	112 (79–145)
Midfoot fusion	19	94.7	91 (85–98)
Ankle fracture nonunion	4	75.0	93 (75–112)
Talar neck fracture nonunion/revision	3	100	103 (52–154)
Fifth metatarsal fracture nonunion	3	100	96 (0–213)
Distal tibia osteotomy	2	100	96 (83–109)
Calcaneal osteotomy nonunion	1	100	104
First metatarsal osteotomy nonunion	1	100	102

Abbreviations: CI, confidence interval; rhBMP-2, recombinant human bone morphogenetic protein-2.
Source: Data from Rearick et al.[24]

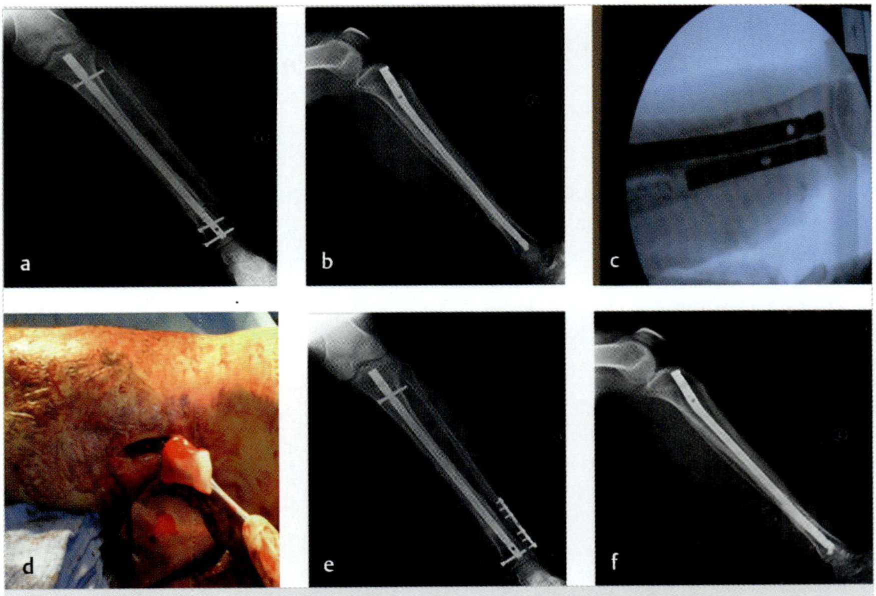

Fig. 25.2 Bone morphogenetic protein-2 (BMP-2) case study. A 36-year-old man who underwent open reduction and internal fixation of a left open distal tibia–fibula fracture with a free flap. The patient presented with a malunion/nonunion at 1 year postoperatively, as seen on the **(a)** anteroposterior and **(b)** lateral views of the ankle. **(c,d)** Nonunion treatment included placement of recombinant human bone morphogenetic protein-2 on an absorbable collagen sponge with plating of the fibula. Follow-up films demonstrate union of the tibia and fibula at 1 month after revision surgery, as seen on **(e)** anteroposterior and **(f)** lateral views of the ankle.

  - There has not been any reported evidence of cancer after BMP use in foot and ankle fusion surgery.
- *Pregnant women:* The potential effects of BMP on the human fetus have not been evaluated.
- Active infection due to BMP proinflammatory properties.
- Individuals younger than 18 years or with no radiographic evidence of closure of epiphyses.
- Individuals with allergy to bovine type I collagen or rhBMP-2.

25.2.5 Conclusion

- While evidence supports favorable results for the use of BMPs in foot and ankle applications, additional level I clinical studies are necessary to correctly evaluate the efficacy and safety of BMPs.

25.3 Platelet-Rich Plasma

25.3.1 Introduction

- Platelet-rich plasma (PRP) is an autologous growth factor therapy containing a platelet concentration greater than that of whole blood.
- Centrifugation and separation techniques are used to prepare PRP.[27]
- PRP accelerates tissue regeneration via three distinct mechanisms: anabolic, anti-inflammatory, and scaffolding.[28,29]
- *Anabolic mechanism:* Platelets secrete growth factors including TGF-β, insulinlike growth factor-1 (IGF-1), and vascular endothelial growth factor (VEGF) promoting mitosis, angiogenesis, and cell migration leading to increased tissue regeneration.
- *Anti-inflammatory mechanism:* Platelets release anti-inflammatory cytokines such as interleukin-1 (IL-1) receptor antagonist, IL-4, IL-10, and IL-13, which preserve cartilage indirectly by limiting the catabolic effects of proinflammatory cytokines.[30,31]
- Scaffolding mechanism is triggered by PRP's plasma proteins. Fibrinogen, along with other clotting factors, forms a fibrin matrix that allows for cell adherence and proliferation.[31]
- The composition of PRP varies due to its autologous nature and differences in preparation methods:[32,33]
  - *Numerous PRP preparations can be used clinically because the FDA regulates the machines producing PRP and exempts autologously derived blood products from regulation since this is human tissue.*
- Typical composition contains platelets, leukocytes, and thrombin or calcium chloride for platelet activation.[27,32]
- The resulting disparity among PRP samples reduces the credibility of generalizations about PRP from the literature.

25.3.2 Platelet-Rich Plasma for Osseous Healing

- PRP is commonly mixed with bone grafts to enhance the grafts' effects.[34]
- Evaluated in use for talus osteochondral lesions during arthroscopic debridement and microfracture procedure:
  - Equivalent healing rates with significantly better pain and function compared to non-PRP groups.[35]
- Evaluated in use for displaced intra-articular calcaneus fracture healing:[36]
  - PRP mixed allograft results in significantly improved function and union rates compared to allograft alone.
  - Equivalent function and union rates between allograft with PRP and autograft alone, without donor site morbidity.[37]

25.3.3 Platelet-Rich Plasma for Achilles Tendinopathy

- Achilles tendinopathy is a common musculoskeletal complaint and often occurs due to overuse of the Achilles tendon.[38,39]
- PRP is one of several conservative treatments applicable to this injury.[38]
- *Method of use:* direct injection at the site of injury.
- In setting of ruptured Achilles tendon, use of PRP results in decreased pain, decreased stiffness, and improved strength compared to repair without use of PRP.
- The long-term effects of PRP on Achilles tendinopathy show overall decreased pain and increased activity compared to non-PRP intervention.
- No associated tendon ruptures with use of PRP.

25.3.4 Platelet-Rich Plasma for Ankle Osteoarthritis

- Ankle osteoarthritis is a relatively infrequent degenerative joint disorder with limited treatment options.[40]
- Surgery is mainly preferred for late stage and advanced cases.
- Less invasive options, including PRP injections, are being researched to treat mild to moderate forms of ankle osteoarthritis.[37]
- Short-term results support PRP's use in modulating osteoarthritic ankle pain via PRP injections.
- Additional clinical studies are necessary to correctly evaluate the efficacy and safety of PRP use for ankle osteoarthritis.

25.3.5 Contraindications/ Limitations

- Thrombocytopenia.
- Platelet dysfunction syndromes.
- Patients with malignancies.
- *Pregnant women:* The potential effects of PRP on the human fetus have not been evaluated.
- Active infection due to PRP proinflammatory properties.

25.3.6 Conclusion

- PRP injections are low cost and less invasive than surgical alternatives, making them accessible and low risk.[32]
- The criteria needed to create the optimal PRP preparation still remain inconclusive. More level I clinical studies and meta-analyses are needed to compare the efficacies of different PRP preparations on foot and ankle pathologies (▶ Fig. 25.3 and ▶ Table 25.2).[40]

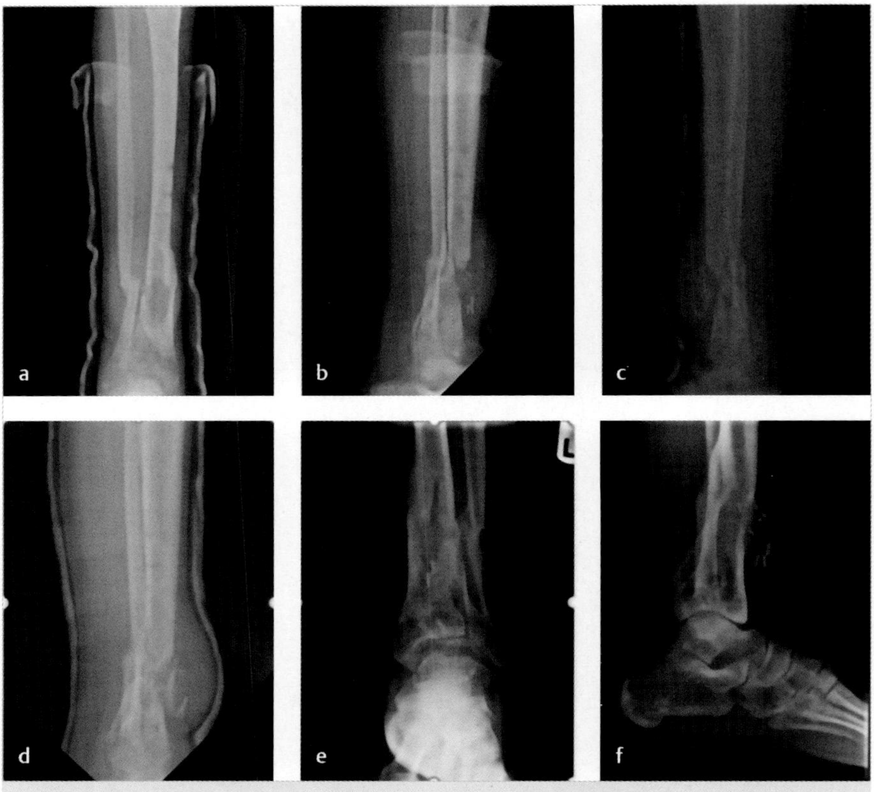

Fig. 25.3 Platelet-rich plasma (PRP) case study. A 43-year-old man with a nonunion segmental tibia defect was treated using a bone graft and PRP adjunct. The patient had a history of methicillin-resistant *Staphylococcus aureus* (MRSA) osteomyelitis for which intravenous (IV) vancomycin was administered. **(a)** Preoperative lateral and **(b)** anteroposterior views of the ankle display nonunion of tibia. Radiographs taken **(c)** immediately postoperation and **(d)** 2 weeks after surgery. **(e)** Anteroposterior and **(f)** lateral views of the ankle taken at 6 months postoperation show union of the tibia.

Table 25.2 Summary of selected studies reviewed

Agent	Study (level of evidence)	Procedure and disease	PRP preparation method (kit manufacturer)	Application	Activation method	Combined treatments	Comparison group	Outcome
rhPDGF (Augment Bone Graft, BioMimetic Therapeutics)	DiGiovanni et al[5] (I)	Ankle or hindfoot arthrodesis	NA	Surgical	NA	No	Yes (ABG)	Union rate comparable between groups
	DiGiovanni et al[6] (I)	Ankle or hindfoot arthrodesis	NA	Surgical	NA	No	Yes (ABG)	Significant for equivalence between rhPDGF and ABG groups. No adverse events observed in the PDGF group
	Daniels et al[4] (I)	Ankle or hindfoot arthrodesis	NA	Surgical	NA	No	Yes (ABG)	Significantly higher joint fusion rate in the rhPDGF group than in the ABG group. Significantly lower mean time to fusion in the rhPDGF group than in the ABG group
	Younger et al[41] (IV)	Arthroscopic debridement of talus	NA	Surgical	NA	No	Yes (ABG)	Significant decreases in VAS, AOS, and SF-36 scores upon addition of rhPDGF
BMP	Bibbo et al[18] (II)	Ankle or hindfoot arthrodesis	NA	Surgical	NA	No	Yes (historical controls)	Higher union rate (96%) than historical controls (48%)

(Continued)

Table 25.2 (*Continued*) Summary of selected studies reviewed

Agent	Study (level of evidence)	Procedure and disease	PRP preparation method (kit manufacturer)	Application	Activation method	Combined treatments	Comparison group	Outcome
	Fourman et al[19] (II)	Ankle arthrodesis	NA	Surgical	NA	Yes (Ilizarov type frame)	Yes (no BMP)	Significantly higher union rate (92%) than control (53%)
	DeVries et al[20] (II)	Revision tibiocalcaneal arthrodesis	NA	Surgical	NA	Yes (procedures were highly variable)	Yes (no BMP)	Higher union rate (71.4%) than control (56.3%), but slower time to radiographic union (184 vs. 115 d)
	Kanakaris et al[21] (IV)	Ankle, subtalar, talonavicular, pubic or sacroiliac failed arthrodesis	NA	Surgical	NA	Bone graft (11 cases)	No	Clinical and radiographic improvement in 17 cases
	Schuberth et al[22] (IV)	Forefoot procedures, tibiotalar or tibiotalocalcaneal arthrodesis, or distal tibial osteotomy	NA	Surgical	NA	Yes (procedures were highly variable)	No	Significant difference in union between patients < 50 y of age (100%) and patients > 50 (73%)
PRP	Görmeli et al[35] (I)	OCLs of the talus	(SmartPrep 2 system, Harvest Autologous Hemobiologics)	Single injection occurred 24–36 h after surgery	No	Arthroscopic debridement and microfracture techniques	Yes (HA and saline)	Pain and function in the PRP group were significantly better than in the HA or saline group

(Continued)

Table 25.2 (*Continued*) Summary of selected studies reviewed

Agent	Study (level of evidence)	Procedure and disease	PRP preparation method (kit manufacturer)	Application	Activation method	Combined treatments	Comparison group	Outcome
	Wei et al[36] (I)	Displaced intra-articular calcaneal fractures	Double centrifugation (laboratory made)	Surgical	10% calcium chloride and bovine thrombin solution	Allograft	Yes (ABG, allograft alone)	Function and radiographic parameters in allograft with the PRP group were significantly greater than in the allograft alone group
	Zou et al[39] (I)	Ruptured Achilles tendons	Double centrifugation (WEGO PRP preparation kit)	Surgical	No	Krackow's suture technique to repair ruptured tendon	Yes (no PRP injection)	Pain, stiffness, and general health in the PRP group were significantly better than in the control group
	Fukawa et al[37] (IV)	Ankle osteoarthritis	Double centrifugation (laboratory-made blood separation pack)	Three 2-mL injections were given at 2-wk intervals	Calcium chloride	No	No	Pain and health showed significant improvement at 12 mo postinjection

Abbreviations: AOS, Ankle Osteoarthritis Scale; BMP, bone morphogenetic protein; HA, hyaluronic acid; PDGF, platelet-derived growth factor; PRP, platelet-rich plasma; rhPDGF, recombinant human PDGF; SF-36, 36-Item Short Form Health Survey; VAS, visual analog scale.

25.4 Key Testing Facts

- Augment Bone Graft (Stryker., Memphis, TN) is a formulation of rhPDGF-BB,consisting of a 0.3 mg/mL solution of rhPDGF-BB combined with a β-tricalcium phosphate (β-TCP) carrier. Meta-analysis of the three foot ankle arthrodesis studies showed that treatment with rhPDGF-BB and ABG yielded comparable outcomes in terms of short-term and long-term follow ups.
- While favorable results exist for the use of BMPs in non foot and ankle applications, additional level 1 clinical studies are necessary to correctly evaluate the efficacy and safety of BMPs on foot ankle pathology
- While the small series of PRP's effectiveness continues to grow, criteria needed to create the optimal PRP preparation still remains inconclusive. Additional level I clinical studies and meta-analyses are needed to compare the efficacies of different PRP preparations on foot and ankle pathologies prior to its routine clinical application.

References

[1] Alvarez RH, Kantarjian HM, Cortes JE. Biology of platelet-derived growth factor and its involvement in disease. Mayo Clin Proc. 2006; 81(9):1241–1257

[2] Hollinger JO, Hart CE, Hirsch SN, Lynch S, Friedlaender GE. Recombinant human platelet-derived growth factor: biology and clinical applications. J Bone Joint Surg Am. 2008; 90 Suppl 1:48–54

[3] Daniels T, DiGiovanni C, Lau JT, Wing K, Younger A. Prospective clinical pilot trial in a single cohort group of rhPDGF in foot arthrodeses. Foot Ankle Int. 2010; 31(6):473–479

[4] Daniels TR, Younger ASE, Penner MJ, et al. Prospective randomized controlled trial of hindfoot and ankle fusions treated with rhPDGF-BB in combination with a β-TCP-collagen matrix. Foot Ankle Int. 2015; 36(7):739–748

[5] Digiovanni CW, Baumhauer J, Lin SS, et al. Prospective, randomized, multi-center feasibility trial of rhPDGF-BB versus autologous bone graft in a foot and ankle fusion model. Foot Ankle Int. 2011; 32(4):344–354

[6] DiGiovanni CW, Lin SS, Baumhauer JF, et al. North American Orthopedic Foot and Ankle Study Group. Recombinant human platelet-derived growth factor-BB and beta-tricalcium phosphate (rhPDGF-BB/β-TCP): an alternative to autogenous bone graft. J Bone Joint Surg Am. 2013; 95(13):1184–1192

[7] Sun H, Lu PP, Zhou PH, et al. Recombinant human platelet-derived growth factor-BB versus autologous bone graft in foot and ankle fusion: a systematic review and meta-analysis. Foot Ankle Surg. 2017; 23 (1):32–39

[8] Solchaga LA, Hee CK, Roach S, Snel LB. Safety of recombinant human platelet-derived growth factor-BB in Augment(®) Bone Graft. J Tissue Eng. 2012; 3(1):2041731412442668

[9] Wang EA, Rosen V, D'Alessandro JS, et al. Recombinant human bone morphogenetic protein induces bone formation. Proc Natl Acad Sci U S A. 1990; 87(6):2220–2224

[10] Miyazono K, Kamiya Y, Morikawa M. Bone morphogenetic protein receptors and signal transduction. J Biochem. 2010; 147(1):35–51

[11] Nohe A, Keating E, Knaus P, Petersen NO. Signal transduction of bone morphogenetic protein receptors. Cell Signal. 2004; 16(3):291–299

[12] Groppe J, Greenwald J, Wiater E, et al. Structural basis of BMP signaling inhibition by Noggin, a novel twelve-membered cystine knot protein. J Bone Joint Surg Am. 2003; 85-A Suppl 3:52–58

[13] Rosen V. BMP and BMP inhibitors in bone. Ann N Y Acad Sci. 2006; 1068:19–25

[14] Cheng H, Jiang W, Phillips FM, et al. Osteogenic activity of the fourteen types of human bone morphogenetic proteins (BMPs). J Bone Joint Surg Am. 2003; 85(8):1544–1552

[15] Alt V, Donell ST, Chhabra A, Bentley A, Eicher A, Schnettler R. A health economic analysis of the use of rhBMP-2 in Gustilo-Anderson grade III open tibial fractures for the UK, Germany, and France. Injury. 2009; 40(12):1269–1275

[16] Dahabreh Z, Calori GM, Kanakaris NK, Nikolaou VS, Giannoudis PV. A cost analysis of treatment of tibial fracture nonunion by bone grafting or bone morphogenetic protein-7. Int Orthop. 2009; 33(5): 1407–1414

[17] Haubruck P, Tanner MC, Vlachopoulos W, et al. Comparison of the clinical effectiveness of bone morphogenic protein (BMP) -2 and -7 in the adjunct treatment of lower limb nonunions. Orthop Traumatol Surg Res. 2018; 104(8):1241–1248

[18] Bibbo C, Patel DV, Haskell MD. Recombinant bone morphogenetic protein-2 (rhBMP-2) in high-risk ankle and hindfoot fusions. Foot Ankle Int. 2009; 30(7):597–603

[19] Fourman MS, Borst EW, Bogner E, Rozbruch SR, Fragomen AT. Recombinant human BMP-2 increases the incidence and rate of healing in complex ankle arthrodesis. Clin Orthop Relat Res. 2014; 472(2):732–739

[20] DeVries JG, Nguyen M, Berlet GC, Hyer CF. The effect of recombinant bone morphogenetic protein-2 in revision tibiotalocalcaneal arthrodesis: utilization of the Retrograde Arthrodesis Intramedullary Nail database. J Foot Ankle Surg. 2012; 51(4):426–432

[21] Kanakaris NK, Mallina R, Calori GM, Kontakis G, Giannoudis PV. Use of bone morphogenetic proteins

in arthrodesis: clinical results. Injury. 2009; 40 Suppl 3:S62–S66

[22] Schuberth JM, DiDomenico LA, Mendicino RW. The utility and effectiveness of bone morphogenetic protein in foot and ankle surgery. J Foot Ankle Surg. 2009; 48(3):309–314

[23] Coughlin MJ, Grimes JS, Traughber PD, Jones CP. Comparison of radiographs and CT scans in the prospective evaluation of the fusion of hindfoot arthrodesis. Foot Ankle Int. 2006; 27(10): 780–787

[24] Rearick T, Charlton TP, Thordarson D. Effectiveness and complications associated with recombinant human bone morphogenetic protein-2 augmentation of foot and ankle fusions and fracture nonunions. Foot Ankle Int. 2014; 35(8):783–788

[25] Bentley H, Hamdy FC, Hart KA, et al. Expression of bone morphogenetic proteins in human prostatic adenocarcinoma and benign prostatic hyperplasia. Br J Cancer. 1992; 66(6):1159–1163

[26] Papanagiotou M, Dailiana ZH, Karachalios T, et al. Heterotopic ossification after the use of recombinant human bone morphogenetic protein-7. World J Orthop. 2017; 8(1):36–41

[27] Navani A, Li G, Chrystal J. Platelet rich plasma in musculoskeletal pathology: a necessary rescue or a lost cause? Pain Physician. 2017; 20(3):E345–E356

[28] Beitzel K, Allen D, Apostolakos J, et al. US definitions, current use, and FDA stance on use of platelet-rich plasma in sports medicine. J Knee Surg. 2015; 28(1):29–34

[29] Cavallo C, Roffi A, Grigolo B, et al. Platelet-rich plasma: the choice of activation method affects the release of bioactive molecules. BioMed Res Int. 2016; 2016:6591717

[30] Wojdasiewicz P, Poniatowski ŁA, Szukiewicz D. The role of inflammatory and anti-inflammatory cytokines in the pathogenesis of osteoarthritis. Mediators Inflamm. 2014; 2014:561459

[31] Xie X, Zhang C, Tuan RS. Biology of platelet-rich plasma and its clinical application in cartilage repair. Arthritis Res Ther. 2014; 16(1):204–218

[32] Dhurat R, Sukesh M. Principles and methods of preparation of platelet-rich plasma: A review and author's perspective. J Cutan Aesthet Surg. 2014; 7 (4):189–197

[33] Russell RP, Apostolakos J, Hirose T, Cote MP, Mazzocca AD. Variability of platelet-rich plasma preparations. Sports Med Arthrosc Rev. 2013; 21 (4):186–190

[34] Gu W, Li T, Shi Z, et al. Management of Hepple stage V osteochondral lesion of the talus with a platelet-rich plasma scaffold. BioMed Res Int. 2017; 2017:6525373

[35] Görmeli G, Karakaplan M, Görmeli CA, Sarıkaya B, Elmalı N, Ersoy Y. Clinical effects of platelet-rich plasma and hyaluronic acid as an additional therapy for talar osteochondral lesions treated with microfracture surgery: a prospective randomized clinical trial. Foot Ankle Int. 2015; 36(8):891–900

[36] Wei L-C, Lei G-H, Sheng P-Y, et al. Efficacy of platelet-rich plasma combined with allograft bone in the management of displaced intra-articular calcaneal fractures: a prospective cohort study. J Orthop Res. 2012; 30(10):1570–1576

[37] Fukawa T, Yamaguchi S, Akatsu Y, Yamamoto Y, Akagi R, Sasho T. Safety and efficacy of intra-articular injection of platelet-rich plasma in patients with ankle osteoarthritis. Foot Ankle Int. 2017; 38 (6):596–604

[38] Guelfi M, Pantalone A, Vanni D, Abate M, Guelfi MG, Salini V. Long-term beneficial effects of platelet-rich plasma for non-insertional Achilles tendinopathy. Foot Ankle Surg. 2015; 21(3):178–181

[39] Zou J, Mo X, Shi Z, et al. A prospective study of platelet-rich plasma as biological augmentation for acute Achilles tendon rupture repair. BioMed Res Int. 2016; 2016:9364170

[40] Repetto I, Biti B, Cerruti P, Trentini R, Felli L. Conservative treatment of ankle osteoarthritis: can platelet-rich plasma effectively postpone surgery? J Foot Ankle Surg. 2017; 56(2):362–365

[41] Younger A, Wing K, Penner M, Cresswell M. A study to evaluate the safety of platelet-derived growth factor for treatment of osteochondral defects of the talus. Knee Surg Sports Traumatol Arthrosc. 2016; 24(4):1250–1258

Index

Note: Page numbers set **bold** or *italic* indicate headings or figures, respectively.

A

D

E

I

J

K

L

R

S

U

V

W